Endoscopic Control of Gastrointestinal Hemorrhage

Editor

John P. Papp, M.D.

Associate Clinical Professor of Medicine
Michigan State University College of Human Medicine
and
Chairman, Section of Gastroenterology
Department of Medicine
Blodgett Memorial Medical Center
Grand Rapids, Michigan

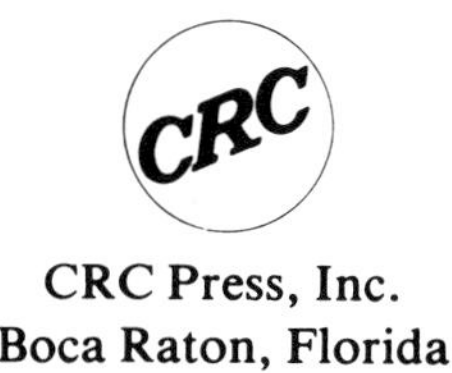

CRC Press, Inc.
Boca Raton, Florida

Library of Congress Cataloging in Publication Data
Main entry under title:

Endoscopic control of gastrointestinal hemorrhage.

Includes bibliographies and index.
1. Gastrointestinal hemorrhage. 2. Gastroscope and gastroscopy. 3. Electrocoagulation. I. Papp, John P., 1938- . [DNLM: 1. Electrocoagulation. 2. Endoscopy. 3. Hemorrhage, Gastrointestinal—Therapy. WI 143 E56]
RC802.E52 616.3′3 81-455
ISBN 0-8493-6295-4 AACR1

This book represents information obtained from authentic and highly regarded sources. Reprinted material is quoted with permission, and sources are indicated. A wide variety of references are listed. Every reasonable effort has been made to give reliable data and information, but the author and the publisher cannot assume reponsibility for the validity of all materials or for the consequences of their use.

Direct all inquiries to CRC Press, Inc., 2000 N.W. 24th Street, Boca Raton, Florida, 33431.

International Standard Book number 0-8493-6295-4

Library of Congress Card Number 81-455
Printed in the United States

PREFACE

Gastrointestinal bleeding is a common clinical problem in medicine. It is estimated that 100 patients per 100,000 patient population will be admitted to a hospital for the management of upper gastrointestinal bleeding this year. The mortality from gastrointestinal bleeding has remained approximately 10% for nearly three decades despite advances in critical care, blood replacement, and surgery. However, there has been a change in the proportion of patients over sixty from 8% in 1937 to 45% in 1976.

With the development of fiberoptic technology and electrocoagulation electrodes and power units, an era of therapeutic gastrointestinal endoscopy became a reality in 1970. A decade of endoscopic electrocoagulation research has been directed to producing a safe and effective modality to stop arterial bleeding in the gastrointestinal tract.

This book has been written to present the state of the art on endoscopic control of gastrointestinal hemorrhage with emphasis on combining the clinical approach to the patient while reviewing the experimental data which has resulted in the availability of various modalities of therapy.

I wish to express my appreciation to the several authors of this book, to the Blodgett Memorial Medical Center Research Fund for its financial support, to my colleagues for referring their patients, and to my endoscopy assistants for their clinical and research support. Lastly, I wish to express my gratitude to my parents, my wife, Mary Ann, and children, Mary Lynn, John, and James for their loving patience and emotional support while preparing this book. To them, I dedicate this book.

THE EDITOR

John P. Papp, M.D., is a Senior Attending Gastroenterologist at Blodgett Memorial Medical Center, Grand Rapids, Michigan, and Director of the Gastrointestinal Endoscopy unit. He is also an Associate Clinical Professor in the Department of Medicine, College of Human Medicine, Michigan State University. He was born in Cleveland, Ohio, on August 28, 1938. In 1960, he received his B.A. from The College of Wooster, Wooster, Ohio, and his M.D. in 1964 from The Ohio State University College of Medicine. He is married to Mary Ann Papp and has three children, a girl and two boys.

In 1964 he began an internship at The Cleveland Clinic, Cleveland, Ohio. From 1965 to 1967 he was a Lieutenant in the Medical Corps of the U.S. Navy stationed at Charleston, South Carolina and served as an Executive Officer in the Naval Station Dispensary. From 1967 to 1969 he was a resident in Internal Medicine at the University of Michigan Medical Center, Ann Arbor, Michigan. In 1969 he became a Fellow in Gastroenterology under Dr. H. Marvin Pollard at the University of Michigan Medical Center, and a National Institute of Health Trainee at Michigan from 1970 to 1971. In 1971 he became a Diplomate of the American Board of Internal Medicine and a Diplomate in Gastroenterology in 1972. He is also a Fellow in the American College of Physicians and the American College of Gastroenterology. He has over 100 publications and is a pioneer in the field of electrocoagulation.

He is a Trustee of the American College of Gastroenterology and is serving his second two-year term as Councilor of the American Society for Gastrointestinal Endoscopy. He is also Past-President of the Michigan Society for Gastrointestinal Endoscopy and is currently Secretary-Treasurer of the Michigan Society of Internal Medicine.

CONTRIBUTORS

David C. Auth, Ph.D., P.E.
Professor of Electrical
Engineering and Adjunct Professor
of Bioengineering
University of Washington
Seattle, Washington

H. Worth Boyce, Jr., M.D.
Professor of Medicine
Director, Division of Digestive
Diseases and Nutrition
University of South Florida
College of Medicine
Tampa, Florida

Peter B. Cotton, M.D., F.R.C.P.
Consultant Gastroenterologist
The Middlesex Hospital and
Medical School
London, England

Andrew D. Feld, M.D.
Senior Fellow in Gastroenterology
University of Washington
Seattle, Washington

Wolfgang E. Fleig, M.D.
Gastroenterologist
Division of Metabolism, Nutrition,
and Gastroenterology
Department of Internal Medicine
University of Ulm
Ulm, Germany

David A. Gilbert, M.D.
Assistant Professor of Medicine
Co-director, Gastrointestinal
Endoscopy Service
University of Washington
Seattle, Washington

Frank W. Harris, M.D.
TAG Medical Corporation
Boulder, Colorado

John P. Papp, M.D.
Associate Clinical Professor
of Medicine
Michigan State University
College of Human Medicine and
Chairman, Section of Gastroenterology
Blodgett Memorial Medical Center

Karl J. Paquet, M.D.
Professor of Surgery
Department of Surgery
University of Bonn
Bonn, Germany

Robert L. Protell, M.D.
Clinical Assistant Professor of Medicine
University of Washington
Seattle, Washington

B. H. Gerald Rogers, M.D.
Clinical Associate in Medicine
University of Chicago
Pritzker School of Medicine
Chicago, Illinois

Fred E. Silverstein, M.D.
Associate Professor of Medicine
Director, Gastrointestinal Endoscopy
Service
University of Washington
Seattle, Washington

Stephen E. Silvis, M.D.
Professor Medicine
Veterans Administration Medical
Center and University of Minnesota
Minneapolis, Minnesota

Alan G. Vallon, M.D.
Research Assistant, Department of
Gastroenterology
The Middlesex Hospital and
Medical School
London, England

Jerome D. Waye, M.D.
Associate Clinical Professor of Medicine
Mount Sinai School of Medicine
of the City University of New York
Chief, Gastrointestinal Endoscopy Unit
Mount Sinai Hospital, New York

TABLE OF CONTENTS

Chapter 1

GENERAL APPROACH TO UPPER GASTROINTESTINAL BLEEDING

H. Worth Boyce, Jr.

TABLE OF CONTENTS

I. INTRODUCTION

Acute upper gastrointestinal bleeding may prove to be the final medical problem in a person's life or it only may be a sign of an otherwise transient, one time insult to the esophageal, gastric, or duodenal mucosa. Neither patient nor physician can predict from the first sign of bleeding whether the bleeding will persist, stop in response to medical therapy, or simply cease spontaneously. The management scheme in this discussion will be directed toward the person who presents with bright red blood by hematemesis or nasogastric aspiration with or without melena or bright red blood per rectum. When first seen by the physician, the patient with active bleeding is in a high-risk category that will require a prompt, efficient management scheme and an orderly decision-making process if morbidity and mortality are to be minimized. Obviously, persons who have a history of hematemesis or melena before presentation, a stable pulse, and blood pressure without signs of hypovolemia, and only "coffee ground" material or minimal bright red blood on gastric aspiration, need a thoughtful evaluation and observation. This group usually does not require either major resuscitative measures, prompt endoscopy, or direct attempts at medical or surgical therapy for the bleeding lesion. If acute rebleeding occurs in this group, the person must immediately be considered at high risk and placed into the scheme of immediate diagnostic study and prompt therapeutic decision making.

Today, there is general agreement among gastroenterologists and surgeons that the acutely bleeding patient is better served if those responsible for his care obtain an early, accurate diagnosis of the bleeding lesion. This knowledge permits decisions regarding the type and timing of treatment aimed either at eliminating the cause or producing hemostasis. Adherence to this philosophy will prevent needless prolongation of medical therapy in high-risk patients and obviate disasters from premature or inappropriate surgical procedures.

The philosophy of early diagnosis of the bleeding lesion by endoscopy has been supported by observations that bleeding patients managed by general supportive measures without accurate diagnosis or specific therapy do not fare well when compared with those managed selectively for a specific diagnosis. It also has been shown that patients requiring surgery for bleeding lesions do best when an accurate preoperative diagnosis has been made.[10]

The need for prompt diagnosis has become more logical and appropriate with the development of nonsurgical, transendoscopic therapeutic measures that appear safe and effective in stopping bleeding from certain upper gastrointestinal lesions. These techniques may convert an emergent condition to a stable one and thereby either resolve the problem or permit a specific elective therapy to be applied with reduced risk to the patient. Accurate diagnosis unquestionably is the key to success of this approach.

II. THE BLEEDING PATIENT

Upper gastrointestinal bleeding may present to the physician under almost any situation and in any type of specialty practice. About three-fourths of persons have never bled before and obviously are extremely frightened to see their life's blood being lost. Having no idea of its origin or extent, usually they promptly will report or be brought for medical attention. These people are ready and eager to cooperate in most instances, the inebriated person being the classical exception. The bleeding patient is acutely aware and sometimes confused by the medical actions and conversations around him but he wants things done for and to him to treat his problem. He readily accepts needles, gastric tubes, and endoscopy when these management steps are offered. If properly explained and applied, these procedures rarely generate any complaints from the patient. The physician must be aware that there are rare patients who become uncooperative merely because of their extreme anxiety. Usually, the experienced clinician can help the patient relax and accept the situation if he remains compassionate, calm, and confident.

We should emphasize here that management of acute upper gastrointentional bleeding is best managed by a team, including an internist/gastroenterologist and a surgeon, who should be notified promptly of the patient's admission and status.

A. The Elderly Patient

There is general belief that the patient over 60 years of age is at greater risk from gastrointestinal bleeding. This susceptibility is accentuated if bleeding is massive in degree. Recently, Chang et al. have reported a series of 66 massively bleeding elderly patients.[4] Significant associated medical illness was found in 82%, 70% had hypovolemic shock. The mean blood transfusion requirement was 7.8 units. Of the 66, 49 had peptic ulcer disease. The diagnostic accuracy of endoscopy was 93% in this series compared to 46% for barium contrast radiography.

Elderly patients are at greater risk from the bleeding problem, as well as the diagnostic approach. Major diseases are more common. Older people take more drugs and the physician must take this into consideration when ordering medications that could have adverse effect in this emergent situation. The important message here is to have as much information about the patient's medical history as possible to minimize errors of pharmacologic omission and commission.

An early diagnosis permits prompt decisions regarding therapy. Elective surgery repeatedly has been shown to have a mortality rate considerably lower than that of emergency operation.[15] Gastric surgery in elderly patients has a high rate of complications, a remarkable 35% in one recent report.[4] The high risk, both from emergency surgery and bleeding, underscore the importance of prompt resuscitation, early endoscopic diagnosis, and any rational effort to convert an emergent situation for operative intervention to one of an elective nature.

B. The Pediatric Patient

As with many other diagnostic and therapeutic measures, the young bleeding patient may be effectively and safely treated in a fashion quite similar to that employed in adults.[1,7,8]

Early endoscopic examination should be employed, if possible, within 24 hours of bleeding onset for optimum diagnostic accuracy. Resuscitation with fluid and blood in proper amounts is just as essential as in adult patients. Gastric lavage is performed using the largest tube possible based on patient size and age.

Preparation in children obviously must be individualized, but is relatively standard, in those over five years of age. Meperidine (1.0 to 2.0 mg/kg) and atropine sulfate (0.01mg/kg) are given intramuscularly 30 to 45 min before the procedure. Diazepam 5 to 15 mg may be given slowly intravenously, judging dosage by clinical titration as needed just before the endoscopy begins. Some prefer also to use promethazine 1 mg/kg and chlorpromazine 1 mg/kg intramuscularly, in addition to the meperidine.[7]

The diagnostic accuracy of early endoscopy in all pediatric ages, the neonate to teenagers,[7,18] has proven equal to that in adults with acute upper gastrointestinal bleedng. The newer small (8 mm) and intermediate diameter (11 mm) forward viewing endoscopes are excellent for this purpose. The older model Olympus ® GIF-P endoscope (7.2-mm diameter) has been preferred in the neonate.[9]

The bleeding lesions encountered in children are similar in type to those found in adults. Peptic ulcers, gastritis, and varices are the most common.

III. INITIAL MANAGEMENT

It must be emphasized that several activities must occur simultaneously when the bleeding patient first is seen. The responsible physician ideally will be one of a team of medical personnel available to assist the patient. *First things first* should be the philosophy and must be remembered throughout the management process. This means that resuscitation and support of essential body functions are paramount. Consequently, initial management must be oriented toward restoring or sustaining these functions while simultaneously proceeding with acquisition of a data base via pertinent history (including prior medical records, if possible), physical examination, and gastric lavage to clean the stomach and, hopefully, slow the rate of bleeding.

A. Immediate Status Evaluation

In most instances, the reason for the patient's presentation to the medical facility, i.e., upper gastrointestinal bleeding, either will be obvious or strongly suggested by the circumstances. The first order of business is to determine the status of essential body functions, primarily cardiovascular and pulmonary.

The general appearance of the patient tells the story in most instances, but in some, additional maneuvers may be needed to adequately evaluate the degree of systemic distress that exists. The facial expression of fear and anxiety, skin color, perspiration, restlessness or overt hypoxia with flaring nares and tachypnea, any or all, indicate a problem with oxygenation of the tissues likely due to the hypovolemia of acute blood loss.

The pulse rate provides a reliable index of hypovolemia in most instances. However, if the patient is taking atropinelike drugs, the pulse may be falsely rapid and unreliable as a guide. The opposite may be true when an appropriately increased pulse rate is prevented by such drugs as digitalis preparations and reserpine. In general, the pulse rate is reliable to monitor acute intravascular volume depletion and hypoxia and is a far more reliable sign than the hematocrit which may require one to two days to equilibrate following acute blood loss. The hematocrit remains falsely high early after bleeding and does not reflect the reduction in oxygen carrying capacity of the blood that requires prompt correction. A low hematocrit may be the result of chronic anemia and not a reflection of acute blood loss. The history and a later glance at red cell morphology on the stained blood smear or red cell indices will help in this regard.

The blood pressure, especially if taken in a recumbent position, may not reflect the degree of hypovolemia present. This is especially true in persons whose peripheral cardiovascular compensatory reflexes, i.e., vasoconstriction, are intact. Blood pressure decline is relative and absolute values may be misinterpreted unless the physician is aware of the patient's usual blood pressure level. When patient observation, pulse, and blood pressure values are not considered diagnostic for hypovolemia, it is proper to challenge cardiovascular response to sudden postural change by the so-called tilt test.

The tilt test is an indicator of impending shock as a consequence of significant, usually acute, blood loss. The pulse and blood pressure are taken with the patient supine. The head of the bed is then raised 75 degrees. After one minute in this position, the physician observes for pallor and/or sweating and repeats the pulse and blood pressure determinations. An increase in pulse rate of over 20 beats/min indicates at least a 500 m*l* blood volume deficit. A drop of diastolic blood pressure in excess of 10 mm Hg also indicates significant hypovolemia.

Modest increases in respiratory rate are compatible with the acute anxiety present in many patients in an emergency care setting. The effort used in performing respiration, the flare of the nares, and the patient's facial expression are clues perhaps of equal value to the rate of breathing for detecting hypoxia.

Urinary output provides a valuable index to blood volume and renal perfusion. Accurate monitoring of urinary flow rate often is best done via an indwelling Foley catheter during the acute stages of management.

When the initial appearance of the patient suggests hypovolemia, one member of the team should be establishing intravenous access by one or more routes depending on the apparent severity of the blood loss. A larger bore, #18- or #19-gauge needle or a venous catheter should be used. It is preferable to place the intravenous line in the right arm, since the patient usually is placed on his left side for the endoscopic examination. Placement of a central venous catheter is indicated in patients with severe bleeding to monitor central pressure and for fluid and blood replacement. Baseline blood studies should be obtained from a specimen taken with the initial venipuncture and ideally include a complete blood count, platelet estimate, blood urea nitrogen, glucose, prothrombin time, partial thromboplastin time, electrolytes, and chemistry profile (SMA 12). The first portion of the blood sample obtained should be sent immediately to the blood bank for typing and cross-match for four units of whole blood. Packed red blood cells may be indicated in certain situations such as congestive heart failure.

While this initial assessment and immediate therapy is being accomplished, an assistant should be dispatched to obtain prior records and x-rays if available. The history and physical examination should also be underway.

B. Pertinent Historical Data

Appropriate historical information is no less important, perhaps more important, here than with other acute medical emergencies. Prior illness, operations, and drug therapy all may play a conclusive role in decisions regarding both surgical and nonsurgical therapy. A history of recent aspirin ingestion is relatively common and, likely, is etiologically related to the onset of bleeding and the bleeding lesion in some cases.

There are several disorders that are known to place the bleeding patient in a high-risk group. The necessary information can be obtained from the patient, prior medical records, family members, and by a call to the patient's physician. It is important to know if any emergency treatment was given before the patient's arrival, i.e., drugs, intravenous fluids, blood, etc. Significant risk factors include age over 60, hematemesis in excess of melena, hemoglobin below 8 g/d*l* on admission, jaundice, recurrent bleeding during the same admission, and onset of bleeding during hospitalization.[17] A past history of congestive heart failure, chronic renal insufficiency, chronic obstructive pulmonary disease, diabetes mellitus, myocardial infarction, or graft replacement of an aortic abdominal aneurysm are all exceedingly important risk factors.[2,6,17] A history of a previous bleeding lesion or the color of blood vomited are of relatively little help in assessing the cause, the degree of bleeding, or the prognosis. A history of proven esophageal varices places the patient with alcoholic cirrhosis in a high-risk category, but that information is of relatively little benefit in predicting the bleeding source. Less than one third of patients known to have esophageal varices will be proven to be bleeding from varices on admission.[8]

C. Physical Examination

The initial assessment of physical status provides an objective measure of the patient's cardiovascular compensation and a basis for urgent therapy. This data base should be broadened as the management sequence proceeds.

The patient's temperature should be measured. Gastrointestinal bleeding has been said to be related to mild temperature elevations not exceeding 100°F.

A general physical examination should be done as soon as possible. Special care should be taken with the cardiovascular and pulmonary examinations. Skin and mucosal lesions of mouth and nose may provide clues to potential bleeding lesions, as with Osler—Weber—Rendu disease, but can by no means be considered diagnostic of the source. Examination of the palmar creases with the fingers hyperextended provides a reasonable clinical measure of the hemoglobin level. The color in these creases will be a bright red color with hemoglobin levels greater than 7.5 gm/dl. Careful abdominal examination and testing for stool blood always should be done. Hyperactive bowel sounds often are associated with moderate to severe gastrointestinal hemorrhage.

D. Laboratory Studies

The essential blood studies should be obtained during the initial venipuncture as previously mentioned. As more historical and physical data are collected, there often is a need for additional studies.

Hemoglobin and hematocrit repeated every six to eight hours or less provide more help in assessment by serial values than by being done on a random basis.

A normal serum creatinine will permit the conclusion that any blood urea nitrogen elevation is likely due to hypovolemia with reduced renal perfusion, absorption of urea from the small bowel, or both. The blood urea nitrogen value due to blood in the small bowel ranges from 20 to 80 mg/d*l*, but usually is less than 35mg/d*l*. Values in excess of 100 mg/d*l* are indicative of intrinsic renal disease in addition to blood in the gut.

The electrocardiogram is an important study, especially in the elderly, in those with a history of coronary artery disease or in the patient who has had recent chest pain. The clinician must be aware of the fact that myocardial infarction during acute gastrointestinal bleeding may not be associated with chest pain. Any patient with shock or pulmonary edema must be suspected of having a myocardial infarction. This is especially important in order to prevent rapid fluid overload in the hypotensive patient who fails to respond to volume expansion because of myocardial failure.

E. Ongoing Resuscitation

The patient suffering from acute gastrointestinal bleeding is best treated by whole blood replacement as soon as it is available. Initial volume replacement consists of saline, Ringer's lactate solution or a plasma expander, i.e., albumin solution or fresh frozen plasma. Volume required is determined by response of pulse, blood pressure, and respirations. If bleeding ceases and vital signs return toward normal, packed red cells may be appropriate to reduce the risk of volume overload while maximizing the oxygen carrying capacity. Oxygen should be administered by catheter or mask as indicated.

Vital signs are taken at frequent intervals, fluid intake and output recorded, and an indwelling Foley catheter placed if needed. Urine output should exceed 50 ml/hr if volume replacement and renal function are adequate.

IV. DIAGNOSIS OF THE BLEEDING SOURCE

Resuscitation is paramount for successful diagnosis and treatment. There are some patients who should be taken promptly to the operating room because of massive bleeding and failure of response to resuscitative efforts. In this instance, endoscopy may be done to rule out esophageal disease after the patient is under general anesthesia to reassure the surgeon that an abdominal approach is proper.

There has been much misunderstanding and controversy during the past decade over the indications for emergency endoscopy.[2,19] Palmer's original recommendation was for use of the vigorous diagnostic approach in patients with active and significant upper gastrointestinal bleeding.[13] There is little to be gained by emergent endoscopy in the

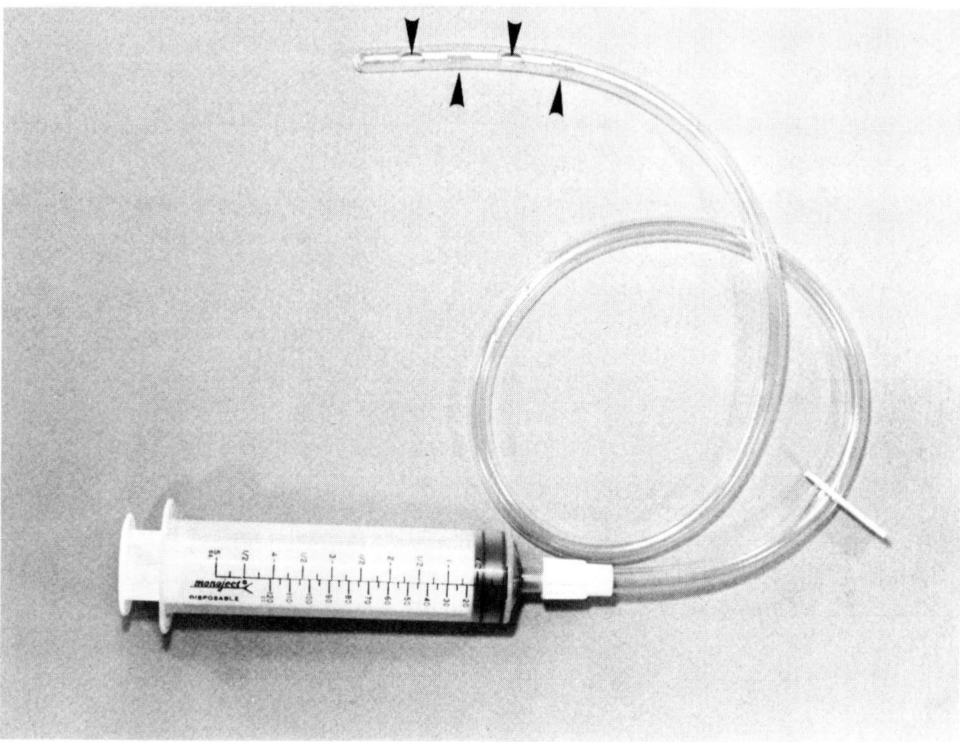

FIGURE 1. The Monoject Adult Gastric Lavage Kit® for gastric lavage consists of a large bore (34 French) tube and a 150 ml syringe with a large nozzle. Arrows indicate large ports on distal end of tube.

patient who is stable and has minimal or no active bleeding.[11] Endoscopic examination in such recent active bleeders may be properly done within 24 hr under ideal medical-technical circumstances and still provide an accurate diagnosis of the bleeding source.[5]

A. Gastric Ice Water Lavage

An essential aspect of the early diagnostic approach is to slow the bleeding rate and evacuate the stomach. Fortunately, over one-half of the patients with active bleeding will cease bleeding completely or slow the rate markedly following ice water lavage. Some have argued that iced saline is preferable because of the potential danger of water overload and hyponatremia. This has rarely been a problem, but caution is in order in patients who have had a gastric resection or pyloroplasty that may permit rapid gastric emptying. Saline solutions are best avoided in patients with congestive heart failure or cirrhotic ascites.

Lavage is performed with a large-bore gastric tube of at least 34 French diameter with several large ports to aid in clot removal. A 150-m*l* syringe wth a large nozzle is essential for optimum results (Figure 1). The tube is passed approximately 55 cm from the incisor teeth and lavage begun with gentle gastric aspiration. Then 200 to 300m*l* of ice water is instilled and either gently aspirated or allowed to drain by gravity. This procedure is repeated until the bleeding ceases or slows to a trickle, usually is less than 30 min. At this point, the patient should be prepared for endoscopy as soon as possible. Hopefully, by this time, the patient has responded sufficiently to resuscitation to permit completion of the diagnostic scheme.

B. Panendoscopy

During resuscitation and gastric lavage, the patient should receive verbal preparation and instruction regarding the indication for, and technique of, peroral panendoscopy. He should receive appropriate reassurance about the safety and tolerability of endoscopy with modern flexible, fiberoptic, intermediate diameter instruments (8 to 11 mm) without pharyngeal anesthesia or sedative-analgesic premedication. The bleeding patient has been shown to accept emergent endoscopy very well without drug preparation.[13,14]

There are few contraindications to endoscopy in the actively bleeding patient. Endoscopy usually should be delayed until the patient recovers from hypovolemic shock. On occasion, as in the torrential bleeder, endoscopy may be done in the operating room to rule out a bleeding lesion in the esophagus. The uncooperative patient perhaps is the only absolute contraindication for endoscopy. Application of these contraindications to the patient with acute upper gastrointestinal bleeding requires careful thought and consideration of relative risk vs. the potential help from accurage diagnosis, plus the possibility of nonsurgical therapy.

The patient is positioned on the left side and a continuous gentle aspiration is made as the gastric lavage tube is removed. An oropharyngeal suction device should be readied to aspirate any regurgitated material at this time. The 8 to 11 mm diameter flexible endoscopes with a standard or larger size suction channel currently are the preferred instruments for emergency endoscopy. These instruments are passed easily and rapidly into the esophagus. The examination should require only 8 to 10 minutes to the descending duodenum, including a retroversion maneuver to examine the gastric fundus and cardia. When forward viewing endoscopes are used, relative blind areas exist in the fornices of the duodenal bulb, the distal antral lesser curvative area, and the posterior wall lesser curvative aspect of the cardia. Although current instruments have excellent tip flexibility and optics, incomplete examinations still occur. The failure rate for diagnosis in acute bleeding is reported as between 7 and 10%.[17] The most common causes for failure are incomplete gastric cleansing because of physician impatience, use of a small bore (16 or 18 Fr) aspiration tube, or continued bleeding. If the endoscopy is not considered adequate, even though a bleeding or potential bleeding lesion is seen, it is important to repeat the examination within 24 hr to be certain no other lesion has been overlooked.

When no lesion is found during emergency endoscopy, most believe the source of upper gastrointestinal bleeding has been mucosal erosions that are too small to identify. Lesions in the distal duodenum proximal to the ligament of Treitz or hemobilia rarely may be the cause. If no source is identified and active bleeding continues, angiography is indicated as the next diagnostic, and potentially therapeutic, step. Barium contrast radiography should not be done at this stage.

C. Angiography

Selective celiac and superior mesenteric angiography may be used to localize a bleeding site in the upper tract, but rarely can identify the exact type of lesion. When endoscopy has failed and bleeding continues at least moderately active, there is a good chance of diagnostic success. In one report, visceral angiography documented a bleeding site in 22 of 23 cases.[3] Such success requires a minimum bleeding rate of 0.5 to 1 m*l*/min which is considerable, i.e., 720 to 1440 m*l*/24 hr. Arteriography obviously has one major disadvantage, i.e., a marked reduction in diagnostic accuracy when bleeding slows. When a bleeding site is identified, the angiographer has the capability to treat the bleeding by infusion of vasoconstricting drugs, or injection of gelfoam or autologous clot in an attempt to embolize the bleeding vessel.

D. Barium Contrast Radiography

Several reports clearly have shown that barium contrast radiography of the upper digestive tract is grossly inaccurate for diagnosis of bleeding lesions. The method as usually performed is rarely, if ever, capable of diagnosing the erosive mucosal disorders and fails to document from 30 to 50% of chronic peptic ulcers and varices. One report indicates an overall diagnostic accuracy for barium contrast study of 30% compared to 83% for endoscopy and 95% for a subgroup studied by angiography.[3] Barium given before endoscopy and angiography greatly reduces or eliminates their diagnostic accuracy. If barium contrast study has any role in acute upper gastrointestinal bleeding, it is best done several days after the acute bleeding episode has resolved.

V. PROGNOSIS OF THE BLEEDING PATIENT

There is no symptom or sign known to the clinician to permit an accurate prediction as to the duration, degree, and effect of acute upper gastrointestinal bleeding. Certain observations have been made that provide clues to permit categorization of the higher-risk patient but, in any single case, a number of these risk factors must be present to allow some accuracy in predicting the outcome. The recently reported prospective A/S/G/E National Survey of Upper Gastrointestinal Bleeding involved 2428 consecutive patients.[17] Endoscopy was performed in 94 percent with a 1 percent complication rate. The overall mortality in the series was 10.8% with a range of 2.5% for those who received no blood transfusion to 34.2% mortality for those who received in excess of ten units. Surgery was performed in 15.6% of patients.

VI. THERAPEUTIC DECISION MAKING

The practice of early, precise diagnosis of the type and location of a bleeding lesion, plus historical and physical information, provide the clinician with the optimum data base upon which to make timely therapeutic judgements. In some instances, the need for immediate surgery is obvious and the patient is spared the risk, inconvenience, and cost of an unnecessary delay. This option provided by early endoscopic diagnosis proves especially valuable in the elderly and those with severe associated disease. The importance of an accurate preoperative diagnosis is dramatically illustrated in the report of Mackie and Gent.[10] These authors observed an operative mortality of 32% in bleeding patients who had no preoperative diagnosis of a specific bleeding site compared to 9.5% mortality in those with a precise preoperative diagnosis. A prompt accurate diagnosis then appears both to reduce delay either in a decision to operate or not operate and to decrease the mortality rate in such patients compared with those not having a precise preoperative diagnosis of the bleeding site.

In patients who are proven to be bleeding from esophageal varices, the institution of vasopressin infusion and properly applied balloon tamponade can be expected to result in at least temporary cessation of bleeding in over 80%.[16] There is no justification for balloon tamponade based on a presumptive diagnosis, since it has been shown that less than 30% of patients who present with bleeding and known esophageal varices will be bleeding from the varices.[8] The decision for balloon tamponade therapy then is dependent upon the endoscopic confirmation of bleeding from an esophageal or gastric varix. Experience indicates that it is best to use a balloon tamponade tube modified by addition of nasogastric tube for constant hypopharyngeal aspiration.[16]

Decisions regarding therapy need to be based on the patient's immediate status, bleeding rate, bleeding source, and other risk factors listed above. This decision should be made by the team responsible for the patient's care. Joint decisions by physician and surgeon team members unquestionably are the most appropriate.

A decision on the most appropriate treatment usually is based on multiple factors including:

1. The patient's general health, i.e., associated diseases
2. Confirmation of the bleeding site
3. Previous proven bleeding from the same or a similar lesion
4. Rate of bleeding
5. Continuous bleeding requiring five units of blood transfusion but no stability of vital signs
6. Recurrent bleeding from the same lesion during the same hospitalization, especially from peptic ulcer disease
7. Availability of nonsurgical methods of proven safety and effectiveness that may stop bleeding completely or permit surgery to be done on an elective rather than an emergent basis.

REFERENCES

1. **Ament, M. E., Gans, S. L., and Christie, D. L.,** Experience with esophago-gastro-duodenoscopy in diagnosis of 79 pediatric patients with hematemesis, melena or chronic abdominal pain, *Gastroenterology,* 68, 858, 1975.
2. **Baker, M. S., Fisher, J. H., van der Reis, L., and Baker, B. H.,** The endoscopic diagnosis of an aortoduodenal fistual, *Arch. Surg.,* 111, 304, 1976.
3. **Butler, M. L. Johnson, L. F., and Clark, R.,** Diagnostic accuracy of fiberoptic panendoscopy and visceral angiography in acute upper gastrointestinal bleeding, *Am. J. Gastroenterol.,* 65, 501, 1976.
4. **Chang, F. C., Drake, J. E., and Fasha, G. J.** Massive upper gastrointestinal hemorrhage in the elderly, *Am. J. Surg.,* 134, 721, 1977.
5. **Cotton, P. B., Rosenburg, M. T., Waldram, R. P. L., and Axon, A. T. R.,** Early endoscopy of esophagus, stomach, and duodenal bulb in patients with hematemesis and melena, *Br. Med. J.,* 2, 505, 1973.
6. **Dean, R. H., Allen, T. R., Foster, J. H., Mattingly, S., Clayson, K. R., and Edwards, E. H.** Aortoduodenal fistula: an uncommon but correctable cause of upper gastrointestinal bleeding, *Am. Surg.,* 44, 37, 1978.
7. **Graham, D. Y., Klish, W. J., Ferry, G. D., and Sabel, J. S.,** Value of fiberoptic gastrointestinal endoscopy in infants and children, *South. Med. J.,* 71, 558, 1978.
8. **Josen, A. S., Givliani, E., Voorhees, A. B., and Ferrer, J. M.,** Immediate endoscopic diagnosis of upper gastrointestinal bleeding, *Arch. Surg.,* 111, 980, 1976.
9. **Liebman, W.N., Thaler, M. M., and Bujanover, Y.,** Endoscopic evaluation of upper gastrointestinal bleeding in the newborn, *Am. J. Gastroenterol.,* 69, 607, 1978.
10. **Mackie, D. E. and Gent, A. E.,** Management of upper gastrointestinal hemorrhage, *Ann. R. Coll. Surg. Engl.,* 59, 56, 1977.
11. **Morris, D. W., Levine, G. M., Soloway, R. D., et al.** Prospective randomized study of diagnosis and outcome in acute upper-gastrointestinal bleeding: endoscopy versus conventional radiography, *Dig. Dis.,* 20, 1103, 1975.
12. **Morrissey, J. F.** Early endoscopy for major gastrointestinal bleeding—it should be done, *Dig. Dis.,* 22, 534, 1977.
13. **Palmer, E. D.** Observations on the vigorous diagnostic approach to severe upper gastrointestinal hemorrhage, *Ann. Intern. Med.,* 36, 1484, 1952.
14. **Palmer, E. D.,** The vigorous diagnostic approach to upper gastrointestinal tract hemorrhage, *JAMA,* 207, 1477, 1969.

15. **Palumbo, L. J., Sharpe, W. S., Lube, D. J., et al.** Distal antrectomy with vagectomy for duodenal ulcer. Sixteen year review of our results in 510 cases, *Arch. Surg.,* 106, 469, 1973.
16. **Pitcher, J. L.** Safety and effectiveness of the modified Sengstaken-Blakemore tube: a prospective study, *Gastroenterology,* 61, 291, 1971.
17. **Silverstein, F. E., Gilbert, D. A., Tedesco, F. J., et al.** Upper gastrointestinal bleeding: results of the A/S/G/E National Survey, *Gastrointest. Endosc.,* 26 (Abstr.), 77, 1980.
18. **Tedesco, F. J., Goldstein, P. D., Gleason, W. A., and Keating, J. P.** Upper gastrointestinal endoscopy in the pediatric patient, *Gastroenterology,* 70, 492, 1976.
19. **Winans, C. S.** Emergency upper gastrointestinal endoscopy: does haste make waste? *Dig. Dis.,* 22, 536, 1977.

Chapter 2

ELECTROSURGICAL PRINCIPLES IN GASTROINTESTINAL ENDOSCOPY

Frank W. Harris

TABLE OF CONTENTS

I. INTRODUCTION

Electrosurgery is the direct application of electricity to tissue for the purpose of cutting or controlling bleeding. Physicians rarely understand electrosurgery because they are uncomfortable with the concepts behind basic electricity. This Chapter will attempt to give an overview of these concepts as they apply to electrosurgery.

II. BASIC ELECTRICITY

Electricity consists of congregations of electrons. Electrons carry a negative charge which attracts them to positively charged atoms which have lost their outer shell valence electrons. This attraction is a force called *voltage.* Voltage pushes electrons through conductive solids like metals and tissue. Under certain circumstances, voltage can also push electrons through less substantial mediums like air or the vacuum in a TV picture tube.

A good analogy for electron flow through a solid conductor would be billiard balls richocheting around a crowded table. However, even small electrical currents consist of so many billions of individual electrons that the *electrical current* as a whole better resembles water flowing through a pipe.

The electrons flow in a current when they are pushed into flowing by a *voltage* (Table 1). Electrons are attracted to positive voltages and are repelled by negative voltages. How many electrons will flow through a conductor, such as a wire, depends on how much opposition or *resistance* the conductor has to current flowing through it. Resistance is measured in *ohms.* Voltage is measured in *volts.* Current is measured in *amperes.* One ampere is 6.2 billion-billion electrons which is why we can disregard the discrete nature of the electrons. One volt will force one ampere of current to flow through a one ohm resistance. This relationship is called *Ohm's Law.*

Perhaps the most basic concept needed to understand electrosurgery is that electricity *always* flows in a complete loop or circular pathway (Figure 1A and 1B). In electrosurgery, that current goes out of the *active electrode* through the patient (the resistive load) and returns to the generator via the *patient* or *return electrode.* It is not always obvious that current flows in a complete circle.

III. AC, DC, AND RF

Electrosurgery uses radio frequency currents. If low-frequency current such as 60 cycles per second household current were used, it would shock and fibrillate the patient. In *direct current* (DC), the electrons flow through the circuit in only one direction. *Alternating current* (AC) is a current which periodically alternates direction around the circuit loop. The amounts of current that flow in each direction, first one way and then the other, are equal. This means the *average* current flow in any one direction is zero. Just because the arithmetic average over time is zero, it does not mean that it is not delivering energy to resistance loads that are in the circuit path. To get around this time-average-equal-to-zero difficulty, AC voltage is often measured as *root mean square voltage* (RMS voltage). RMS means that all current through the load is assumed to be going in the same direction.

We can simulate alternating current by deftly removing the battery from the flashlight circuit in Figure 1 and reversing the polarity. If the battery is reversed back and forth very rapidly, we have generated an AC current (Figure 2). The light bulb will light just as brightly as if the current were DC provided the average current through the bulb is the same regardless of the direction of flow.

Table 1
A GLOSSARY OF ELECTRICAL TERMS

Term	Definition
Current	quantity of electrons flowing past a point each second; e.g., 1A = 6.2×10^{18} electrons/sec.
Voltage	The *force* that pushes electrons through conductors or across an air gap when it makes a spark; 12,000 V makes an electric spark jump roughly 1 cm
Resistance	Opposition to current flow by the material it is passing through; 1 V can drive 1A through 1 Ω of resistance
Power	The *rate* at which heat energy is delivered to tissue or other resistance each second; 1 W of power = 1 V × 1A
Waveform	The variation of voltage (or sometimes current) with time; waveforms can be *seen* when they are plotted on an oscilloscope screen
Capacitance	The storage of opposite electric charges on conductive objects separated by an insulator; high-frequency AC current can pass *through* capacitors even though they block low-frequency and DC current
Electric spark	An electric discharge between the electrode and tissue in electrosurgery; sparks are vital to electrosurgical cutting and fulguration

Tissue membrane potentials can be discharged by voltages at frequencies from DC up to about 50,000 cycles. A DC voltage can discharge the cell membrane potential of a muscle cell or nerve axon if the voltage direction remains the same long enough for the membrane to respond. However, as the frequency is increased, the direction of the voltage is switched back and forth more rapidly and the ions in the membrane have less time to respond. Eventually, the voltage will be unable to move the ions significantly in one direction before the voltage switches back the other way.

To keep electrosurgery from stimulating muscle and nerves, radio frequencies are used. *Radio frequencies* (RF) are very high-frequency AC currents. Radio signals that are actually broadcast over distances range from between 100,000 CPS (alternations) up to 100,000 million c in experimental microwave transmitters. Electrosurgical generator frequencies range from about 400,000 c (just below the AM broadcast band) up to about 3 million c or 3 MHz. Engineers call cycles per second "Hertz" (Hz).

IV. CAPACITANCE

Capacitance is probably the hardest electronic concept to understand in electrosurgery. It is capacitance that makes current flow where common sense tells one there should be no currents. A capacitor is any two pieces of metal or conductor separated by an insulator (Figure 3). Radio frequency current can flow across a capacitor from one conductor to the other almost as if the insulation were not present. For example, a man sitting in a metal dental chair makes a capacitor with respect to the metal chair. His body is a large bag of conductive salt-water and the chair is made of conductive metal. Assuming that his clothes and the plastic upholstery prevent direct contact between his skin and the metal chair, these nonconducting materials comprise a capacitor insulator. Dentists routinely perform electrosurgery on patients without putting a patient electrode on the skin to return the current to the generator. The capacitor couples RF current back to the generator even though there is no direct contact.

In Figure 3, a DC voltage is applied across two parallel metal plates separated with a thin insulator. The electrons will gather on one plate and a positive charge, which is an absence of electrons, gathers on the other. Since each charge is attracted to the opposite polarity of charge, this attraction holds both charges in place on the two metal plates. The *thinner* the insulation between the two plate, *the stronger the attraction and the more charge that can be held on the plates.* Another way to increase the amount of charge that

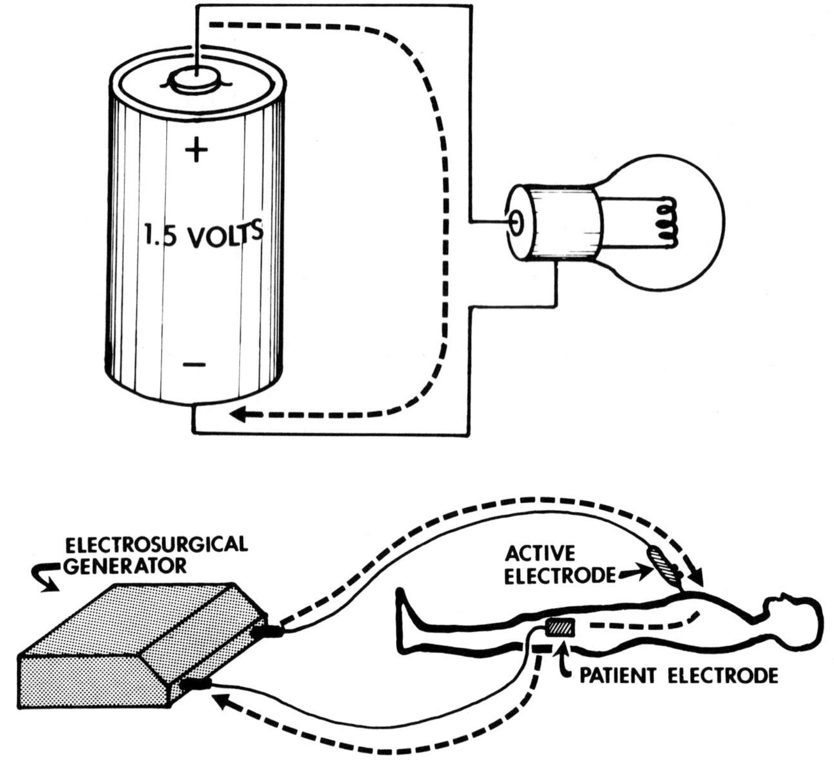

FIGURE 1. Electricity always flows in a complete loop or circular pathway.

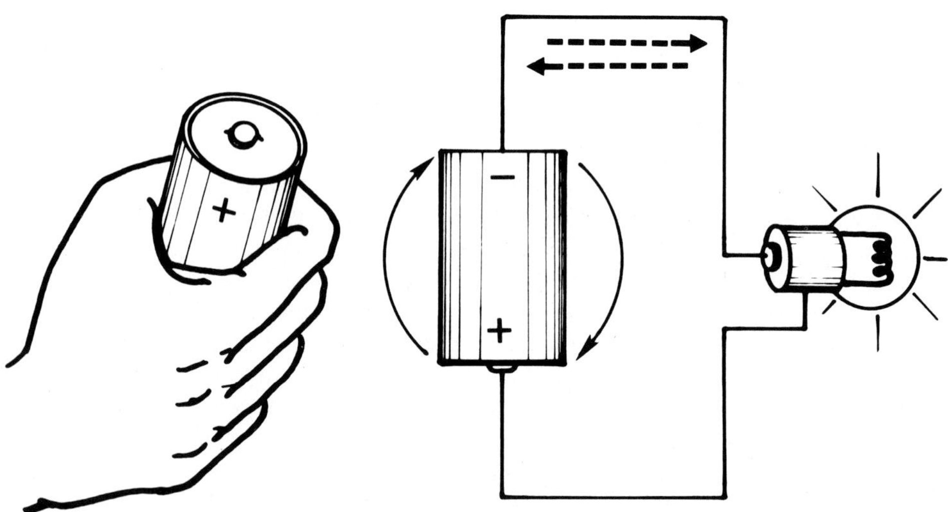

FIGURE 2. Alternating current can be generated by reversing the polarity of the voltage many times per second.

can be held is to increase the *area* of the plates. Once the charge has gathered on capacitor plates, it may stay there indefinitely.

One way to get the charge back out of the capacitor is to short the two plates together (connect them with a conductor) so that the two kinds of charge can get back together.

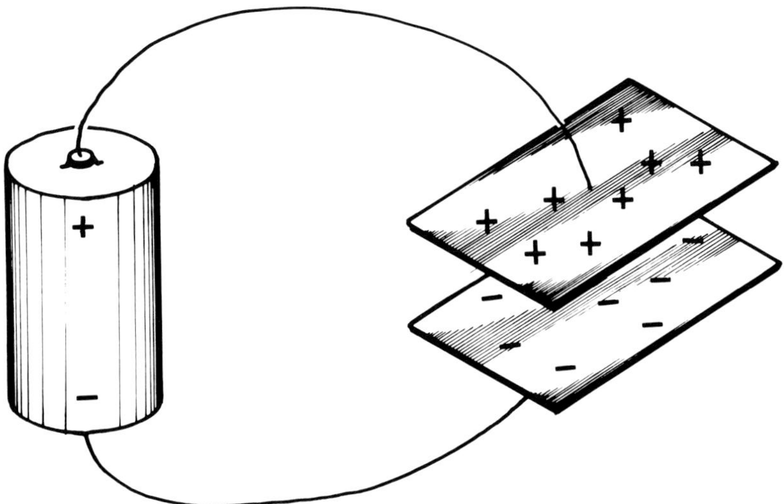

FIGURE 3. Two parallel metal plates separated by an insulator, air.

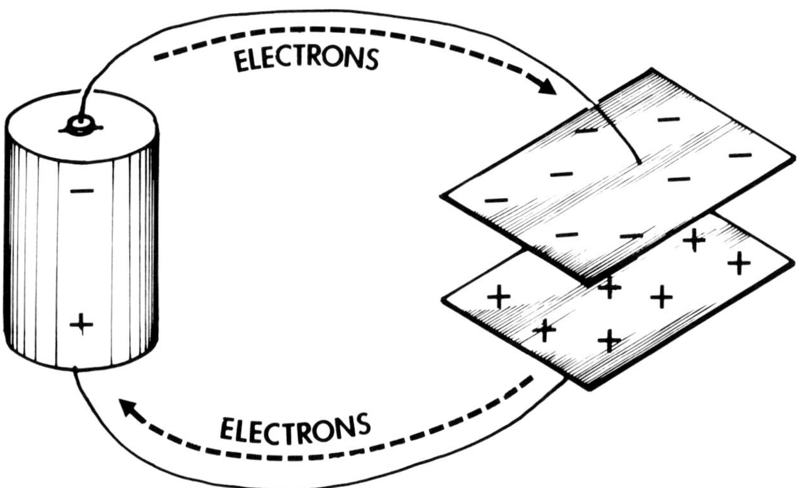

FIGURE 4. Reversing the battery polarity to a charged capacitor. Every time polarity reverses, current travels through the wires to rearrange the charges.

Another way to remove the charge is to reverse the voltage source (the battery) and use the reversed voltage to drive the charge out replacing it with charge of the opposite polarity (Figure 4).

If the battery is reversed back and forth so that the polarity of charges on the capacitor is changed with each reversal of the battery, a current occurs. The current then travels through wires to and from the capacitance.

When an AC voltage is applied to a capacitance, the current flows in wires. No current actually crosses the insulation barrier, but since the currents appear in the wires, it is as though the capacitor were a conductor. The AC current that appears in the wires can do useful work just as DC current. Figure 5 shows a light bulb placed in series with a capacitor. The voltage source is a 60 c household power. The current travels through the light bulb on its way to and from the capacitor plates and lights the light bulb.

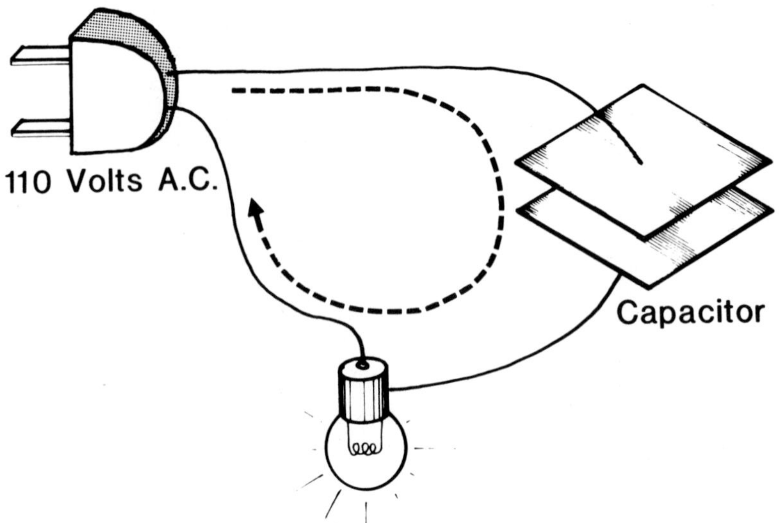

FIGURE 5. AC current can pass "through" a capacitance to light a bulb.

Every time voltage across a capacitor reverses, a small pulse of current goes through the wires to rearrange the charges. The greater the number of reversals per second, the greater the energy conducted "through" the capacitor and into a load such as the light bulb. This means that *low-frequencies require very large capacitors* to conduct significant currents. In contrast, high-radio frequencies can force very large currents through very small capacitors because there are so many small pulses of current per second.

In dental electrosurgery, the active electrode pressed against tissue is analogous to the light bulb. A dental electrosurgical generator usually operates at a relatively high-frequency (3 million HZ) so that the capacitance effect is very significant and the patient plate can be omitted. In medical electrosurgery, which usually has a frequency of about 0.5 million HZ, the body capacitance is insufficient to make a reliable return path and the patient plate cannot be safely omitted.

V. THE ELECTRIC SPARK

The *electric spark* is crucial to electrosurgical cutting and fulguration. It is also fundamental to understanding how physicians and patients are occasionally shocked by high-frequency electrosurgical currents. Electric sparks are like miniature lightning bolts. Air is not normally a conductor. When a large voltage is established across an air gap, the air can break down and become ionized. When air ionizes, it temporarily becomes an ionized fluid much like salt-water. The electrons flow from ionized atom to ionized atom in what physicists call "plasma". Electric sparks evolve through a series of stages that are important to electrosurgery.

High voltages can break down air so that current will flow through the air to make an electric spark. The breakdown of air to form a spark does not occur immediately but occurs in stages (Figure 6). *First,* there is the *glow discharge* which lasts perhaps 10 billionths of a second. This can be seen as a blue or violet glow around the points. If there is not enough voltage to complete the breakdown, this bluish corona glow can go on indefinitely.

In the *second* stage, an electric spark forms. If there is enough voltage to break down air, a glowing, bluish-purple electric pathway appears between the two points. At first

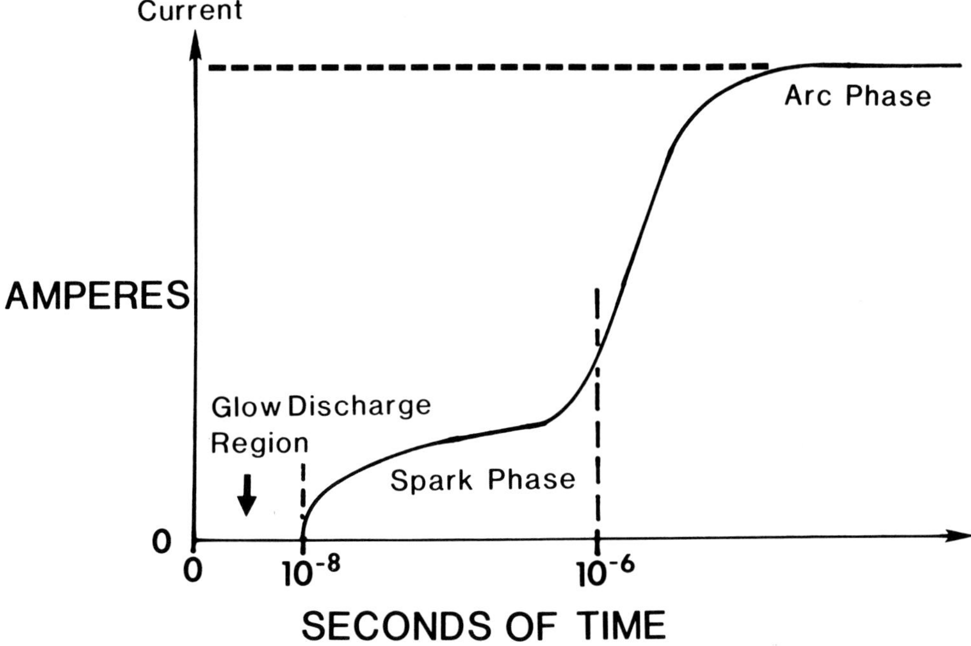

FIGURE 6. Typical evolution of an electric discharge (spark) with time.

the spark path through the air is very narrow, but as more and more current flows down the path, it becomes more established and the spark gets wider and wider and the color turns more yellow.

In the *third stage* after about 1 μsec, the pathway becomes very well established and the resistance of the path suddenly drops down to a few ohms. If the generator is capable of delivering large currents, then large currents will flow down this spark. At this point, the spark enters the *arc phase.*

All of these events from glow discharge to arc take place at a rate proportional to the voltage across the electrodes and proportional to the current that is allowed to flow *through* the spark. The greater the voltage used to start the discharge and the greater the current allowed to flow through the discharge, the faster will the process evolve from glow discharge to spark to arc.

Electric sparks caused by AC voltages are more complicated than they are with DC voltages. Every time the voltage reverses polarity, the ionized air must reorient itself and establish a new spark in the opposite direction. To a large extent, a brand new spark must form in the new direction, but ionized air from previous sparks greatly speeds the process. Sparks from very high-frequency generators (2 MHz) are uniformly blue because they have little time to form. Sparks from low-frequency generators (0.25 MHz) are very yellow and much larger for the same voltage.

The arc phase is often entered by electrosurgical generators in the CUT mode when operating at high power. Tsuzuki[3] claims that arc formation is the basic mechanism of electrosurgical cutting. It is this author's opinion that the association between arcs and cutting is true enough, but this is a coincidence. Arcs are not seen while cutting with high-frequency generators of 2 MHz and above. Arcs would not have time to form at such high-frequencies unless the voltages were much higher and the generator much more powerful than necessary.

VI. HEAT, ENERGY, AND POWER

Physicians are accustomed to dispensing drugs in doses which are carefully thought out beforehand, carefully measured by the pharmacist, and carefully taken by the patient. In contrast, electrosurgery is not calibrated and the physician is left to his judgment and experience about where to set the generator. Usually generator markings are arbitrary numbers from 1 to 10 or 0 to 100. Some of the newer generators are calibrated in watts of power.

Power can be defined as the rate at which energy in the form of heat is delivered to the patient. Quantities of heat energy are measured in *joules.* One joule delivered to a resistance load during 1 sec is defined as 1 W of power. Furthermore, if 1 V forces 1 A of current through a 1 Ω resistance, the power delivered to the resistance will be 1 W.

The watts calibrated on a generator do not correlate very well with the electrosurgical effect because the calibration *assumes* a fixed tissue load resistance, usually some value as 500 Ω. This number has little to do with actual surgery. It an electrode is pressed against tissue, the actual resistance is very dependent on the moisture on the surface of the tissue and the area of contact. To be exact, tissue resistance, often called the tissue impedance, varies as the inverse of the square root of the area.

$$\text{tissue resistance} = \frac{0.8\rho}{\sqrt{2\pi \text{ Area}}}$$

$$\text{where } \rho = \text{tissue resistivity} \approx 460 \text{ ohm-cm}$$

This means that if the electrode has a moist contact area with tissue the size of a pinhead, the resistance will be thousands of ohms. However, if the contact area is a square centimeter, the impedance will be 150 Ω. Generally, *the amount of power a generator will deliver to these different resistances will be much lower than the power it would deliver to a 500 Ω load.* Not only is the actual power delivered different, but the resistance of the tissue increases as the coagulation proceeds.

The most serious shortcoming of calibrating in watts is that it ignores the electric spark. When there is a spark in between the electrode and the tissue, the spark itself has a resistance that also varies. The energy that occurs becomes divided between three places—part of it heats the tissue, part is dissipated in the heat and light of the spark, and part of it heats the electrode.

In summary, generator calibrations in watts gives one a rough ballpark idea about the maximum effect the generator can produce. For example, if the generator calibration says "30 W", it is not realistic to expect to be able to perform a procedure which will require 200 W. On the other hand, one should never assume that 30 W is too little power to cut tissue or to produce unintentional tissue damage. From a safety point of view, what generator mode you are using is usually more important than the power setting.

VII. WAVEFORMS

Whenever electrosurgery is discussed, there is always a lot of talk about *waveforms.* Waveforms are a description of how the radio frequency voltage varies over time. A graph of this variation with time as the variable is a waveform. A typical *cut* waveform is shown in Figure 7. This is just a graph of voltage vs. time as it would be seen on an oscilloscope. In the upper figure, a few microseconds is shown so that the individual cycles of RF voltage can be seen. The waveform in the upper figure is a simple sine

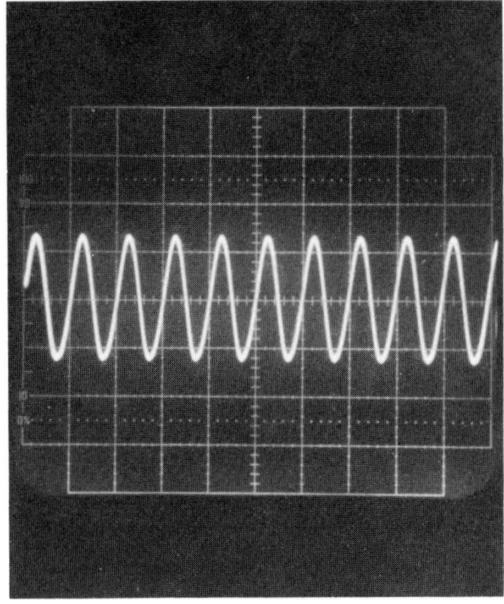

A. CUT waveform over 5 μsec interval.

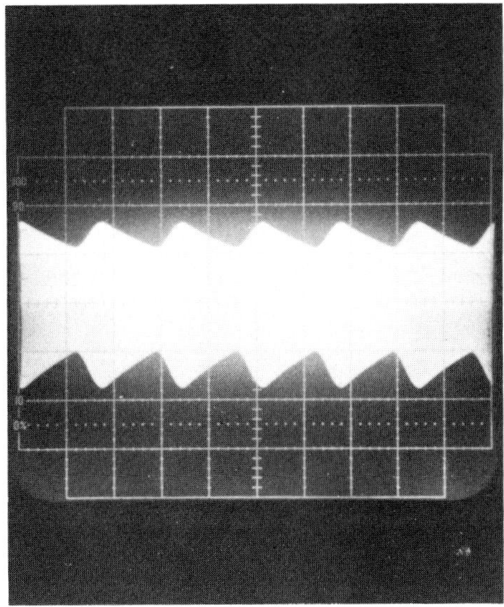

B. CUT waveform over 0.05 sec interval.

FIGURE 7. A typical cut waveform seen on an oscilloscope over a short interval (A) and over a much longer time interval (B). In (B), the Sine waves are too compressed to see. The zig-zag pattern results from a power supply artifact but gives some hemostasis.

wave. In the lower figure, the waveform is looked at over such a "long" period (20 msec) that the individual sine wave cycles are blurred together and can no longer be seen. The whole average level of sine wave cycles of voltage is slowly rising and falling in a saw-tooth shaped amplitude "envelope". This modulation envelope is a common artifact in the power supplies of generators and is derived from the 60 HZ AC power that runs the generator.

The relevance of waveforms is that the higher the voltage, the longer the length of sparks that can be generated. The longer the voltage remains at a high voltage, the more current can flow down through the spark. The length and thickness of the sparks and the current flowing through them is what produces two of the three basic electrosurgical effects, cutting and fulguration.

VIII. ELECTROSURGICAL EFFECTS

Electrosurgery has two basic effects. It can cut tissue and it can coagulate tissue. Since generators are always labeled "cut" and "coag", physicians are lulled into believing that electrosurgery is straightforward. It seems reasonable that whenever the cut light comes on, one should be able to expect the electrode to cut tissue. When the coag light is on, it seems reasonable to expect the tissue to dry and "cook" with little or no tendency to cut. Unfortunately, much more than these simplified concepts is involved.

There are three basic electrosurgical modes; cut, fulgurate, and desiccate. The word "coagulation" or "coag" can mean either fulguration or desiccation. Electrosurgical cutting is defined as sparking to tissue with a cutting effect. Fulguration is defined as sparking to tissue to produce necrosis *without* a cutting effect. Electrosurgical desiccation is defined as necrosing tissue by directly applying the electrosurgical electrode to the tissue so that there is *no sparking* and *no cutting effect.*

The terms "cut" and "coag" as labeled on a generator refer to the voltage waveforms of the generator output in those modes. *The purpose of voltage waveforms is to*

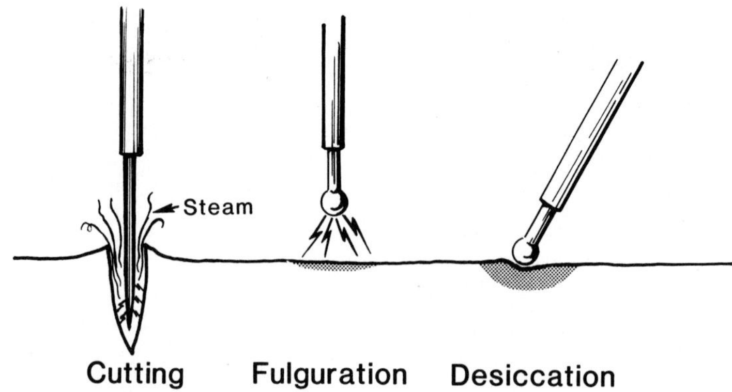

FIGURE 8. Three basic electrosurgical modes: cut, fulguration, desiccation.

determine whether tissue is cut or fulgurated when there is sparking between the electrode and tissue (Figure 8).

For all practical purposes, the voltage waveforms have no effect on an electrode operated in the desiccation mode. When the electrode is in firm contact with the tissue so that there is no sparking, cut and coag waveforms desiccate equally well. A simple step that would eliminate confusion would be to stop using the word "coag". The "coag" knob on generators should really be labeled "fulgurate" if that is what it is designed to do. Similarly, if the generator is designed to desiccate and not fulgurate, then the appropriate knob should be labeled desiccate.

IX. DESICCATION

When the electrode is pressed firmly against moist tissue and there is no sparking, then the electrosurgical effect is always *desiccation.* When the generator is activated, the current flows from the active electrode through the tissue and returns to a large *patient electrode* at some distance away on the patient's skin. The tissue necrosis is controlled by current density. The heating effect of electrosurgical current is always proportional to the current density (Figure 9). At the patient electrode, the current density is very low so that tissue heating is not sufficient to harm the patient's skin. At the small active electrode, the current density is very high so the heating effect is concentrated. As the current travels to the patient electrode, the current spreads out radially away from the active electrode. Therefore, current density falls off very quickly with distance from the electrode site.

Let's examine the events that occur under a desiccation electrode when the generator is turned on and current begins to flow. First, the tissue and moisture in contact with the electrode begin to heat. Protein in the cells begins to denature at about 50°C. This will kill the cell if the heating continues at this temperature. At about 95°C, the tissue turns a light brown color. Usually, the temperature rises swiftly to the boiling point where further temperature climb is temporarily halted by the boiling of water. Steam can be seen leaving the tissue around the electrode. As the water is driven out of the tissue, the tissue loses its electrical conductivity. As the tissue electrical resistance rises, the current through the tissue drops so that the tissue heating decreases. Soon the rise in resistance completely shuts the current off and the desiccation is complete.

The depth of penetration of the necrosis into the tissue is roughly equal to the width of the electrode. If a very large electrode is pressed against tissue, then the generator must supply a very large current to produce a high current density. If a very small electrode is

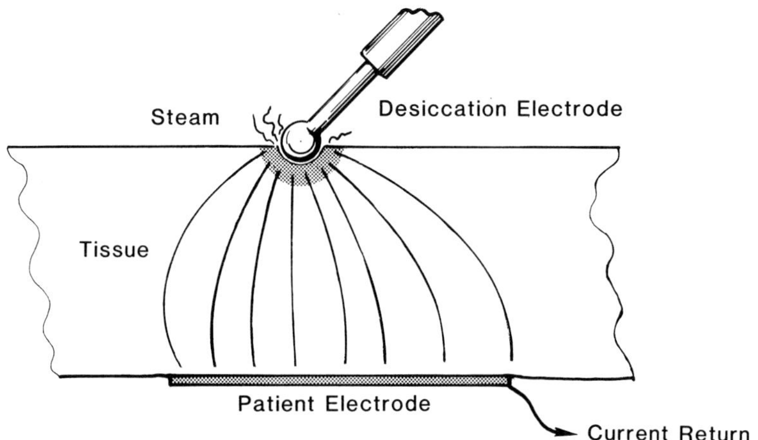

FIGURE 9. Current density in desiccation.

used, the generator need only produce a very small current to produce the same current *density*. A small current will produce small current densities at a very short distance from the electrode contact site, while a large current passed through a large electrode will produce necrosis at a longer range in proportion to the size of the electrode.

When one talks about large and small electrodes contacting tissue, the subject becomes complicated. The larger the electrode, the more tissue it contacts, and the resistance of the tissue as "seen" by the generator decreases. When more tissue is contacted, it is comparable to putting resistors in parallel. To use a water analogy, if one garden hose has a certain amount of resistance to water flow, then a large number of hoses in parallel will have less resistance to water flow. This drop in apparent resistance will coax larger currents from the generator in accordance with Ohm's Law. *The complication is that the generator may or may not be able to supply more current depending on the generator design.* This explains why one generator brand may desiccate better than another. A generator properly designed for desiccation will supply all the current "asked for" by the electrode contact resistance. In fact, it is possible to design a generator so that large and small electrodes will desiccate equally without changing the power control. Ideally, the only effect the power control should have is to increase the *speed* at which the desiccation proceeds.

When desiccation is complete, the surface of the necrotic tissue is dry, so that electrically the generator has been "disconnected" from the tissue. If the action of a generator is to be confined to desiccation, then it is very important that when the desiccation is complete the voltage between the electrode and the tissue not be high enough to allow or cause sparking to the nearest moist tissue.

Desiccation can also play a role in *mechanical* cutting. Desiccation softens collagen fibers. Desiccated tissue is much more easily cut with a blade than fresh tissue. This principle can be used to advantage in polypectomy. The snare is held in firm contact with the polyp which encourages desiccation and discourages sparking. As the desiccation proceeds, the snare is slowly closed and the desiccated stalk is cut off mechanically. The desiccation provides the hemostasis and softens the tissue so that it may be cut mechanically.

X. ELECTROSURGICAL CUTTING

Electrosurgical cutting cuts tissue by means of short intense sparks between the electrode and tissue. Suppose a cut waveform is selected and the generator is turned to a moderate to high setting. The generator is activated and the electrode is held a short distance above the tissue. As the electrode is brought closer and closer to the tissue, eventually an electric spark will jump from the electrode to the tissue. This electric spark is small and "sharp" regardless of the shape of the electrode. If the generator is able to supply enough current to travel down through the spark to the tissue, the current density where the spark lands will be very high. If this current density is high enough, the cells that are struck will be volatilized by the spark so that they burst into steam. The steam not only carries away the water, but the cell contents as well.

The next spark will jump to the tissue at the point closest to the electrode. More cells will be converted to steam. This produces a cushion of escaping steam between the electrode and tissue. For a 500 KHz cut waveform, as many as a million sparks per second are possible, allowing this to be a very smooth process.

The shape of the electrode has only an indirect effect on *electrosurgical* cutting. The larger the *area* of the cutting electrode and the *faster* it is moved through the tissue, the more energetic each spark must be to maintain the steam barrier. In other words, big electrodes with big cutting areas will require higher power settings because each spark must generate more steam to separate the electrode from the tissue.

Suppose an electrode is used that is too big for a given power setting. If the sparks are unable to maintain a steam barrier between the electrode and the tissue, the electrode will "stall" when the electrode contacts the wall of the incision. When this happens, the voltage between the electrode and tissue will be extinguished and large currents will flow directly into the tissue in a desiccation mode. The same electrode cannot desiccate and spark tissue simultaneously.

Frequently, the electrode is applied firmly to the tissue before the generator is turned on. This means that the electrode will begin in a desiccation mode. If the generator is set to a high power setting, the desiccation phase may be completed so quickly that it may not be obvious that it occurred. If a cut waveform at a high setting is used, the voltage will be high when desiccation is complete and sparking will immediately begin to cut tissue.

However, if the power setting is low in comparison with the area of the electrode in contact with the tissue, the cutting mode may not begin at all. At the end of the desiccation phase, the electrode is effectively insulated from the tissue with a layer of dried tissue. This high resistance will allow the voltage to rise between the electrode and tissue, but if the power setting is too low, the voltage may not be high enough to spark to the nearest moist tissue and begin the cutting.

Applying force to an electrode in an attempt to make it begin electrosurgical cutting is exactly the wrong thing to do. The more firmly the electrode is pressed against the tissue, the longer the desiccation phase will be prolonged and the less likely that electrosurgical cutting will begin. It can also happen that pushing down on the electrode can make it burst through the dried crust surrounding the electrode and the depth of electrosurgical cutting can be much deeper than was intended.

If the intention is to cut electrosurgically, then ideally the generator should be activated before the electrode is brought into contact with the tissue. There will never be any difficulty getting the cut started if the spark touches the tissue before the electrode. If the electrode is held lightly so that it has as little contact with the tissue as possible and if the spark is permitted to do the cutting, even a very large electrode can be made to cut its way through tissue provided the electrode is moved very slowly with the sparks leading the way.

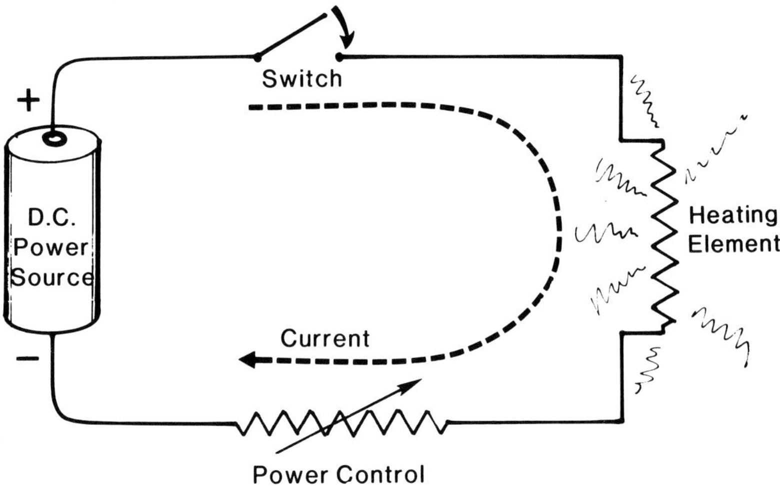

FIGURE 10. Electrically heated cautery iron.

XI. CUTTING BY HEATED ELECTRODE

In the preceding discussion, it has been described how sparks jump from the electrode to the tissue and these sparks heat the tissue so suddenly that the tissue explodes into steam. It should not be a surprise that these sparks are also heating the electrode. If the electrode is small and thin and is made out of a relatively poor heat conductor such as stainless steel, the electrode can become red hot. A hot blade that is heated to well above the boiling point of salt-water can explode tissue into steam when the hot metal makes direct contact with the tissue.

An electrically heated cautery is not the same thing as electrosurgery (Figure 10). In cautery, a hot object such as a branding iron is directly applied to tissue to sear or cut. An electrically heated cautery has a heating element in it that resembles the heating elements on an electric stove. The electrical current is the means of heating the iron, but unlike electrosurgery, the current does not pass through the patient's tissue.

Since the temperature of the cautery iron can be anything, the effect of pressing a hot iron on tissue can range from a superficial soft necrosis resembling desiccation to a superficial hard eschar which resembles fulguration. The coagulation effects of cautery are superficial because heat penetrates tissue by heat conduction alone. In electrosurgery and especially desiccation, the electrical current actually enters the tissue. Heat arises inside the tissue rather than mechanically conducting to the site.

The principle of cutting with a heated blade explains why a stainless steel electrosurgical electrode cuts better than an electrode made out of a good thermal conductor such as silver. A hot steel electrode maintains a high temperature and encourages the formation of a steam barrier. If the tissue is contacted by the hot blade, some vaporization of tissue can be caused by the hot electrode alone. The blade heating complements electrosurgical cutting by sparks because the sparking is needed to maintain an electrode temperature well above the boiling point of tissue fluids. In fact, electrode temperatures as high as 500°C have been measured in surgery during sparking to the electrode.

Desiccation alone does not heat the electrode to greater than the boiling point because the blade temperature is limited to the temperature of the tissue it is heating. The tissue temperature is locked to the temperature of the steam which is being driven off the tissue. When the steam stops, the water is gone from the tissue so the tissue

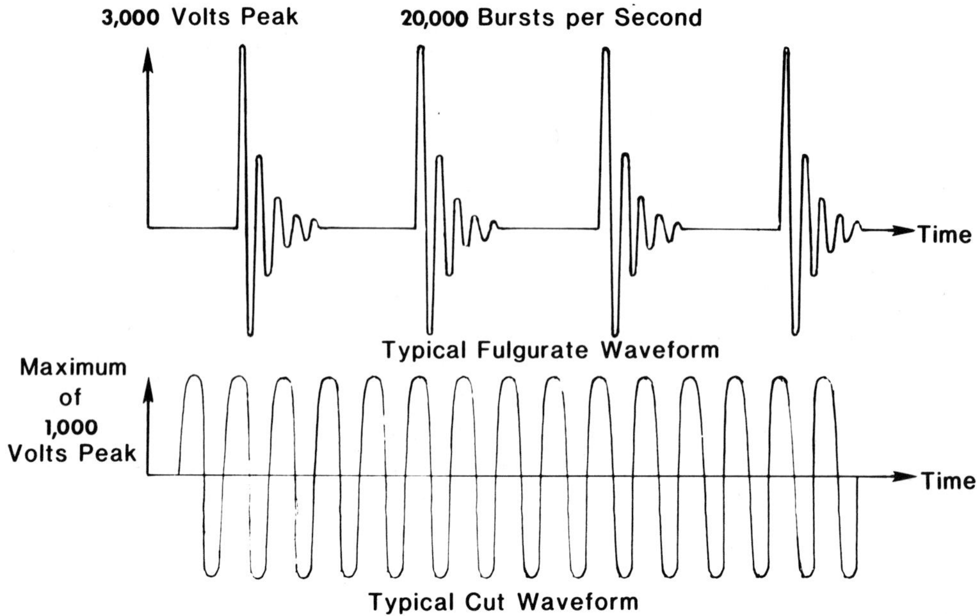

FIGURE 11. Cut and fulgurate waveforms.

electrical resistance is very high. This high resistance turns off the current and stops the desiccation as the last of the water is converted into steam. The temperature of the tissue and electrode never rises above boiling unless sparking begins. In summary, sparking to the electrode heats the electrode. Hot electrodes help maintain the steam barrier which encourages sparking and prevents electrode stalling.

In contrast, a cold electrode is better for desiccation because it collapses the steam barrier and helps to keep the electrode in direct contact with the tissue. This principle is used in neurosurgery where electrode tips are often gold plated or made of silver in an attempt to keep the electrode tip cool. Even if some sparking should occur, the silver electrode conducts the heat away quickly and is less likely to form a steam barrier.

The other advantage of a silver electrode is that a cool electrode is less likely to stick to tissue. Using desiccation for stopping bleeders is frequently frustrated by tissue sticking. Often the bleeding is controlled, but the electrode is stuck fast to the coagulum. When the electrode is pulled free, the crust comes off with it and the bleeding resumes. As tissue is heated and proteins are broken down, there is a point at which the denatured proteins and the remaining water make a sticky glue. By keeping the temperature of the electrode below the optimum temperature for this glue formation, electrode sticking can be prevented.[1]

XII. FULGURATION

Fulguration is sparking to tissue *without* a cutting effect. The cutting effect is caused by short intense sparks causing a high current density on the tissue where they land. If the spark can be modified so that it lands on the tissue but does not produce a high current density, the effect can resemble desiccation with no cutting. In generators now in use, the spark current density is decreased primarily by using a *different voltage waveform* (Figure 11).

The current density of the sparks landing on tissue can be decreased by limiting the current passing through individual sparks. However, the easiest way to have less current density is to have *fewer sparks* per second. The fulguration waveforms achieve this by having fewer voltage cycles per second. This does not mean using a lower frequency. It means leaving out most of the sine wave cycles so that the voltage cycles just occur in short bursts. By limiting the large voltage cycles to perhaps one cycle in ten, there will be only one tenth as many cycles which produce sparks as compared with the cut waveform.

Voltage is the force that makes sparks jump to the tissue. Therefore, the area covered by the sparks can be increased by using a higher voltage than used for the cut waveform. In this way, the area covered is increased which lowers the current density on the tissue and discourages cutting.

In spite of the radically different shape of cut and fulgurate waveforms, the *power* that they can deliver to tissue in direct ohmic contact (desiccation) is the same provided that the average voltage over time, called the RMS voltage, is equal. This means that these two waveforms can desiccate identically provided that sparking does not begin. Since the fulguration waveforms have higher voltage peaks, it is more likely to spark to nearby moist tissue at the completion of desiccation than is the cut waveform. For this reason, *a cut waveform is preferred for desiccation* because the cut waveform is less likely to begin sparking when the desiccation is completed as voltage rises between the tissue and the electrode.

XIII. THE ADVANTAGES OF FULGURATION

Most "coagulation" in general surgery is done with fulguration. If sparks occur and it did not cut, the mode was fulguration. In contrast, pure desiccation is routinely used only in opthalmology, neurosurgery, and in laparoscopic sterilization procedures. Fulguration has several advantages over desiccation.

1. The electrode does not have to have contact with tissue while fulgurating.
2. Because the fulguration process is not limited to the temperature of boiling water, the tissue can be pyrolyzed to a tough strong eschar.
3. High quality fulguration can penetrate a swiftly moving layer of blood to stop brisk arterial bleeders up to 1.5 mm in diameter.
4. Fulguration has the potential to provide better hemostasis for most applications with *less depth of penetration* than desiccation.

Fulguration also has disadvantages compared with desiccation.

1. The high voltages used in fulguration are more likely to break down insulation on forceps, probes, and cables. This can lead to accidental burns to the physician and patient.
2. Fulguration and electrosurgical cutting to a lesser degree generate electrical low-frequency noise which can occasionally cause muscle stimulation and "shocks" to both the physician and patient. This is especially severe any time there is sparking between two metal objects as might occur with a loose connector.
3. Fulguration of neural tissue causes as much bleeding as it stops, due to shrinking of the eschar and the weakness of the tissue. This is why desiccation is preferred in neurosurgery.
4. After 10 years of development, the fulguration produced by the average solid state generator is good, but not excellent. The result is that there is still too much cutting in "coag". In the best transistorized generators, fulguration leaves a shallow crater at the fulguration site which is more tissue destruction than necessary. The best available fulguration is still found in some, but not all, of the old spark gap generators.

XIV. BLEND WAVEFORMS

Blend waveforms are a mixture of cut and fulgurate waveforms (Figure 12). They do not cut cleanly, but they do leave the walls of the incision fulgurated so that as the electrode passes through, some hemostasis can be obtained along with the incision. "Blend" is a relative term. On a typical generator the blend waveform is somewhere between the best fulguration waveform and the best cut waveform that the generator has to offer. With all of the early transistorized generators, the fulguration was so poor that it should really have been labeled "blend".

What is needed is a numerical rating that will evaluate any generator output to assess how easily it will cut and how much hemostasis can be expected when used to fulgurate tissue. This number could be related directly to the current density of the sparks it produces. Perhaps, it would be even better to rate it in terms of mm of arteriole bleeder diameter size that it could control in some standard animal preparation.

The term *crest factor* is a poor substitute for a direct measurement of current density, but is the only specification that directly relates to the quality of fulguration performance. Crest factor is defined as the ratio of peak voltage divided by RMS voltage.

$$\text{Crest factor} = \frac{\text{peak voltage}}{\text{RMS voltage}}$$

At first look, crest factor looks like an adequate indicator of waveform performance. The peak voltage relates directly to how far sparks will jump so this relates well to the area covered. The RMS voltage is related to the *average current delivered.* Unfortunately, the measurement is not made while actually sparking to tissue. In spite of this, crest factor usually relates to cutting and fulgurating as follows.

Crest factor	Description	Hemostasis
1.4	Clean cut	No hemostasis
3.0	Typical blended cut	Light hemostasis on incision wall
6.0	Typical fulguration of transistorized generator cutting is still possible	0.75 mm arteriole bleeder
10.0	Best transistorized fulguration waveform.	1.25 mm arteriole bleeder.
10—15	Best spark gap generator waveforms	1.5 mm arteriole; some authors say up to 2 mm

The reason that the old generators fulgurate better than the modern ones is not just crest factor. It is the author's opinion that a low fulguration frequency is the primary reason. Sparks become fatter and longer at lower frequencies and spread the current density over a wider area. The old generators used fulguration frequencies as low as 250 KHz. In contrast, high-frequencies like 2 MHz produce very thin, "sharp" sparks that are best for cutting. For this reason, the old tube-spark gap machines used this high-frequency for their cut waveform.

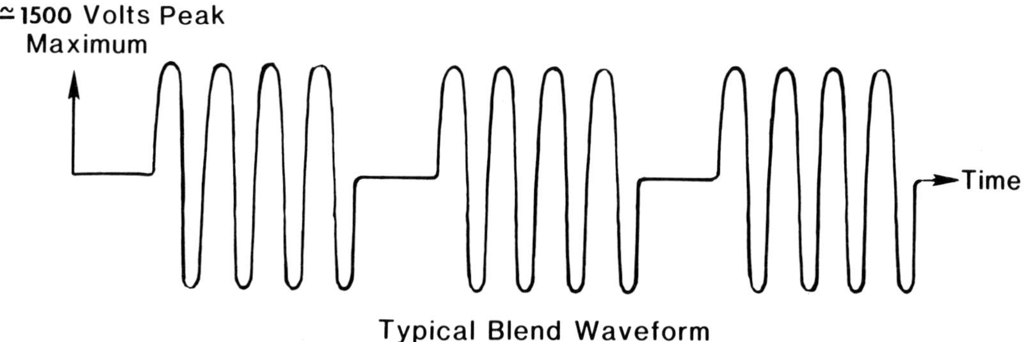

FIGURE 12. Blend waveforms are a mixture of cut and fulgurate waveforms.

REFERENCES

1. **Morrison, C. F., Jr.,** U.S. Patent 4,074,718.
2. **Shinya, H.,** Personal Interview, New York, March 28, 1978.
3. **Tsuzuki, M. and Utashiro, I.,** Theoretical analysis on cutting and coagulating effect of electrosurgical devices, Paper given at AAMI meeting, March 1978.
4. **Williams, C.,** Lecture, Medical College of Wisconsin G. I. Endoscopy Seminar, Canary Islands, Spain, February 1977.

Chapter 3

ELECTROCOAGULATION

John P. Papp

TABLE OF CONTENTS

I. INTRODUCTION

The 1970's saw the birth of therapeutic endoscopic electrocoagulation in the gastrointestinal tract. This new technology was preceded by the development of flexible fiberoptic endoscopes able to visualize the esophagus, stomach, and duodenum. With the introduction of monopolar electrodes to assist the colonoscopist in achieving hemostasis after electrosurgical polypectomy, an era of ten years has been spent in experimental evaluation of electrocoagulation in the control of gastrointestinal bleeding.

Radio frequency electrical current has been used by surgeons to produce tissue heating, coagulation, and hemostasis for many years. Therefore, once the technology of fiberoptics became available in the gastrointestinal tract, it seemed logical to try to use radio frequency electrical current via the endoscope to control bleeding. Three methods of electrocoagulation have been experimentally studied: (1) monopolar electrocoagulation; (2) bipolar electrocoagulation; and (3) fulguration.

The mechanism of blood vessel closure by high-frequency electrocoagulation (coaptation) has been described by Sigel and Dunn[1] and the physical features involved by Sigel and Hatke.[2] Factors that influence coaptation of vessels by electrocoagulation include: (1) length of coagulation; (2) setting of power source; (3) pressure of contact; (4) milieu of activation of probe; and (5) amount of impedence.

II. MONOPOLAR ELECTROCOAGULATION

Monopolar electrocoagulation involves the use of an active electrode held in contact with tissue during treatment. Current flows through the subject to a ground plate.

Blackwood and Silvis[3] were the first to report attempts to quantitate the effects of electrocoagulation on the canine stomach with a Bovie® electrosurgical unit.[3] They concluded that the technique of endoscopic electrosurgery was possible and that a lesion of known diameter could be produced accurately at a setting of 50 or less. Coagulation depth was said to correlate with the diameter of the mucosal defect. Subsequently, they attempted to control depth of tissue necrosis in the canine stomach by controlling amperage and application[4]. They used the Cameron-Miller® electrosurgical unit model 26-265G in their studies. Numerous lesions were produced at varying times and settings. A single application with a monopolar electrode for 1 to 1.5 sec with an amperage of 400 to 425 mA produced mucosal necrosis, but no muscle necrosis. Prolonging the time or increasing amperage to 500 mA resulted in muscle necrosis of the wall of the stomach. Several applications in exactly the same or immediately adjacent location increased the depth of necrosis by 70 to 80%. They concluded that there was difficulty in standardizing the technique of electrocoagulation.

Papp et al.[5] further amplified upon Blackwood and Silvis' studies using a Cameron-Miller® flexible suction coagulator electrode (Model 80-7051) and coagulator unit (Model 80-7910) in dog gastric mucosa. The safest electrocoagulation settings were 5 to 5.5 for a one second application. As opposed to Blackwood and Silvis' findings,[3] the size of the ulcer produced by electrocoagulation did not correlate with depth of injury at the higher settings of 6.5 and 7 on the coagulator unit. Otherwise, the studies of Papp et al.[5] supported the conclusions of Blackwood and Silvis[4].

Lesions were produced in the dog esophagus and duodenal bulb using the Cameron-Miller® electrocoagulation electrode and coagulator unit by Papp et al.[6] to evaluate size of ulceration and depth of coagulation at varying times and power settings. They found the safest settings were 4.5 to 5.5 for 1 to 3 sec in the duodenal bulb and 4.5 to 6 for 1 sec in the esophagus. More than 3 sec electrocoagulation at a setting of five or higher resulted in transmural necrosis. The size of ulceration did not correlate with depth of injury. Hyperamylasemia was noted after duodenal electrocoagulation, but did not correlate with extent of coagulation necrosis. Contrary, Sugawa et al.[7] reported electrocoagulation could be safely used in the dog esophagus using the Cameron-Miller® coagulator unit (Model 80-7910) for 5 to 7 sec at dial settings three, five, and seven. Mann and Mann[8] using the Cameron-Miller® suction electrode (Model 80-7960) found no transmural injury in the esophagus at settings five, six, and seven for 1, 3, and 5 sec. They found the gastric mucosa to be more sensitive to electrocoagulation injury than the esophagus and duodenum. No serosal injury occurred at settings five, six, and seven at 1 and 3 sec. Sugawa et al.[7] found settings of three and five for 3, 5, 7, and 10 sec resulted in muscular layer coagulation necrosis, but no serosal injury in the stomach. The different conclusions by the three investigative groups can only be explained by differences in technique.

Despite efforts to lower time of coagulation and power in monopolar electrocoagulation computer-assisted electrocoagulation in canine gastric bleeding ulcers, excessively deep injury to the gastric wall was reported by Piercey et al.[9]

III. ELECTROFULGURATION

The safety and efficacy of electrofulguration control of bleeding from standard canine experimental gastric ulcers was studied by Dennis et al.[10] At settings two, five, and eight on the Valleylab SSE-3 generator, 0.5 sec applications resulted in effective hemostasis, but on the setting two, an excessive number of applications were required for hemostasis. At settings five and eight, deep injury to the muscularis externa was seen on histological examination at seven days postinjury. An attempt to reduce depth of injury by using an ionizable gas mixture of 50% argon gas and 50% CO_2 was tried and compared to CO_2 alone. No significant difference occurred. They concluded that electrofulguration was effective in stopping bleeding, but tissue injury was unpredictable and deep.

IV. BIPOLAR ELECTROCOAGULATION

Experiments in dogs using bipolar electrocoagulation have shown reduced depth of injury compared to monopolar electrocoagulation.[11,12] However, available bipolar probes have required precise placement of two electrode tips on the target tissue during electrocoagulation. An exciting new multipolar probe (ACMI®) has been developed consisting of an array of six equally spaced longitudinal electrodes along the side and over the rounded tip of a cylindrical probe (Figure 1). The probe is 2.6 mm in diameter and 5.9 mm long located on the end of a catheter passed through a routine biopsy channel. A central opening allows water to be irrigated to clear blood away from a lesion. The power pack and irrigator system is shown in Figure 2. At a setting of seven, the unit will deliver 20 W of power into a standard 100 Ω resistor. Auth et al.[13] reported effective hemostasis in experimental canine gastric ulcers with limited depth of injury at a setting of seven for 1 sec. The appealing features of this new probe are as follows:

1. Low power at the tip of the probe allowing direct placement on a vessel
2. Capability of irrigating immediately prior to electrocoagulation
3. End-on, oblique, or lateral probe application
4. Limited depth of injury
5. The ability to compress an artery by the probe tip

Clinical trials are in progress.

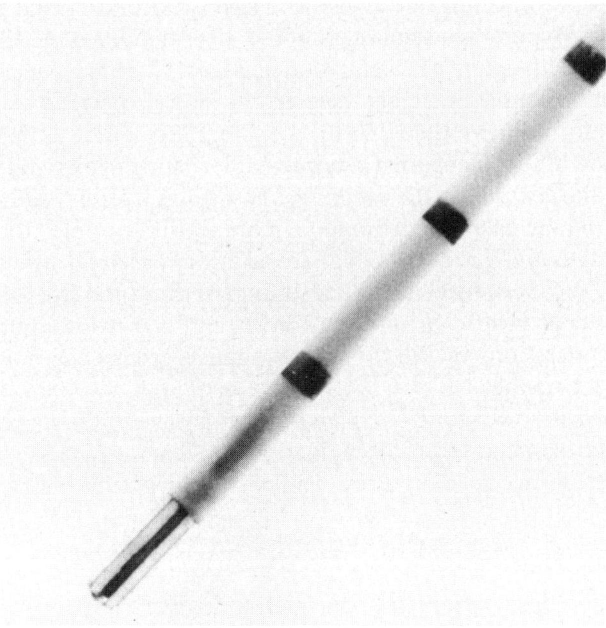

FIGURE 1. A view of the tip of the ACMI® multipolar probe.

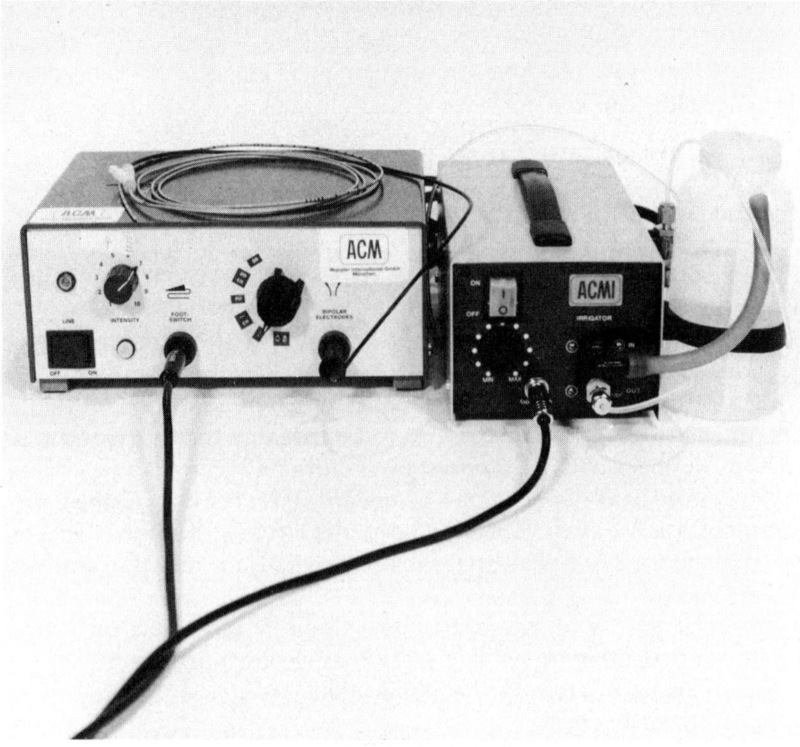

FIGURE 2. The ACMI® power pack (left) and water pump (right) is shown connected to the multipolar probe. The power setting is on seven and the time on one second.

V. HEATER PROBE

The heater probe was developed in Seattle, Washington, in Dr. Rubin's laboratory.[14] Its probe tip is an aluminum cylinder covered with Teflon® and measures 6.4 mm in diameter. A smaller 3.2 mm probe has also been developed. Both have stopped all experimental ulcers made by the standard ulcer maker after a mean of four 1-sec applications and a mean of twelve 1-sec applications, respectively. The smaller probe has resulted in fewer full-thickness gastric wall injuries. Studies are in process to improve its efficacy and safety.

VI. ELECTROCOAGULATION AND FULGURATION IN DOG COLON

Monopolar electrocoagulation and fulguration using the Cameron-Miller® and Valleylab units has been studied in the colon of dogs.[15] The Cameron-Miller® electrode and Olympus® hot biopsy forcep were used at different settings and times. Submucosal and muscular injury occurred at setting 4.5 to 6 Cameron-Miller® and 3 to 6 Valleylab for a 1-sec application. At all other settings and times, transmural injury occurred. The size of the lesion did not correlate with depth of injury.

VII. TECHNIQUES

The secret to therapeutic endoscopy is to get the stomach clear of blood clots. An Edlich gastric lavage tube is passed into the stomach and lavage with two or more units of saline instituted. Thereafter, the patient is sedated as necessary with intravenous diazepam. If no lesion is seen in the esophagus, the endoscope is passed along the lesser curvature of the stomach into the duodenum. If no duodenal site of bleeding is found, the endoscope is withdrawn into the stomach for delineation of the cause of bleeding. If an arterial vessel is seen actively bleeding, or if a vessel is seen, one may use one of three techniques in applying electrocoagulation. Electrocoagulation should not be attempted if torrential bleeding is present nor in esophageal varices.

Gaisford's technique is to irrigate with saline via an irrigator electrode cannula followed by, and sometimes simultaneously using, monopolar electrocoagulation to the bleeding vessel.[16] He uses several short applications of 0.5 to 2 sec with the Valleylab SSE-2 coagulation unit set on five to seven.

Fruhmorgen et al.[17] uses an electro-hydro-thermo-electrode (EHT electrode). The technique is similar to Gaisford's except distilled water is used before and during electrocoagulation. Fruhmorgen et al.[17] reported lower levels of energy used, less depth of injury, lengthened coagulation time, improved visability at the bleeding site, and avoidance of accumulation of coagulum on the electrode. It is not clear whether he places the electrode on a vessel or whether the immediate area surrounding the vessel is electrocoagulated. The EHT electrode is inexpensive, portable, and controls bleeding.

Matek et al.[18] modified the EHT electrode by adding a spring mechanism allowing the contact pressure of the electrode to remain almost constant. The commercial electrocautery unit used is the Martin Elektrotom 170 RF. The spark gap generated coagulation current mode is used at settings six, seven, and eight. By activating a foot switch, water is pumped through the electrode out its tip at about 20 m*l*/min.

My technique differs from the above physicians. Once the actively bleeding vessel is seen, the Cameron-Miller® monopolar electrocoagulation electrode is positioned 2 to 3 mm near the vessel and moved around the vessel in a circular manner applying electrocoagulation at 2 to 2.5 sec until the bleeding stops. Usually four to five applications are necessary at a setting of five on the Cameron-Miller® electrocoagulation unit (Model 80-7910). The amount of joules used varies with the size of the vessel, the amount of impedence, how often the electrode is cleaned, and whether the electrode is activated while going through blood to touch the area around the vessel or whether it is activate when on tissue. Vessels of 1 mm or less usually require four applications of between 60 and 80 J per application. Vessels between 1 and 2 mm require four to five or more applications ranging from 104 to 134 J of energy per application.[19] The principle in my method is that electrocoagulation causes coaptation in the muscular and submucosal layer in contrast to the multipolar probe which can directly coagulate vessels because of the low output of 14 J per application. It is important not to electrocoagulate the vessel directly using my method; for destruction of the vessel occurs resulting in more bleeding.

VIII. CLINICAL EXPERIENCE

Youmans, et al.[20] used a cystoscope through a gastrostomy to cauterize a bleeding vessel in a malignant ulcer in one patient and multiple "stress ulcerations" in another patient in 1970, beginning an era of electrocoagulation in the gastrointestinal tract. Shortly afterwards, Blackwood and Silvis[21] voiced concern that cauterization with the Bovie® electrosurgical generator may actually cause an increase in bleeding. With technological improvements in flexible fiberoptic endoscopes, the availability of electrocoagulation probes, and the improvement in coagulation power units, experimental evaluation of electrocoagulation has been pursued, as has been discussed earlier, in the hope that gastrointestinal hemorrhage can be controlled by electrocoagulation.

Since 1971, 570 patients with acute upper gastrointestinal bleeding have had endoscopy by the author within six hours of their admission to Blodgett Memorial Medical Center to evaluate the cause of their bleeding. Of these patients, 299 had ulcer disease as follows: 165 duodenal, 114 gastric, 18 marginal, and 2 esophageal. There were 32 patients (19%) with active duodenal ulcer bleeding and 30 patients (26.4%) with active gastric ulcer bleeding. The percent of actively bleeding lesions is very similar to the ASGE national study on upper gastrointestinal bleeding where 29.8% had actively bleeding duodenal ulcers and 22.5% gastric ulcers actively bleeding. Five patients had actively bleeding marginal ulcers and two esophageal ulcers.

A. Uncontrolled Studies

In an uncontrolled consecutive series, all patients with actively bleeding lesions had an attempt at control of their hemorrhage by endoscopic monopolar electrocoagulation if bleeding did not stop with conservative management.[22-24] A total of 81 patients have had endoscopic electrocoagulation. In addition to the actively bleeding lesions above, 12 of 30 patients (40%) had Mallory-Weiss tears actively bleeding. While the number of actively bleeding tears may seem high, it is very similar to the findings of the national ASGE study, which reported that 42.4% of Mallory-Weiss tears were bleeding actively. Ten of the 12 patients were successfully electrocoagulated. In a miscellaneous group, there was a patient with a gastric varix, one with hemorrhagic antral gastritis with seven distinct bleeding points, and three with duodenal or gastric arteriovenous malformations.

Of the 81 patients, eight had unsuccessful attempts at electrocoagulation (two Mallory-Weiss tears and six duodenal ulcers) because of torrential hemorrhage obscuring vision or because of inability to place the probe near the bleeding vessel. They all had surgical treatment after endoscopy had identified their site of bleeding. Of 73

Table 1
COST ANALYSIS

A cost comparison is made between patients treated by electrocoagulation and surgery.

	Hosp. days	Electro-coagulated	Hosp. days	Surgical
Mallory Weiss tear				
Total	11	$1400	29	$5311
Lab.		330		1175
Gastric ulcer				
Total	11	$1202	16	$1778
Lab.		214		306
Marginal ulcer				
Total	5	$ 641	16	$3662
Lab.		221		665
Duodenal ulcer				
Total	11	$1463	9.5	$2188
Lab.		532		869

patients with cessation of bleeding by electrocoagulation, ten patients rebled (five duodenal and five gastric ulcers). Five patients had surgery with one postoperative death. Four had successful reelectrocoagulation. One patient had a cardiac arrest prior to surgery and died.

The average age of the patients with gastric ulcers was 64 years of age and 70 for patients with duodenal ulcers. Many of these patients had multiple other problems and were hospitalized in various intensive care units. Nine of the 81 patients died, but none from the lesion causing their bleeding. Six died during their hospitalization (6 of 81) resulting in a mortality rate of 7.4%. Three died several months later from carcinomatosis. The mortality rate compares favorably to other reports, which show a mortality of 20 to 50% in patients older than 60.[25] No morbidity nor mortality occurred as a result of electrocoagulation. It is important to point out that all of the patients would have had surgery had not electrocoagulation been available.

Not only was there a significant reduction in mortality in the older age groups above, but days and cost of hospitalization was found to be reduced in a retrospective analysis (Table 1). The only exception was for patients with duodenal ulcers treated surgically. They had a shorter stay by 1½ days, but their cost averaged $700 more per hospitalization. There was a substantial reduction in hospital stay for the patients with Mallory-Weiss tears treated with electrocoagulation and almost a $4000 less cost per patient. The patients with gastric ulcers electrocoagulated were hospitalized five days less than those surgically treated at about $500 less cost. The patients with marginal ulcers electrocoagulated were hospitalized three times shorter at five to six times less cost when compared to surgical treatment. Physician fees are not included in the above cost data.

Gaisford[16] has reported treating 71 patients by endoscopic electrocoagulation with 92% permanent hemostasis after one treatment. No complications occurred as a result of electrocoagulation. Six patients rebled. Four had repeated successful electrocoagulation for bleeding benign gastric ulcers. One patient with a Mallory-Weiss tear and one with a gastric leiomyosarcoma went to surgery because of persistent bleeding. The lesions electrocoagulated by Gaisford are as follows: esophageal ulcers—4; Mallory-Weiss tears—6; gastric varices—2; gastric ulcers—29; erosive gastritis—8; gastric polyps—2; gastric leiomyomas—2; pyloric channel ulcers—3; duodenal ulcers—13, and jejunal ulcers—8.

Sugawa et al.[7] has treated six patients with electrocoagulation with initial success in all. The lesions were as follows: Mallory-Weiss tear—1; gastric ulcer—1; gastric erosions—3; and gastric polyp—1. One patient with gastric erosions and one with a gastric ulcer rebled and required surgical treatment.

Volpicelli et al.[26] has had success in stopping active bleeding in 12 patients initially (duodenal—6; gastric—5; and esophageal ulcer—1). One patient rebled from a gastric ulcer and was successfully reelectrocoagulated. Elective surgery was performed without difficulty one day later.

The above uncontrolled series numbers 170 patients. The first attempt at electrocoagulation resulted in a combined success of 88%. If rebleeding occurred, reelectrocoagulation was successful in another 2%. Ten percent of the total series had unsuccessful electrocoagulation and required surgery.

In a survey of European endoscopists using monopolar electrocoagulation in uncontrolled series, a 70% success rate was reported in 314 patients with active bleeding. Five perforations were reported. Wara et al.[27] reported recently an 81% (56/69) permanent hemostasis in patients with active bleeding. They used an Olympus® cannula (CD-3L and 4L) allowing simultaneous irrigation and coagulation of the bleeding site. The cannula was passed through one of two channels of the Olympus® TGF endoscope. The power source was an Erbotom F2. Forty to 60 percent of the maximum 170 W power was used in electrocoagulation. Electrocoagulation failed to control bleeding in five patients (7%) and could not be applied in six patients (9%). No complications from electrocautery was reprted. They concluded that endoscopic electrocoagulation was successful, especially if used in the quiescent phase of massive hemorrhage, and that it should be considered before emergency operation. Koch et al.[28] early in the development of electrocoagulation reported one death in a group of 15 bleeding patients treated with monopolar electrocoagulation and three perforations.

B. The Visible Vessel (Figure 3)

It is not surprising that some patients rebleed after initial cessation despite medical management. Rebleeding in nonsurgically treated patients has been reported to range from 25 to 77%.[29,30]

Why do patients rebleed? I reviewed my early experience in patients having rebled after initial cessation and found that four of five patients with a visible vessel in an ulcer bed rebled. Therefore, a randomized prospective study was initiated.[31] A control group of five gastric and eight duodenal ulcer vessels was treated medically. Four of the five gastric ulcer vessels rebled from 8 hours to 20 days. Six of the duodenal ulcer vessels rebled from five hours to five days. All ten patients having rebled were treated surgically. Another 13 patients randomly selected were immediately electrocoagulated with the Cameron-Miller® electrode upon observation of their vessels. Nine vessels were in gastric ulcers and four in duodenal ulcers. One gastric ulcer vessel rebled three days after electrocoagulation and surgery was performed. None of the other vessels rebled nor required surgery.

Of the three patients who stopped bleeding spontaneously in the control group, they were hospitalized 8.3 days with an average cost of hospitalization of $2323. The ten other control patients that had surgery after rebleeding were hospitalized an average of 15.2 days at an average cost of $5042. Those patients immediately electrocoagulated had an average hospitalization of 8.3 days and an average cost of $3152. Their hospitalization was not only about one half the control group, but also cost an average of 48% less. Physician fees are not included in the costs cited above.

Griffiths et al.[32] in a retrospective review of their bleeding patients found 28 patients with a visible vessel. All 28 were recommended for operation because of recurrent

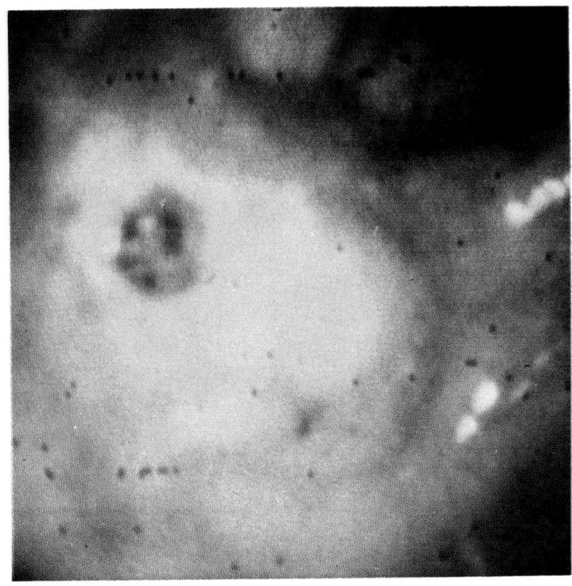

FIGURE 3. A 2 mm visible vessel in a 1.5 cm duodenal ulcer is seen not bleeding.

(86%) or uncontrolled (14%) hemorrhage. They recommended that surgical treatment be considered at the time of identification at endoscopy. The study of Papp[31] would suggest that electrocoagulation be first considered as a treatment modality of choice.

Vallon et al.[33] reported a randomized study of endoscopic argon laser photocoagulation in bleeding peptic ulcers. In their patients (332) with upper gastrointestinal bleeding, 28 had spurting vessels and 35 other ulcers protruding nonbleeding vessels. Of the latter group, 50% (8 of 16) in the control group rebled, while 8 of 19 rebled despite treatment prophylactically with argon photocoagulation. They concluded that argon prophylactic treatment of nonbleeding lesions is not worthwhile.

The cost of an electrocoagulation probe and coagulation unit is about $1500. The unit is small and can easily be moved from area to area. Most power sources have an isolated ground lessening the risk of an electrical accident. The power units can also be used for electrosurgical polypectomy. The electrocoagulation probe (Cameron-Miller®) will allow fluid for irrigation, but is not adequate for suctioning blood. The probe should always be carefully examined prior to electrocoagulation to make sure the metal tip is not loose and that its wire connection is not broken. The entire electrosurgical system must always be checked prior to its use to confirm it is adequately functioning.

IX. CONCLUSION

A full decade of endoscopic research has past since the availability of electrocoagulation electrodes. Extensive research efforts in animal models using mono and bipolar electrocoagulation, electrofulguration, and heater probe modalities have provided general guidelines as to possible modes of application in treating bleeding in patients. While monopolar electrocoagulation in numerous uncontrolled studies and one controlled study has been shown to be effective in stopping arterial bleeding in the majority of instances, a new multipolar probe may prove to be safer and as effective.

Whether one uses the EHT electrode technique or monopolar electrocoagulation with or without irrigation, succesful cessation of bleeding occurs. No morbidity nor mortality has been reported in the American literature.

That the visible vessel will likely bleed profusely and/or rebleed requiring either surgical or endoscopic therapy has recently become appreciated. In a randomized prospective study, prophylactic electrocoagulation of the visible vessel resulted in almost no rebleeding, reduced cost, and length of hospitalization.

Monopolar electrocoagulation is no longer experimental. It is an investigative modality and should be studied in a randomized prospective clinical trial as soon as possible.

ACKNOWLEDGMENTS

I am most grateful for financial support provided to me by the Blodgett Memorial Medical Center Hospital Research Fund over the past several years and for the support of the Research Department and its Chairman, Dr. Walter D. Meester.

I am indebted to Laurel Van Til for her faithful enthusiastic assistance in the research laboratory and in several clinical research projects described in this Chapter and to Nancy Chevepton, Marilyn Frasier, and Pat Young.

REFERENCES

1. **Sigel, B. and Dunn, M. R.,** The mechanism of blood vessel closure by high-frequency electrocoagulation, *Surg. Gynecol. Obstet.*, 121, 823, 1965.
2. **Sigel, B. and Hatke, F. L.,** Physical factors in electrocoagulation of blood vessels, *Arch. Surg.*, 95, 54, 1967.
3. **Blackwood, W. D. and Silvis, S. E.,** Gastroscopic electrosurgery, *Gastroenterology*, 61, 305, 1971.
4. **Blackwood, W. D. and Silvis, S. E.,** Standardization of electrosurgical lesions, *Gastrointest. Endosc.* 21, 22, 1974.
5. **Papp, J. P., Fox, J. M., and Wilks, H. S.,** Experimental electrocoagulation of dog gastric mucosa, *Gastrointest. Endosc.*, 22, 27, 1975.
6. **Papp, J. P., Fox, J. M., and Nalbandian, R. M.,** Experimental electrocoagulation of dog esophageal and duodenal mucosa, *Gastrointest. Endosc.*, 23, 27, 1976.
7. **Sugawa, C., Shier, M., Lucas, C. E., and Walt, A. J.,** Electrocoagulation of bleeding in the upper part of the gastrointestinal tract, *Arch. Surg.*, 110, 975, 1975.
8. **Mann, S. K., and Mann, N. S.,** Effect of monopolar electrocoagulation on esophagus, stomach and duodenum in dogs, *Am. J. Gastroenterol.*, 71, 568, 1979.
9. **Piercey, J. R. A., Auth, D. C., Silverstein, F. E., Willard, H. R., Dennis, M. B., Ellefson, D. M., Davis, D. M., Protell, R. L., and Rubin, C. E.,** Electrosurgical treatment of experimental bleeding canine gastric ulcers: development and testing of a computer control and better electrode, *Gastroenterology*, 74, 527, 1978.
10. **Dennis, M. B., Peoples, J., Hulett, R., Auth, D. C., Protell, R. L., Rubin, C. E., and Silverstein, F. E.,** Evaluation of electrofulguration in control of bleeding of experimental gastric ulcers, *Dig. Dis. Sci.*, 24, 845, 1979.
11. **Moore, J. P., Silvis, S. E., and Vennes, J. A.,** Evaluation of bipolar electrocoagulation in canine stomachs, *Gastrointest. Endosc.*, 24, 148, 1978.
12. **Protell, R. L., Gilbert, D. A., Jensen, D. M., Silverstein, F. E., Hulett, R., and Auth, D. C.,** Computer assisted electrocoagulations: bipolar vs. monopolar in the treatment of experimental gastric ulcer bleeding, *Gastroenterology*, 76 (Abstr.), 1221, 1979.
13. **Auth, D. C., Gilbert, D. A., Opie, E. A., and Silverstein, F. E.,** The multipolar probe—a new endoscopic technique to control gastrointestinal bleeding, *Gastrointest. Endosc.* 26 (Abstr.), 63, 1980.
14. **Protell, R. L., Rubin, C. E., Auth, D. C., Silverstein, F. E., Terou, F., Dennis, M., and Piercey, J. R. A.,** The heater probe—a new endoscopic method for stopping massive gastrointestinal bleeding, *Gastroenterology*, 74, 257, 1978.
15. **Papp, J. P., Nalbandian, R. M., Wilcox, R. M., and Ludwig, E. E.,** Experimental evaluation of electrocoagulation and fulguration of dog colon mucosa, *Gastrointest. Endosc.*, 25, 140, 1979.
16. **Gaisford, W. D.,** Endoscopic electrohemostasis of active upper gastrointestinal bleeding, *Am. J. Surg.*, 137, 47, 1979.
17. **Fruhmorgen, W. M., Kaduk, B., Reidenback, H.-D., Bodem, F., and Demling, L.,** Modified electrocoagulation and its possibilities in the control of gastrointestinal bleeding, *Endoscopy*, 4, 253, 1979.
18. **Matek, W., Fruhmorgen, P., Kaduk, B., Reidenback, H.-D., Bodem, F., and Demling, L.,** The healing process of experimentally produced bleeding lesions after hemostasis electrocoagulation with simultaneous instillation of water, *Endoscopy*, 12, 231, 1980.
19. **Papp, J. P., Auth, D. C., and Silverstein, F. E.,** Analog computer evaluation of monopolar electrocoagulation in patients having had UGI bleeding, *Gastrointest. Endosc.*, 26 (Abstr.), 73, 1980.
20. **Youmans, C. R., Patterson, M., McDonald, D. F., and Derrick, J. R.,** Cystoscopic control of gastric hemorrhage, *Arch. Surg.*, 100, 721, 1970.
21. **Blackwood, W. D., and Silvis, S. E.,** Electrocoagulation of hemorrhagic gastritis, *Gastrointest. Endosc.*, 18, 53, 1971.
22. **Papp, J. P.,** Endoscopic electrocoagulation in upper gastrointestinal hemorrhage: a preliminary report, *JAMA*, 230, 1172, 1974.
23. **Papp, J. P.,** Endoscopic electrocoagulation of upper gastrointestinal hemorrhage, *JAMA*, 236, 2076, 1976.
24. **Papp, J. P.,** Endoscopic electrocoagulation of actively bleeding arterial upper gastrointestinal lesions, *Am. J. Gastroenterol.*, 71, 516, 1979.
25. **Himal, H. S., Watson, W., Jones, C. W., Miller, L., and MacLean, L. D.,** The management of upper gastrointestinal hemorrhage, *Ann. Surg.*, 179, 489, 1972.
26. **Volpicelli, N. A., McCarthy, J. D., Bartlett, J. D., and Bager, W. E.,** Endoscopic electrocoagulation: an alternative to operative therapy in bleeding peptic ulcer disease, *Arch. Surg.* 113, 483, 1978.

27. **Wara, P., Hojsgaard, A., and Amdrup, E.,** Endoscopic electrocoagulation—an alternative to operative hemostasis in active gastroduodenal bleeding?, *Endoscopy,* 12, 237, 1980.
28. **Koch, H., Pesch, H. J., Bauerle, H., Fruhmorgen, P., Rosch, W., and Classen, M.,** Experimentelle Untersuchungen und Klinische Erfahrungen zur Electrokoagulation blutende Lasionen im oberen Gastrointestinaltrakt., *Fortschr. Endoskop.,* 10, 67, 71, 1972.
29. **Malt, R. A.,** Control of massive upper gastrointestinal hemorrhage, *N. Engl. J. Med.,* 286, 1043, 1972.
30. **Donaldson, R. M., Jr., Hardy, J., and Papper, S.,** Five-year follow-up study of patients with bleeding duodenal ulcer with and without surgery, *N. Engl. J. Med.,* 259, 201, 1958.
31. **Papp, J. P.,** Endoscopic electrocoagulation of the nonbleeding visible ulcer vessel, *Gastrointest. Endosc.,* 25 (Abstr.), 45, 1979.
32. **Griffiths, W. J., Neumann, D. A., and Welsh, J. D.,** The visible vessel as an indicator of uncontrolled or recurrent gastrointestinal hemorrhage, *N. Engl. J. Med.,* 300, 1411, 1979.
33. **Vallon, A. G., Cotton, P. B., Armengol Miro, J. R., Laurence, B. H., and Salord Oses, J. C.,** Randomized study of endoscopic argon laser photocoagulation in bleeding peptic ulcers, *Gastrointest. Endosc.,* 26 (Abstr.), 70, 1980.

Chapter 4

SCLEROTHERAPY OF ESOPHAGEAL VARICES

K. J. Paquet and W. E. Fleig

TABLE OF CONTENTS

I. HISTORICAL INTRODUCTION

Throughout this century, clinicians have been challenged by the problem of effectively treating complications of portal hypertension. The idea of obliterating esophageal varices via the endoscope originated in 1939 when Crafoord and Frenckner[1] reported on a single patient treated by injection sclerotherapy after an episode of upper gastrointestinal hemorrhage. They used a rigid esophagoscope. The varices were injected with a sclerosing agent during general anesthesia. Since portal-systemic shunting became established in the 1940s and was subsequently accepted to be the method of choice in patients with bleeding esophageal varices, sclerotherapy was set back by most groups focusing on portal hypertension. During these years, sporadic but enthusiastic reports by Moersch[2-4] Patterson and Rouse,[5] and Kempe and Koch[6] dealt with this new method.

In view of the doubts about portocaval shunt operations that arose from first controlled studies by Jackson et al.[7] and Resnick and associates,[8] interest in endoscopic sclerotherapy was renewed. This trend was intensified by the disappointing results of emergency shunting procedures, which were hampered by mortality rates of 40 to 60% and an excessive postoperative morbidity demonstrated by Mikkelsen and Pattison,[9] Guetgemann and Esser,[10] Wantz and Payne,[11] and several others. Macbeth[12] presented first results on a larger series of patients with cirrhotic and noncirrhotic portal hypertension, who were treated by injecting subepithelial and submucous varices with a sclerosing agent. Several of his cirrhotic patients were alive for more than seven years after initiation of sclerotherapy. Hunt, Johnston, and Rogers [13] treated 53 acutely bleeding patients by injection sclerotherapy subsequent to Sengstaken-Blakemore tube tamponade. In their series, 23 out of 32 cirrhotic patients left the hospital (28% admission mortality) and mortality was only 15% in patients suffering from portal thrombosis without evidence of liver disease. Control of hemorrhage was achieved in 82%. In a retrospective analysis of 15 years of injection sclerotherapy,[14] the same group was able to stop variceal bleeding in 93% out of 113 patients admitted to their clinic. Total admission mortality was 18%. Several groups in Europe, South Africa, and the U.S. have adopted this method.

In 1956, Wodak created a different endoscopic approach to manage acute variceal hemorrhage and to prevent recurrent bleeds.[15] The sclerosing agent is injected paravariceally by his technique, therefore, it does not obliterate the portosystemic collaterals. Denck[16,17] and Paquet[18,19] have propagated and modified this method. More than 1000 patients have been treated by each of these groups to date. Mortality and complication rates are comparably low. Acute hemorrhage is effectively controlled in 87 to 92%[20,21] even in patients not responding to balloon tamponade.[22,26]

Despite obvious success, endoscopic sclerotherapy has been attacked for many years because of a lack of controlled studies. This omission is partly due to the fact that sclerotherapy had to be proven effective and safe prior to initiating controlled trials. On the other hand, experienced advocates of this method felt unable to clear themselves from withholding effective treatment from vitally threatened patients. Similar arguments have been used against controlled trials on laser photocoagulation for gastrointestinal hemorrhage.[23] Since Terblanche and co-workers[24] have published a limited, but very promising, controlled study of elective sclerotherapy, and because noninvasive means are effective in many variceal bleeds, carefully proposed controlled studies of endoscopic sclerotherapy for various indications should no longer be denied. Facing this factual situation, which is comparable to the state of portal-systemic shunt operations 15 years ago, this Chapter attempts to critically review the state of the art concerning techniques, indications, and clinical results of endoscopic sclerotherapy.

Table 1
ETIOLOGY OF PORTAL HYPERTENSION

Posthepatic	Intrahepatic		Prehepatic
Postsinusoidal	Parasinusoidal		Presinusoidal
Constrictive pericarditis, chronic right-sided heart failure	Liver cirrhosis		Portal Thrombosis Inborn abnormalities of the portal vien
Budd-Chiari disease		Arterio-portal shunting	
		Schistosomiasis Sarcoidosis Lymphomas Osteomyelosclerosis Congenital hepatic fibrosis	

II. PATHOPHYSIOLOGICAL CONSIDERATIONS AND TECHNIQUES OF ENDOSCOPIC SCLEROTHERAPY

A. Pathological Physiology

Esophageal varices are a common feature of portal hypertension due to various etiologies (Table 1). Hepatofugal blood flow through different portal-systemic collaterals is predominantly caused by liver cirrhosis in adults, whereas pediatric patients almost exclusively suffer from prehepatic portal obstruction. Hepatopetal gastric and duodenal collaterals sometimes occur in lienal vein thrombosis, while proximal-distal flow through esophageal varices is found in patients with huge goiters and fibrosis or tumors of the mediastinum. Hemorrhage from such "downhill" esophageal varices is extremely rare and can usually be controlled by conservative methods.[25]

Fifty percent of patients with esophageal varices have gastric varices as well. Surprisingly, only about 5% of variceal bleeds originate from these vessels. By contrast, varices of the distal esophagus and of the esophagogastric junction contribute to more than 90% of bleeding episodes observed endoscopically.[26] This is due to the topography of the portal-systemic collaterals within the gastric and esophageal wall. Stelzner and Lierse[27] demonstrated that varicose veins of the stomach and the proximal part of the esophagus are defined to the submucosal layer. By contrast, the bulk of varices of the distal esophagus and of the esophagogastric junction is located subepithelially (Figure 1). The esophageal epithelium may be directly attached to the wall of these dilated veins without any intermediate fibrous stratum seen on histological sections.[28] Lesions of the epithelium may damage the vessel. Massive hemorrhage may result.

The factors leading to the onset of hemorrhage from esophageal varices remain controversial. Several authors[29,30] suggest that increased portal pressure causes varix rupture, while others fail to correlate portal pressure measured laparoscopically with the probability of future hemorrhage.[31] Endoscopic diagnosis of esophagitis is made in the majority of patients within two weeks after variceal hemorrhage.[32] This is consistent with the extensive experience of many endoscopists. The intriguing hypothesis of

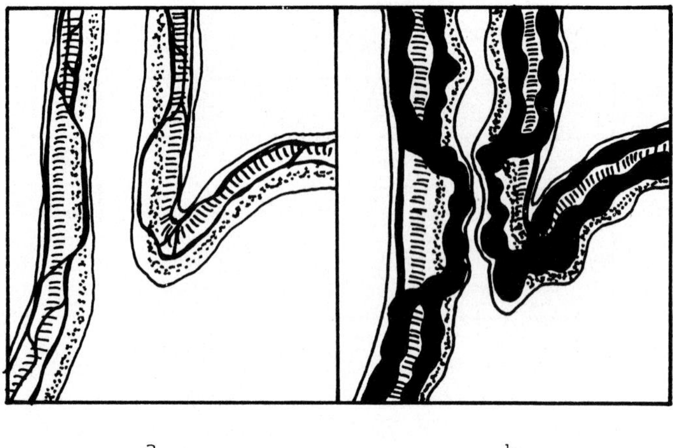

FIGURE 1. Anatomical situation at the gastroesophageal junction according to Stelzner and Lierse.[27] (A) Normal circulatory situation; (B) esophageal varices in portal hypertension. :::: Muscularis mucosae; ///// Muscularis propria.

reflux-induced lesions resulting in hemorrhage is not supported by the experiments of Eckardt and co-workers.[32a,32b] They investigated esophageal pH and resting lower esophageal sphincter pressure. No difference between cirrhotic patients with previous variceal hemorrhage and healthy controls was detected. Nevertheless, antireflux management remains essential in the treatment of bleeding esophageal varices.

B. Techniques of Endoscopic Sclerotherapy and Mechanism of Action

Considering the above pathophysiological situation, control of acute hemorrhage and prevention of recurrent bleeding can be achieved by two different therapeutic principles: (1) obliterating the varices, and (2) covering patent varices with a fibrous layer. Both techniques are used by several groups competitively and will be described and discussed further.

1. Endoscopic Obliteration of Esophageal varices

To date, the original technique of Crafoord and Frenckner[1] is still used without any principal modifications. The idea of this method is to acutely induce thrombosis of the respective varix by injecting a sclerosing agent intra-variceally (Figure 2). This should efficiently stop acute bleeding and prevent recurrent hemorrhage, if all exposed varices are obliterated.

Patients bleeding acutely are admitted to the intensive care unit and resuscitated. Several authors include vasopressin/pitressin infusion in emergency treatment.[32] After endoscopic diagnosis of variceal hemorrhage is made, a Sengstaken-Blakemore or Linton® tube is inserted.[12-14, 32-34] The patient is allowed to recover. At a convenient time up to 36 hours after initiation of balloon tamponade, sclerotherapy is performed. Subsequent to premedication with atropine and diazepam,[32,33] general anesthesia is induced if the procedure is to be performed via the rigid instrument.[12-14, 32] With a flexible endoscope, general anesthesia is favored[35] or omitted[33,36] by different authors.

The Sengstaken or Linton® tube is removed. Subsequently, the endoscope is introduced into the esophagus. The varices are readily visible at this point. A needle is then passed down the instrument and directed into one of the distended varices. Three

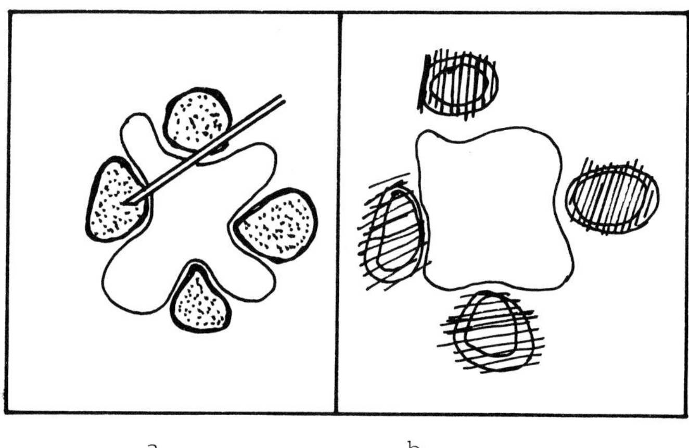

FIGURE 2. Technique of intravariceally injecting esophageal varices. (A) Situation at the onset of therapy; (B) Thrombosed varices and augmented fibrous submucous tissue due to leakage of sclerosing agent out of the injected vein.

to ten m*l* of the sclerosing agent is injected. Thereafter, the needle is removed, and the injection site is compressed by either rotating[32] or further advancing[14] the endoscope over the puncture wound. Additional varices are treated in like manner. The instrument is left in position to compress the injected veins for another 5 to 10 min. When the instrument is finally withdrawn, several authors prefer to reinsert a Sengstaken tube and leave it inflated for an additional 6 to 30 hr.[13,14,32,34] It is argued[34] that this compression is essential to completely obliterate injected varices as the vein walls become adherent. Others[33] are aware of erosions caused by the inflated balloon, and therefore, do not reinsert the tube routinely.

The aim of the method described is to thrombose injected varices. To do so, the sclerosing agent should be retained within the respective vein. However, radiological studies of Johnson[34] and of Barsoum and collaborators[37] have clearly demonstrated that the sclerosant solution is rapidly released from the injected varix into periesophageal vessels and finally into systemic circulation, whether a flexible fiberscope or the wide-bore rigid instrument is used. In addition, the sclerosing agent escapes into the perivariceal tissue and induces submucosal fibrosis and thickening of variceal walls, as shown from histological specimens in man[34] and in experimental esophageal varices in dogs.[38] Recently, Soehendra's group[39] has reported severe cardiovascular reactions and even anaphylactic shock in several of their patients injected intravariceally. This may also argue for the sclerosing agent being quickly disseminated into the circulation. Nevertheless, the method is capable of effectively controlling variceal bleeding, probably by combined action of thrombosing the veins and inducing perivascular inflammation and subsequent fibrosis. Since distal esophageal varices are mainly confined to the mucosa,[27] the portal-systemic collateral system is significantly reduced by this technique.

Barsoum and associates[37] also investigated questionable obliteration of gastric varices by injecting collaterals at the esophageal level. Using a sclerosing agent with contrast, they were not able to force the injected solution downwards across the cardia, even when the injected varix was compressed by the rigid esophagoscope proximally to the puncture site. Therefore, obliteration of gastric varices is unlikely to result from this procedure.

2. Endoscopic Paravariceal Injection Sclerotherapy

The technique presently used by the authors[40,41] Figure 3 (a and b) is based on that described by Wodak[15] and has been modified by Paquet.[18-20] After resuscitation of the bleeding patient with blood and fresh frozen plasma, gastric lavage via a large-bore tube and emergency endoscopy are performed. If a diagnosis of bleeding esophageal varices is made, the patient is immediately subjected to sclerotherapy. Preliminary balloon tamponade is only performed when general anesthesia cannot be initiated without delay. After premedication with atropine and diazepam, anesthesia is performed using thiopental sodium, suxamethonium chloride, and nitrous oxide/oxygen. A 50cm rigid, large-bore esophagoscope is passed down to the esophagogastric junction, thereby compressing the bleeding site. Blood is removed from the stomach by suction. Sclerotherapy is initiated at the level of the cardia. Injections are made strictly paravariceally and subepithelially. Injection into the submucosa is to be avoided. Correct subepithelial position of the needle tip results in a pale weal arising at the onset of injection—0.5 to 2.0 m*l* aliquots into one site. This procedure is repeated 30 to 40 times, producing a helical arrangement of weals while slowly removing the endoscope. Treatment is confined to the distal esophagus. Additional injections are only needed for proximal bleeding sites. A maximum of 40 to 60 m*l* of the sclerosant solution is utilized. The massive edema resulting from confluent weals occludes the ruptured varix mechanically. After endoscopic control of the injected region, a gastric tube is passed down the instrument and the endoscope is removed. The stomach is washed free of blood and the tube is withdrawn. Nasogastric tubes or balloon tamponade are not used after sclerotherapy.

In patients treated electively, identical injections are performed. Denck,[42] Haslhofer,[43] and Wodak[28] have reported extensive histological studies in patients who died at various times after the onset of sclerotherapy. They found marked inflammation around the injected material with granulomas, which lead to the formation of a fibrous subepithelial layer, covering the nonoccluded portosystemic collaterals (Figure 4). Effects on gastric varices are unlikely to occur. To obtain a smooth esophagus lacking previously prominent varices, sclerotherapy has to be repeated two to three times at four to seven days intervals.

C. Instruments

The rigid esophagoscope primarily used by Crafoord and Frenckner[1] is still a valuable device in endoscopic sclerotherapy. Since a small-bore instrument fails to distend the varices, the largest esophagoscope which can be introduced safely should be used. Suction is performed by tubes that can be passed down the instrument on demand.

Macbeth[12] created an offset injection needle that exceeds the esophagoscope several centimeters in length. Because of the inadequate distance judgement when looking down the endoscope without an additional optical device, the cannula's proximal end is marked at a position when the tip exceeds the distal end of the endoscope by 1 cm. The proximal offset allows for adequate handling of needle and syringe without impending the view down the esophagoscope. This instrumental setup has been used by Hunt, Johnston, and Rodgers.[13,14] Wodak[28] and Denck[42] still employ this device with slight modifications.

As the intravariceal injection is sometimes difficult to control from an optical distance of 50 cm, Bailey and Dawson[44] designated a minor, but very helpful modification, in 1975. A lateral slot opposite to the beak of the instrument allows a single varix to protrude into the lumen, while the others are compressed outside the instrument. It is now easily injected, and after the needle has been withdrawn possible bleeding can be stopped by simply rotating the esophagoscope. The injected varix is compressed and a

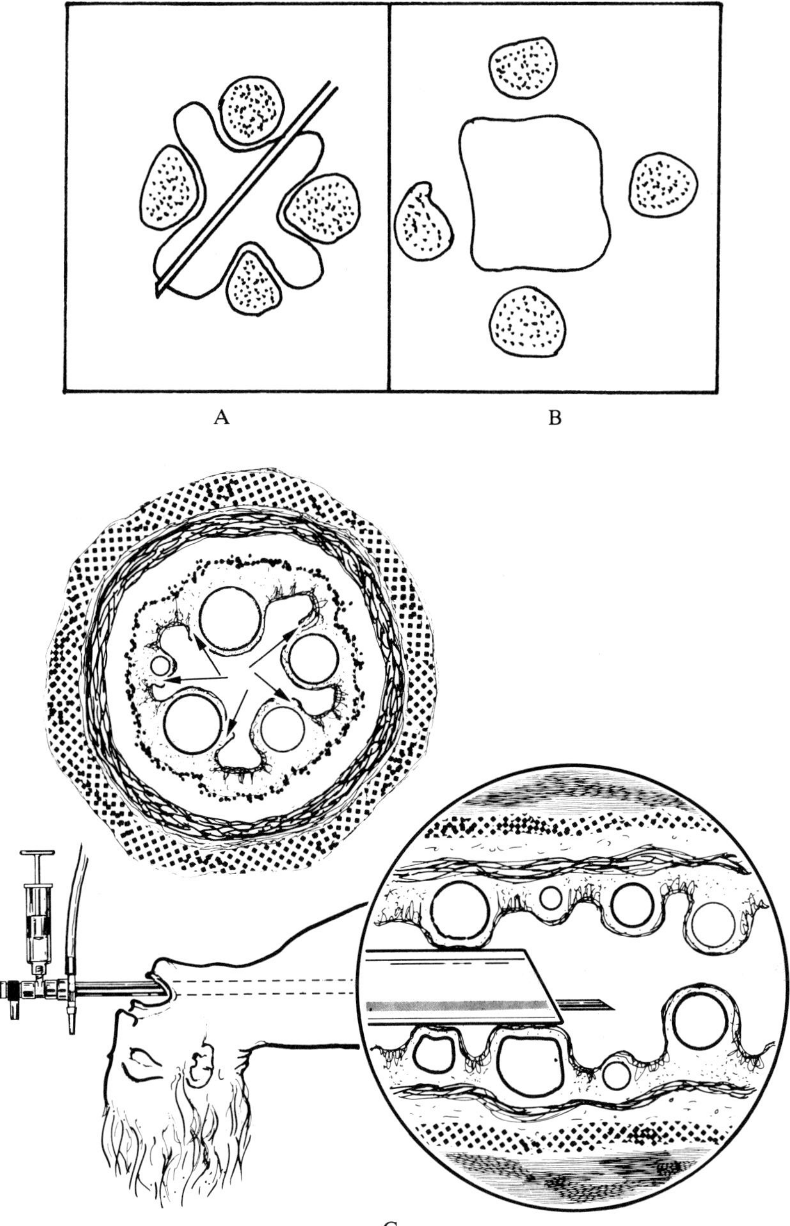

FIGURE 3. Technique of paravariceally injecting the esophageal wall. (A) Situation at the onset of therapy. Note the exact subepithelial and paravariceal position of the cannula; (B) situation after sclerotherapy. The patent varices are covered by a strong fibrous layer; (C) technique and site of injection in paravariceal sclerotherapy of esophageal varices. (Figure 3C from Paquet, K. J., in *Percutaneous Biopsy and Therapeutic Vascular Occlusion,* Anacker, H., Gulotta, V., and Rupp. N.;, eds., Thieme-Stratton, New York, 1980. With Permission.)

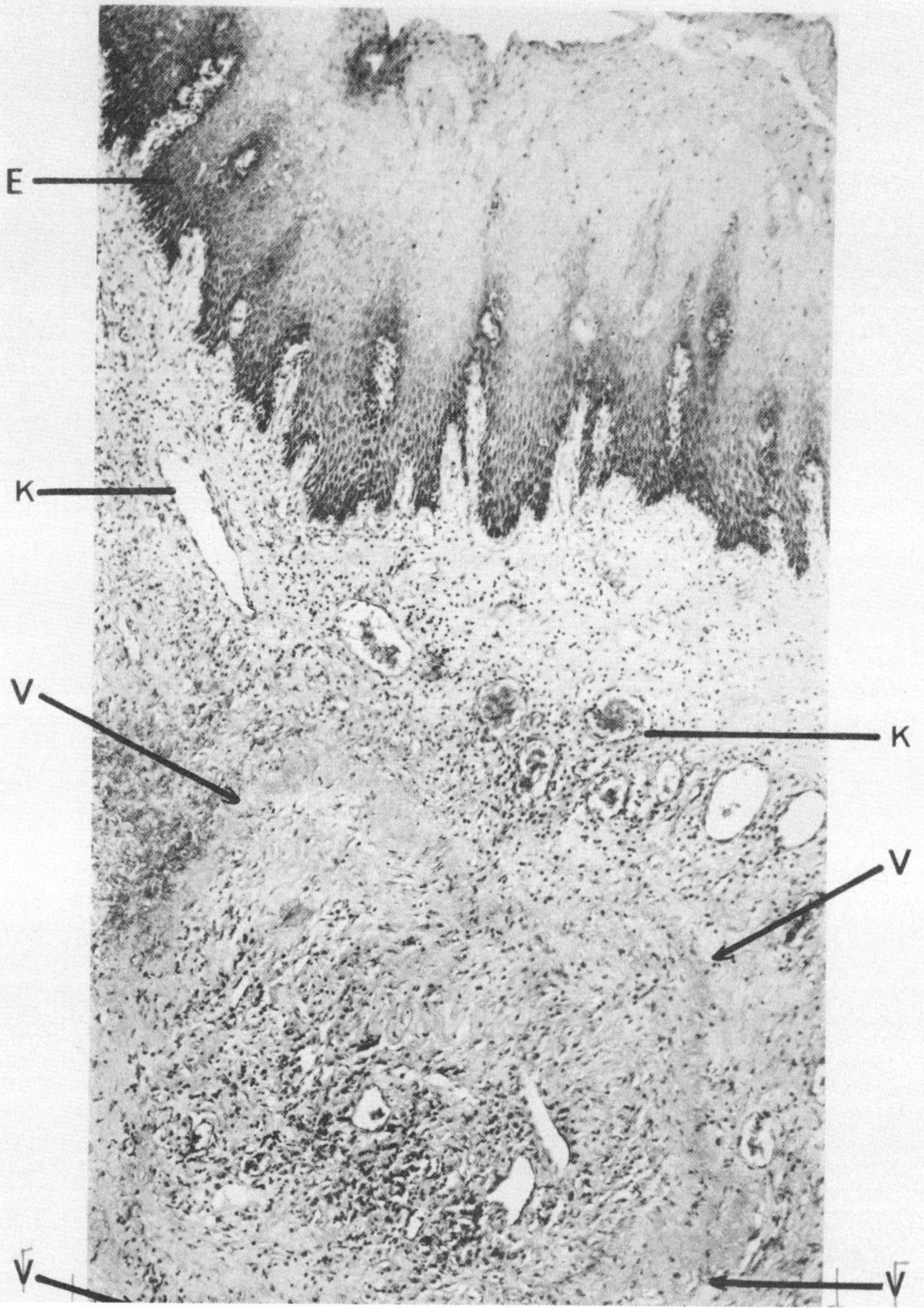

FIGURE 4. Micrograph of an autopsy specimen of an esophagus treated by paravariceal sclerotherapy for acute variceal hemorrhage, E = epithelium; K = collaterals; V = giant varix, partially perfused. (From Paquet, K. J., Lindecken, K. D., and Göcke, H., *Ztschr. Kinderchir.*, 27, 303, 1979. With permission.)

new one is presented inside the slot. This instrument with the Macbeth needle is used by Johnson,[34] Terblanche and co-workers, [24,32] and most groups performing intravariceal injections.

Important modifications to optimally adapt the rigid 50-cm esophagoscope with distal fiber lighting to paravariceal injection have been designed by Paquet.[19,45] A large-bore suction channel was mounted inside the endoscope to facilitate identification of the bleeding site in a clean esophagus. A wide-angle rigid 60-cm fiberscope (Hopkins type, Storz, Tuttlingen, Germany) with additional distal high-power fiber lighting is fixed inside a metal tube, which can be freely rotated with the large-bore esophagoscope. After passing the instrument down to the cardia, the metal tube coaxially covering the small diameter fiberscope is exchanged. A 2.0 cm long, 12-gauze cannula is fixed at the distal end of a second tube. When this tube is tilted over the fiberscope, the optical system exactly focuses the tip of the needle and provides optimal conditions to inject the sclerosant solution (Figure 5).

General anesthesia is argued to affect the outcome of cirrhotic patients presenting with upper gastrointestinal hemorrhage. Therefore, the use of flexible instruments has become popular during recent years.[20,33,36,41,46] Flexible needles which can be extended and retracted mechanically have been developed by Machida and Olympus (Figure 6). They may be passed down any biopsy channel of at least 2.8 mm inner diameter. Therefore, any commercial flexible upper GI frontal or oblique viewing fiberscope, except the pediatric instruments, can be used. However, since poor, if any, suction is left with the needle inserted into a single channel instrument, the situation may be insufficiently controlled in bleeding patients. Twin channel surgical fiberscopes are better adapted to this method, but harder to swallow.

The risk of bleeding from the injection site is more distressing with the use of flexible instruments, since compression of the injected vein is inadequate by commercial endoscopes. Several modifications to overcome this problem have been tested in recent years.

Williams and Dawson[35] have transferred the Bailey and Dawson[44] modification of the rigid esophagoscope to the flexible instrument. A 50-cm flexible tube of 2-cm inner diameter with a window cut 2 cm from the distal end is threaded over the fiberscope to its proximal end. After the instrument has been inserted into the distal esophagus, the tube is cautiously slid down outside the gastroscope to the cardia. Varices protruding into the window are then easily injected and compressed thereafter by rotating the tube. As general anesthesia is obligatory upon this procedure, no advantage over the rigid instrument becomes evident.

Lewis and co-workers[33] reported on an interesting device consisting of a flexible twin channel fiberscope, a flexible injector with retractable needle, and a 150 cm #7 catheter, which is equipped with a 400 m*l* capacity latex rubber balloon at the tip. This balloon catheter is inserted into the larger biopsy channel in a retrograde fashion before passing the endoscope down to the distal esophagus. After visualizing the varices to be treated, the instrument is advanced into the stomach and the balloon inflated. The endoscope is brought back into the esophagus and the inflated balloon retracted to compress the gastroesophageal junction. Indentical to the action of the Linton-Nachlas tube, the balloon impacted into the cardia reduces the hepatofugal inflow of blood into the varices, thereby minimizing bleeding from the injection site. Two hints may be associated to this technique: (1) blood clots remaining in the distal esophagus may impede the view and traction on the balloon has to be released to wash them down into the stomach; (2) varices may be less tightly filled or even collapsed and thereby be more difficult to inject.

Very recently, Brunner[47] suggested a different approach to prevent bleeding from

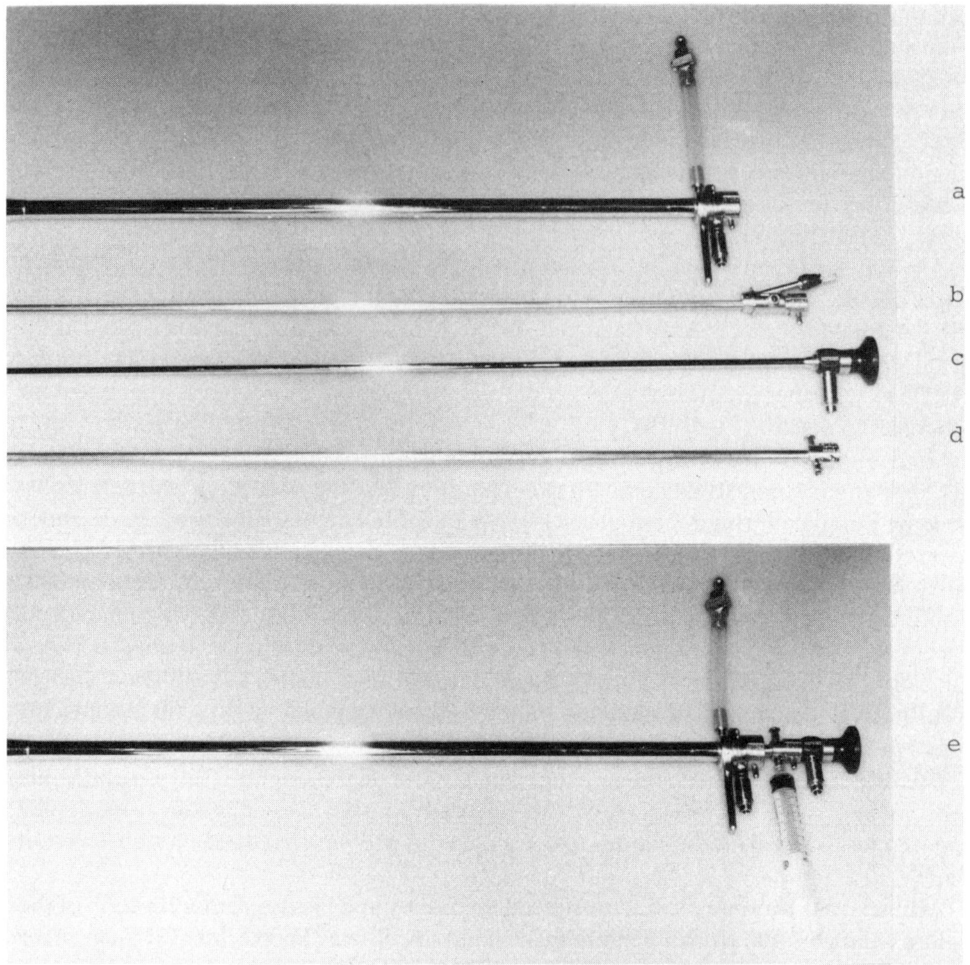

FIGURE 5. Rigid esophagoscope according to Paquet, (A) Large bore esophagoscope with distal fiber lighting and suction channel; (B) metal tube to cover C; (C) Hopkins optical system that focusses the tip of D; (D) metal tube to cover C with soldered cannula; (E) instrument ready for use.

injected varices. An inflatable latex cuff is mounted outside a twin-channel fiberscope several centimeters proximally to the tip. Once a varix is injected as usual, the instrument is propagated and the cuff inflated to compress the puncture site. The same effect results from more extemporized means using a double-latex condom, as designed by Brooks[48] of Galambos' group. He adds a somewhat humoristic modification to a technique classified as a "Mickey Mouse" procedure by Galambos just one year ago.[49]

D. Sclerosing Agents

Two groups of sclerosing agents are used—oleaginous mixtures and aqueous solutions of drugs. The main components of commercially available sclerosing agents (Table 2) are discussed below.

Morrhuate sodium is used by several groups in the U.S.[33,50-52] It is a solution of sodium salts of the fatty acids of cod liver oil. A 5% aqueous solution is commercially available with 2 to 3% benzyl or ethyl alcohol for preservation. The induction of thrombosis when injected intravenously and the fibrogenic effect are sufficient.

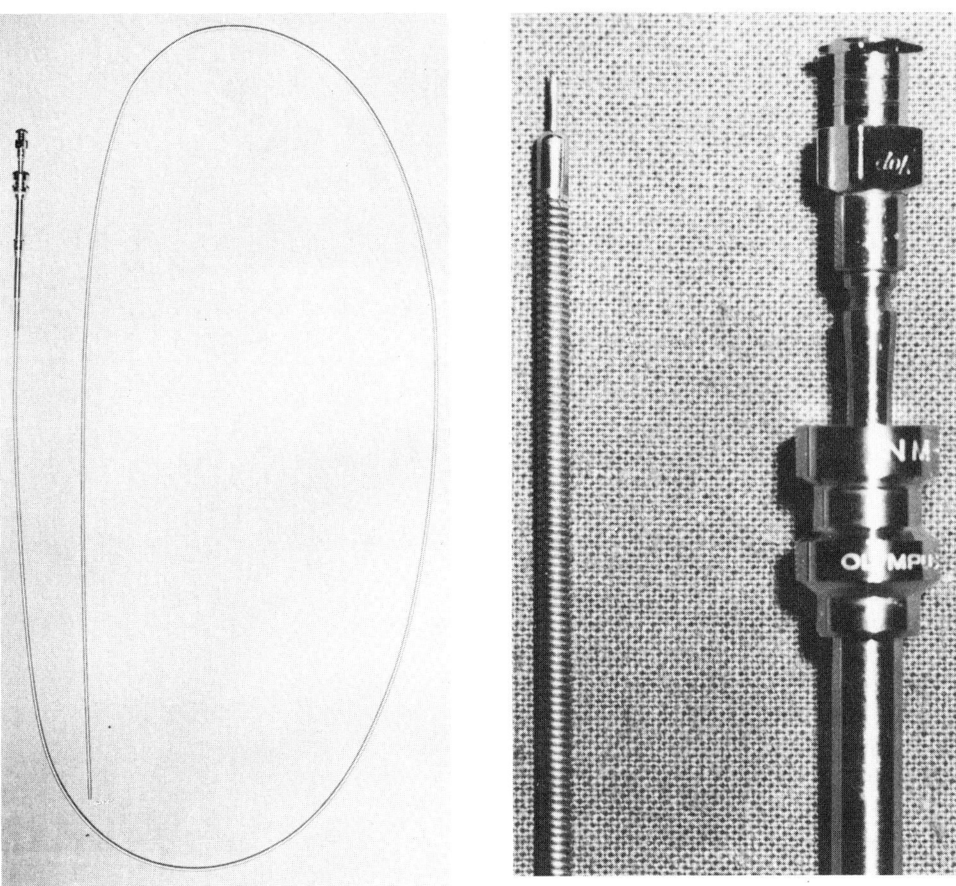

FIGURE 6. Flexible needle for the injection of sclerosing agents via the flexible fiberscope. The cannula can be retracted completely by an operating mechanism attached to the Luer lock at the proximal end.

Polidocanol (hydroxypolyethoxydodecane) had been developed as a local anesthetic. However, the intensive inflammation induced by this drug when injected in effective concentrations prohibited its application in local anesthesia. The sclerosant effect was utilized instead and the agent is now widely accepted in the treatment of varicose veins of the legs. A 0.5 or 1.0% aqueous solution with 5% ethanol is used for sclerotherapy of esophageal varices by intravariceal,[36] as well as paravariceal[20,21] injection. Local toxicity is less pronouned than that of morrhuate sodium, which completely macerates the endothelium when applied intravenously. No allergic reactions have been reported. It has been proven effective and safe in more than 1000 patients treated by the authors.

The effect of *sodium tetradecyl sulfate,* an anionic surfactant agent, is similar to that of morrhuate sodium. Since allergic reactions are known, the drug has not been introduced into the sclerotherapy of esophageal varices.

Ethanolamine oleate is used by Terblanche and co-workers[24,32] and several groups in the U.K.[13,14,34] A 5% sterile solution is convenient. No major untoward reactions have been reported.

Oleagenous solutions have been preferred by Wodak[28] and Denck.[42] A mixture of turpentine oil, liquid paraffin, benzyl alcohol, and an azotoluol derivative has been

Table 2
SCLEROSING AGENTS

Drug	Solution strength	Commercial preparation	Marketed in	Effect on esophageal varices
Morrhuate sodium	5%	Morrhuate sodium inj.,	U.S.	+
		Varicocid®	F.R.G.[a]	
Sodium tetradecyl sulfate	0.1—1.0%	Sotradecol	U.S., F.R.G.	?
Ethanolamine oleate	5%		UK.	+
Polidocanol	0.5—1.0%	Aethoxysclerol	F.R.G.	+
Liquid paraffin	—		Everywhere	+
Phenolized almond oil	—		F.R.G.	?

[a]Federal Republic of Germany.

Table 3
HEMATOLOGICAL AND CHEMICAL PARAMETERS IN MONITORING ACUTE ESOPHAGEAL VARICEAL HEMORRHAGE

Hematocrit
WBC
Thrombocyte count
Blood group
Prothrombin time and partial thrombin time
SGOT, SGPT
Alkaline phosphatase
Bilirubin
Urea
Creatinin
Electrolytes
Albumin
Arterial ammonia
Arterial pH, pO_2, pCO_2, and base excess

retracted because of potential carcinogenecity of the latter. Sterile *liquid paraffin* is used now without any additions.

Phenolized almond oil is a valuable drug in the sclerotherapy of hemorrhoids. An effective fibrogenic effect with minimal local toxicity is postulated, but no conclusive data are available concerning sclerotherapy of esophageal varices.

III. PATIENT CARE AND MONITORING AND SUPPORTIVE MANAGEMENT IN PARAVARICEAL INJECTION SCLEROTHERAPY

A. Acute Hemorrhage

Patients bleeding acutely are admitted to the intensive care unit. After insertion of intravenous catheters, a series of laboratory evaluations is performed (Table 3) and resuscitation is started. Coagulation defects are corrected and portal-systemic encephalopathy is prevented by:

1. Aspirating all blood from the stomach
2. Cleaning the large bowel from blood and clots by frequent irrigation
3. Inhibiting excessive intraluminal ammonia production and facilitating ammonia rediffusion into the colon by lactulose and/or neomycin[53]
4. Administering branched chain amino acids solutions parenterally[54]

When emergency sclerotherapy is performed and the bleeding is controlled, no nasogastric tube is used further. Blood pressure, heart rate, urine output, and state of consciousness are recorded hourly. Hematocrit is controlled every six hours. Antireflux regimen consists of cimetidine 200 mg i.v. every 4 hr and/or antacids. Calories are administered via the parenteral route by infusing 1000 m*l* of 40% glucose supplemented with insulin. Since alcoholics frequently suffer from malnutrition, vitamins may be added. Diuretics should be used with caution in order not to precipitate portal-systematic encephalopathy. If hemodynamics are stable after 24 hr, sclerotherapy is considered to be effective and the patient is transferred to the intermediate care unit. He is allowed to drink and is fed a mashed protein and sodium-restricted diet. Sclerotherapy is repeated twice at four to seven days intervals to completely submerge the varices. Further management is identical to electively treated patients.

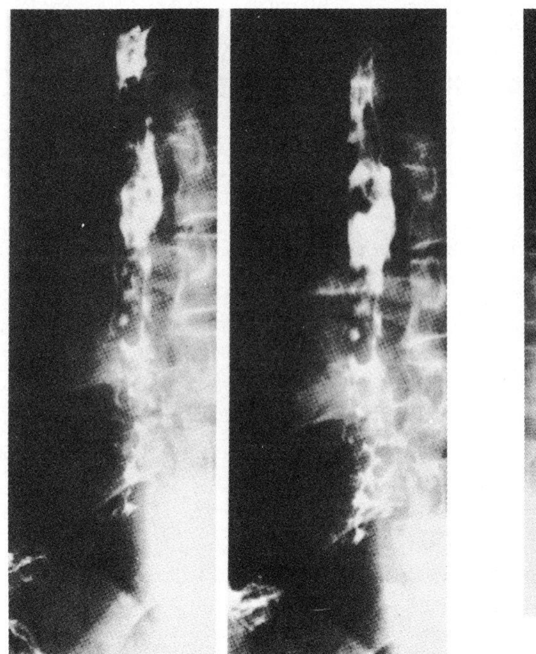
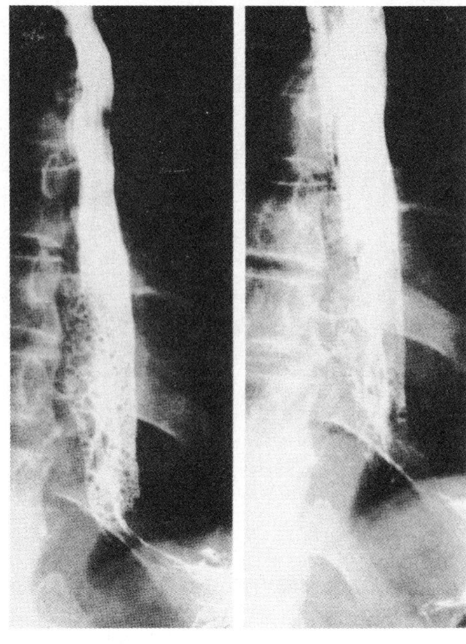

FIGURE 7. Barium swallow demonstrating esophageal status. (A) Before; (B) after paravariceal sclerotherapy in a patient with severe portal hypertension. (From Paquet, K. J. and Oberhammer, E., *Endoscopy,* 10, 7, 1978. With Permission.)

B. Elective Sclerotherapy

Patients elected for sclerotherapy after previous hemorrhage from esophageal varices and after exact diagnosis of the underlying disease are subjected to the following routine investigations before and after treatment: (1) flexible esophagoscopy to photographically document the variceal condition; (2) barium swallow (Figure 7); and (3) evaluation of the lower esophageal sphincter function by pressure and pH recordings. Hepatic vein-wedged pressure is evaluated in elected patients after detailed informed consent is obtained.

Sclerotherapy is performed as described and monitoring at the intermediate care unit equals that mentioned above. The following parameters are recorded daily: hematocrit, thrombocyte count, serum and urine electrolytes, and serum urea. Albumin, aminotransferases, cholinesterase, alkaline phosphatase, bilirubin, prothrombin time, and arterial ammonia are checked weekly. A mashed protein and sodium-restricted diet is prescribed throughout the admission period.

C. Follow-up Protocol

Since the fibrous layer resulting from paravariceal injection sclerotherapy undergoes continuous reconstruction, it will decrease with individual velocity in different patients. Varices may become prominent again with increased risk of recurrent hemorrhage. Therefore, periodical follow-up examinations are essential to achieve satisfactory, long-term results.

After the patient has been dismissed from the hospital for four weeks, a first endoscopic control is performed. Subsequent physical, laboratory, and endoscopic examinations follow at 3- to 6- month intervals (Table 4). Recurrent varices when detected are immediately treated by repeated paravariceal injection via the flexible instrument on an outpatient basis.

Table 4
FOLLOW UP PROTOCOL AFTER PARAVARICEAL INJECTION SCLEROTHERAPY

Interval after discharge	Upper GI endoscopy	Barium swallow	LES function tests	Labor-atory tests	Physical examina-tion and history taking	Abdominal ultra-sound
4 weeks	X	X	X	X	X	
3 months	X			X	X	
6 months	X		X	X	X	
9 months	(X)					
12 months	X			X	X	X
18 months and every further 6 months	X			X	X	

Table 5
ADULT PATIENTS TREATED BY PARAVARICEAL INJECTION SCLEROTHERAPY WITHIN TEN YEARS CLASSIFIED ACCORDING TO CHILD'S CRITERIA (n = 909).

Child's category	A	B	C
Number of patients	72	173	664
% of total	8	19	73

Note: The numerical scoring system of Pugh et al. is used.

IV. INDICATIONS AND RESULTS OF PARAVARICEAL INJECTION SCLEROTHERAPY

Paravariceal injection sclerotherapy of esophageal varices has been used by us since 1969. For the first years, 5% morrhuate sodium (Varicocid®) was the sclerosing agent used. We have favored 0.5 or 1% polidocanol (Aethoxysklerol Kreussler®) for more than six years because of better effects and minor local toxicity. Within the first ten years, a total of 909 patients has been treated by this method at the University Clinics of Bonn and Ulm/Federal Republic of Germany. According to the numerical scoring system of Pugh et al,[55] 73% had to be introduced into Child's C class, 19% into the B, and only 8% into the A category (Table 5). Two thirds of the patients were between 40 and 60 years old. Indications and results vary with patients being treated electively or as an emergency and with the patient's age.

The number of patients admitted for acute massive hemorrhage from esophageal varices not controlled by conservative means (Table 6) was 324. Of these patients, 67% were in the C category, 23% with the B, and 10% with the A class. Bleeding was effectively controlled by emergency paravariceal injection sclerotherapy in 297 patients (92%). In a small prospective study, a similar success rate of 92% was observed in patients who had not responded to 6 hours to 4 days balloon tamponade.

Similar indications occurred in adult patients undergoing sclerotherapy after one or more previous bleeds (Table 7). An even larger portion is attributed to the C category (84%). In 94.1% out of these 540 patients, liver cirrhosis due to various etiologies was

Table 6
INDICATIONS OF EMERGENCY SCLEROTHERAPY IN 324 ADULT PATIENTS NOT RESPONDING TO CONSERVATIVE TREATMENT

Diagnosis	Child A	Child B	Child C	Total
Decompensated cirrhosis and hepatic coma	—	—	216 (67.0%)	216 (67.0%)
Compensated cirrhosis	18 (5.6%)	76 23.0%)	—	94 (28.6%)
Prehepatic portal obstruction	12 (3.7%)	—		12 (3.7%)
Others	(2)	—	—	2
Total	32 (10.0)	76 (23.0)	216 (67.0)	324 (100.0%

Table 7
INDICATIONS OF "ELECTIVE" SCLEROTHERAPY IN 540 PATIENTS AFTER ONE OR MORE PREVIOUS BLEEDS

Diagnosis	Child A	Child B	Child C	Total
Decompensated cirrhosis	—	—	442 (82.0%)	442 (82.0%)
Decompensated or compensated cirrhosis with clotted shunt	5 (1.0%)	11 (2.0%)	12 (2.0%)	28 (5.0%)
Compensated cirrhosis, shunt refused	17 (3.2%)	20 (3.7%)	—	37 (6.9%)
Prehepatic portal obstruction	23 (4.3%)	—	—	23 (4.3%)
Osteomyelosclerosis	5 (1.0%)	3 (0.5%)	—	8 (1.5%)
Others	—	2 (0.3%)	— —	2 (0.3%)
Total	50 (9.5%)	36 (6.5%)	454 (84.0%)	540 (100.0%)

the underlying disease. Only 4.3%, 1.5%, and 0.3% suffered from prehepatic portal obstruction, osteomyelosclerosis, or other diseases, respectively.

Complications due to sclerotherapy occurred in 12% out of 909 patients (Table 8). Marked pleural effusions were detected by routine thorax X-ray 24 hours after sclerotherapy was done in 18 patients (2%). Painful and deep esophageal ulcers that did not perforate into the mediastinum were detected by water soluble contrast in 3.1%, while complete transesophageal necrosis (Figure 8) with mediastinitis and/or pyothorax made up another 2%. Esophageal stenosis resulted from sclerotherapy in 22 patients (2.4%) and could be easily dilated by means of the Eder-Puestow device (Key Med). Hemorrhage from gastric varices was also considered to be a complication of sclerotherapy and is, therefore, listed in this group accounting for 2.4%.

Admission mortality of all adult patients undergoing sclerotherapy (N = 909) amounted to 13.5% (123 patients). Causes of death are given in Table 9. Most patients died from liver failure with portral-systemic coma, which was already present at admission. In 3.4% of patients, failure of sclerotherapy to effectively control

Table 8
COMPLICATIONS OF PARAVARICEAL INJECTION SCLEROTHERAPY IN 909 PATIENTS

Complication	Number of patients	% of total
Esophageal ulcer without transesophageal necrosis	28	3.1
Esophageal stenosis	22	2.4
Hemorrhage from gastric varices	22	2.4
Large pleural effusion	18	2.0
Ulcer with complete trans- esophageal necrosis, mediastinitis, and/or pyothorax	18	2.0
Total	108	11.9

hemorrhage significantly contributed to the fatal outcome, as did complications of sclerotherapy despite effective hemostasis in another 2.4%. Mortality was 20% in emergency treated patients (n = 324) and 11% in 540 patients treated electively after one or more previous bleeds.

Recurrent hemorrhage is one of the parameters that help to estimate the efficacy of therapeutic procedures for variceal bleeding. Minor rebleeds occurred in 23.8% within the primary admission period, and 80% occurred after the first treatment and were easily controlled by repeated sclerotherapy. As one procedure is not sufficient to induce adequate fibrogenesis, this is to be expected when primary treatment is not complete. About 6% of patients rebled within the next four months, 18.8% at some time later in their follow-up, therefore, examinations are crucial in detecting recurrent varices; 40% of all patients were subjected to repeated injections after four months, 40% after one year, while in the remaining 20%, primary sclerotherapy had efficiently covered the portal-systemic collaterals for 2 to 5 years.

Table 10 summarizes the long-term results of 858 patients whose fate is known. Only 51 patients (5.6%) escaped from follow-up; 67% of all patients were alive at the end of the 10-yr treatment period.

Prophylactic sclerotherapy for grade 3 and 4 varices (Figure 9) in patients without a history of previous hemorrhage is controversial. Within a period of two years, 45 patients who were admitted for sclerotherapy by their home physicians were elected for prophylactic sclerotherapy according to the following indications:

1. Decompensated liver cirrhosis plus reflux esophagitis from hiatal hernia
2. Decompensated liver cirrhosis plus grade IV varices with erosions (Figure 9)
3. Decompensated liver cirrhosis with clotting factors below 30% of normal controls

As the effect of prophylactic sclerotherapy was very promising in these patients, Paquet started a prospective controlled trial. Patients who complied with the above indications were assigned by random to groups treated by sclerotherapy or conservatively. Preliminary results of a 17-month trial period are delineated in Table 11. Six hemorrhages and four deaths were observed in the medically treated group (n = 11), while only one bleeding episode and no deaths occurred in 13 patients submitted to sclerotherapy. These results encouraged us to design a multicenter study that is presently being performed.

In pediatric patients, indications for sclerotherapy are markedly different. Until July 1, 1980, we had treated 52 children 1 to 14 years of age by this method. In children

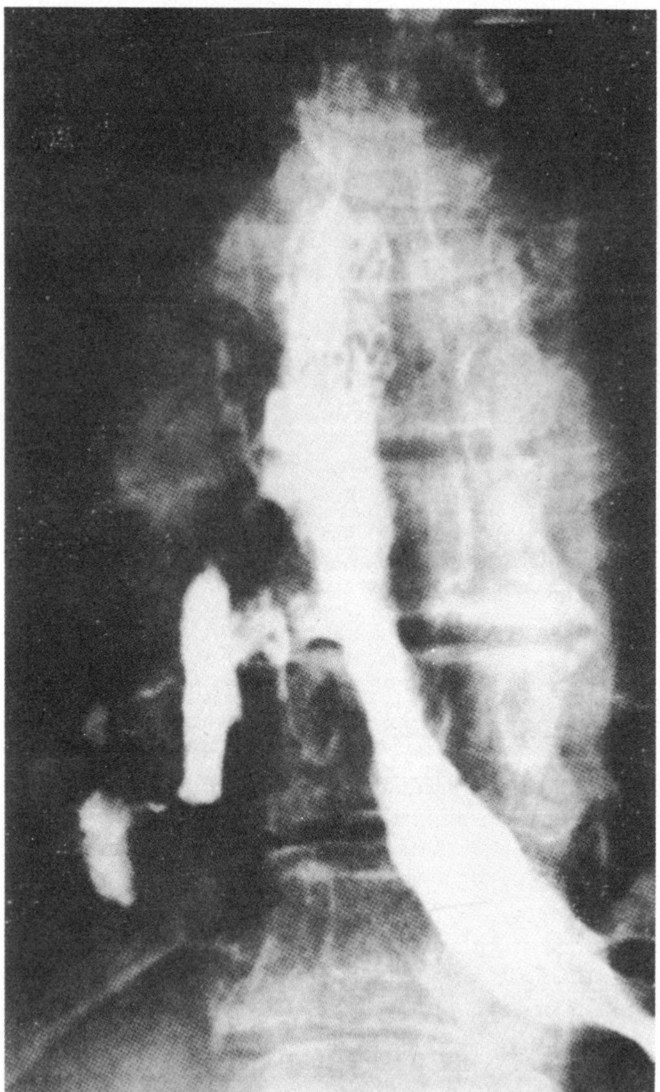

FIGURE 8. Radiological demonstration of complete necrosis of the esophageal wall subsequent to paravariceal sclerotherapy. Water soluble contrast enters the mediastinum and right pleural space. This patient was successfully treated by pleural and mediastinal drainage, nasogastric tube, parenteral nutrition, and antibiotics. (From Paquet, K. J. and Oberhammer, E., *Endoscopy,* 10, 7, 1978. With Permission.)

younger than five years, a special rigid instrument constructed by us is necessary. (Figure 10, from Storz, Tuttlingen, West Germany). In 92% of these 52 patients, prehepatic portal obstruction was found. Patient data are summarized in Table 12. Emergency sclerotherapy effectively stopped variceal hemorrhage in 14 (93%) out of 15 patients who presented with uncontrolled bleeding. One esophageal ulcer without transmural necrosis was observed (Figure11), and two cases of esophageal stenosis had to be bougienated. One of the little patients rebled from esophageal varices three months after initiation of treatment. All others are free of recurrence for up to six years.

Table 9
ADMISSION MORTALITY AND CAUSES OF DEATH AFTER PARAVARICEAL INJECTION SCLEROTHERAPY OF ESOPHAGEAL VARICES (N = 909)

Cause of death	Admission diagnosis	n	% of total
Liver failure	Decompensated hepatic cirrhosis and coma	52	5.7
Liver failure and uncontrolled bleeding	Decompensated cirrhosis	31	3.4
mediastinitis and/or pyothorax	Decompensated cirrhosis (13); portal obstruction (2)	15	1.6
Pneumonia	Decompensated cirrhosis	9	1.0
Heart failure	Decompensated cirrhosis	9	1.0
Uncontrolled hemorrhage from gastric varices	Decompensated cirrhosis	7	0.8
Total		123	13.5

Table 10
LONG TERM RESULTS OF PARAVARICEAL INJECTION SCLEROTHERAPY WITHIN A TEN YEARS PERIOD (1969—1979) (N = 909)

Number of patients	% of total	Fate
611	67.2	Alive
123	13.5	Died during first admission
124	13.7	Died at home or at other hospitals during follow-up
51	5.6	Fate unknown
909	100.0	Total

This contrasts nicely to the failure of various operations that had been done in 30 of these 52 patients prior to endoscopic sclerotherapy. It should be emphasized that none of the 17 portal-systemic shunts was patent for more than 14 months (Table 13). Two cirrhotic children have died at home during follow-up probably from liver failure.

V. DISCUSSION

Esophageal varices are useful portal-systemic collaterals. On the other hand, they may vitally endanger patients when massive hemorrhage arises on occasion of varix rupture. Since conservative treatment has a poor effect on acute variceal bleeding, several semiinvasive approaches have been tested in recent years. Our group has gained adequate experience in treating esophageal varices by paravariceal injection of a sclerosing agent. Based on the data presented here, several questions are to be discussed:

1. Which method is the most effective and safe in controlling acute variceal hemorrhage?
2. Which procedure provides reasonable reliability in preventing further bleed?
3. Which special technique should be used?

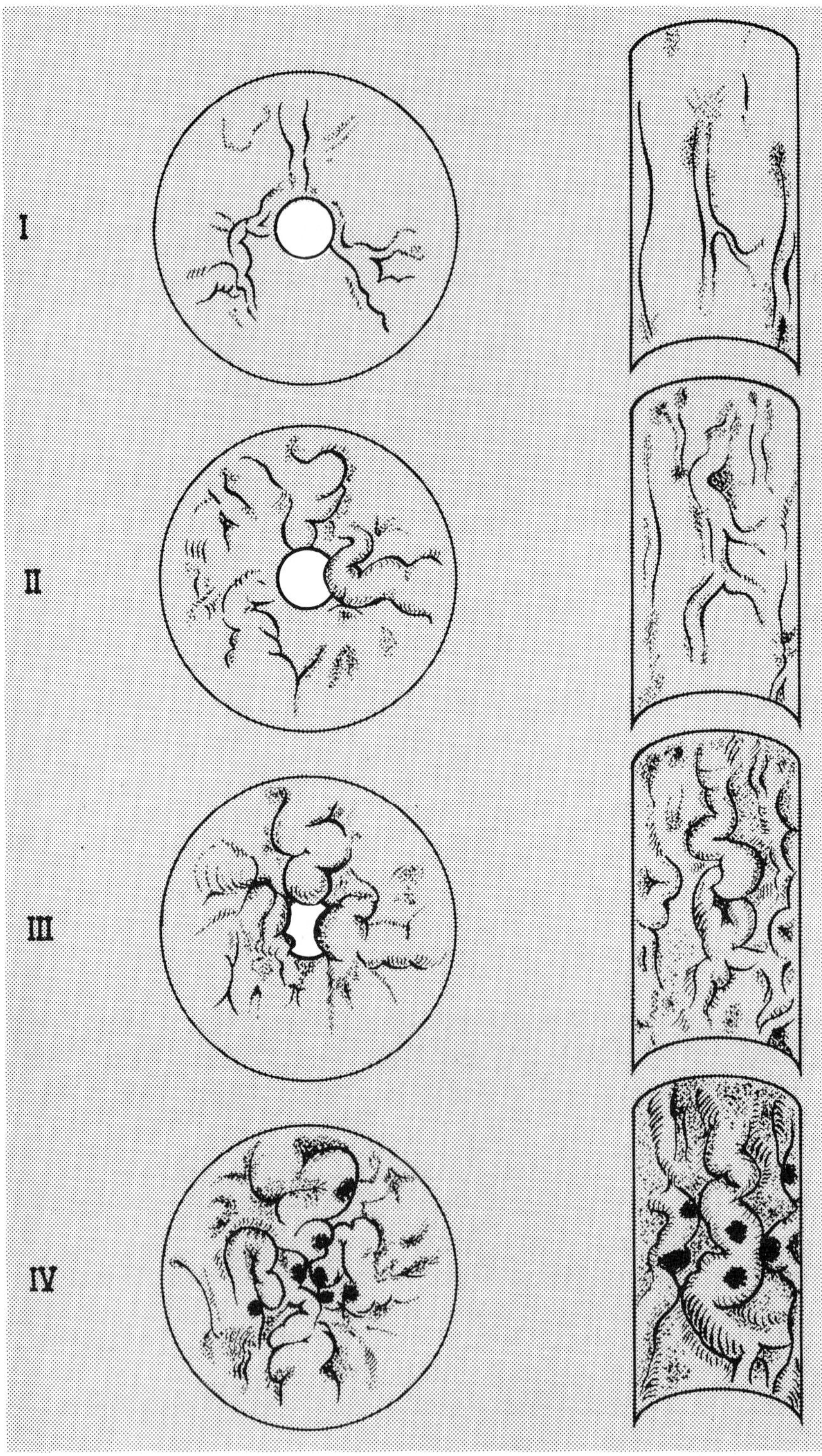

FIGURE 9. Gradual development of esophageal varices in portal hypertension. Superficial erosions (black dotted areas) are a common feature of grade IV varices implying a high risk of hemorrhage.

Table 11
PRELIMINARY RESULTS OF A PROSPECTIVE CONTROLLED RANDOMIZED TRIAL ON PROPHYLACTIC PARAVARICEAL INJECTION SCLEROTHERAPY IN PATIENTS WITH DECOMPENSATED CIRRHOSIS OF THE LIVER (JANUARY 1978—MAY 1979)

Group	Number of patients	Number of therapies	Hemorrhages	Deaths
I	13	27	1 (8%)	—
II	11	—	6 (55%)	4 (36%)

Which Method is the Most Effective and Safe in Controlling Acute Variceal Hemorrhage?

Since effects of pharmacological measures[56,57] and of balloon tamponade[58,59] do not exceed 50 to 80% temporary hemostasis, and rebleeding is as high as 60%,[60] semi-invasive methods appear as the treatment of choice. In our patients, 92% of 324 acute massive bleedings were definitely controlled by solely performing paravariceal sclerotherapy. A prospective evaluation of paravariceal injection in massively bleeding patients who had failed to respond to balloon tamponade of six hours to four days duration revealed a similar rate of 92% hemostasis by this method.[22] This compares favorably with the results recently presented by Terblanche and collaborators.[32] They were able to stop acute hemorrhage by primary Sengstaken tamponade and intravariceal injections in 92% out of 36 hospital admissions in 22 patients. Hunt et al.[13] failed to stop bleeding only 7 times out of 44 injections (84% success rate), and Johnston and Rodgers[14] successfully controlled 93% of 194 bleeding events in 117 patients. By contrast, Soehendra,[61] who has used paravariceal injection sclerotherapy between 1972 and 1978 in 106 mostly electively treated patients with a disastrous admission mortality of 38%, failed to control acute hemorrhage by intravariceal injection in 8 out of 37 patients (22%), and 18 in–hospital deaths (49%) occurred.[61] Presently, he propagates a method of a combined intravariceal and perivariceal injection of 5 m*l* aliquots of 1% polidocanol, and up to 20 injections are made.[39] Since severe cardiovascular reactions have been observed,[39] one is allowed to assume, that the mass of injected sclerosant is washed into systemic circulation. In addition, 5 m*l* aliquots of 1% polidocanol will, in our experience, inevitably result in severe ulceration, if not complete transesophageal necrosis, when applied perivascularly. Therefore, this particular technique should no longer be performed in patients who expect adequate relief from their dangerous situation.

In nearly all other groups, paravariceal and intravariceal injection sclerotherapy reveal a similar efficacy concerning acute hemorrhage from esophageal varices.

Data on recurrent bleeding after primary sclerotherapy are difficult to find. Johnston and Rodgers[14] reported an average relief from hemorrhage of ten months in intrahepatic and of 30 months in extrahepatic obstruction, but no recurrence rates in terms of percent of patients who rebled are given. Terblanche and co-workers reported 51 bleeding episodes during 36 separate hospital admissions in 22 patients.[32] Though no recurrence rates are reported except for three uncontrolled rebleeds, and though the patients were then attributed to chronic treatment groups by random,[24] it may be calculated from the initial numbers that 14 patients had one readmission each for recurrent hemorrhage (64%) and that 15 additional in-hospital rebleds occurred (68%). When random attribution to chronic injection treatment group[24] is taken into account, out of nine acutely, plus chronically injected patients, four (44%) rebled within the two-years' assessment period. Lewis and co-workers[33] reported that two out of their

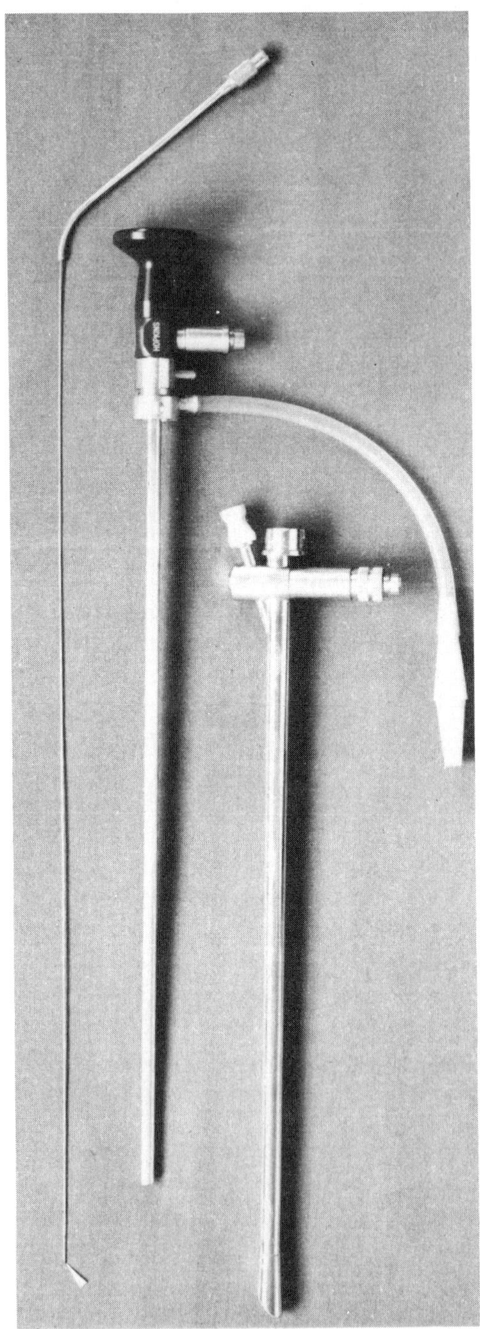

FIGURE 10. Rigid instrument for pediatric patients younger than five years with needle, "HOPKINS" fiberoptic system and suction device.

nine acutely injected patients rebled from esophageal varices (22%) in a mean follow-up period of 4.1 months since last injection. In our 909 patients, 23.8% had minor seeping rebleeds within the primary treatment, 6% within the first four months after initiation of treatment, and an additional 20% had some episode of recurrent hemorrhage within a 10-yr follow-up. If either in-hospital rebleeds from esophageal

Table 12
INDICATIONS AND PATIENT DATA OF 52 PEDIATRIC PATIENTS SUBMITTED TO SCLEROTHERAPY OF ESOPHAGEAL VARICES

Age (years)	Number of patients	Number of Previous bleeds	Admission diagnosis	Treatment: Emergency	Treatment: Elective
1	1	3	Portal Thrombosis	x	
2	1	25	Cirrhosis (CAH)	x	x
2—5	6	2—3	Portal obstruction	x	x
6—9	14	1—4	Portal obstruction	x	x
10—14	27	1—4	Portal obstruction	x	x
10—14	1	2	Cirrhosis and portal obstruction	x	x
10—14	2	0/2	chronic active hepatitis (CAH)		
1—14	52	0—25	Total	15	37

varices or recurrence of bleeding within ten years is compared to other groups, paravariceal injection sclerotherapy seems to be somewhat superior to the intravariceal method, but the data derived from the latter technique may probably improve with larger experience.

Complications were observed in 13.5% of our patients, consisting of severe esophageal ulcers, transesophageal necrosis with mediastinitis, esophageal stenosis, large pleural effusions, and rebleeds from gastric varices; 3 to 4% were considered life-threatening. Small areas of superficial mucosal slough indicate sufficient therapy, do not cause any discomfort, and are not regarded as a complication. Terblanche et al.[32] reported major complications in 12 of their 22 patients treated acutely (54%). They consisted of two periesophageal leaks (9%), two cases of mild esophageal stenosis (9%), two esophageal tears (9%), three severe pneumonias (14%), and two complications due to the Sengstaken tube (9%). The numbers of Lewis and collaborators are too small to draw any conclusions from their complication rates. However, one point must be emphasized—5 of their 18 injected patients developed temperatures greater than 38.5°C, which has been interpreted as being due to pyrogens in the sclerosant. In fact, no such reactions have been reported by groups using ethanolamine oleate or polidocanol. In-hospital mortality is difficult to compare, as it crucially depends on the state of hepatic function. In our series of emergency sclerotherapy, 67% out of 324 patients had to be placed into Child's C category. In-hospital mortality was 20% in these patients. In a prospective trial on poor risk patients who did not respond to Sengstaken tube tamponade, admission mortality approached nearly 40%.[22] Terblanche's group reports a mortality rate per hospital admission of 25% and an overall mortality of 41%.[24] Of their patients, 9% were in the Child A group, 73% with the B group, and only 18% with the C group. Of Lewis' and collaborators', 9 patients were treated acutely (33% Child C, 67% Child B), 2 died within several days (22%), and one 8 months after sclerotherapy was initiated. These results on acute mortality of paravariceal and intravariceal injection sclerotherapy do not differ significantly.

Two additional semiinvasive methods are to be compared to either intravariceal or paravariceal sclerotherapy. Percutaneous transhepatic obliteration has been propagated by Lunderquist.[62] Hemostasis for more than one week is achieved in only 56% of patients, and complications in terms of portal thrombosis frequently occur (36%).[63] Since many of the obliterated veins are recanalized within several months, Lunderquist

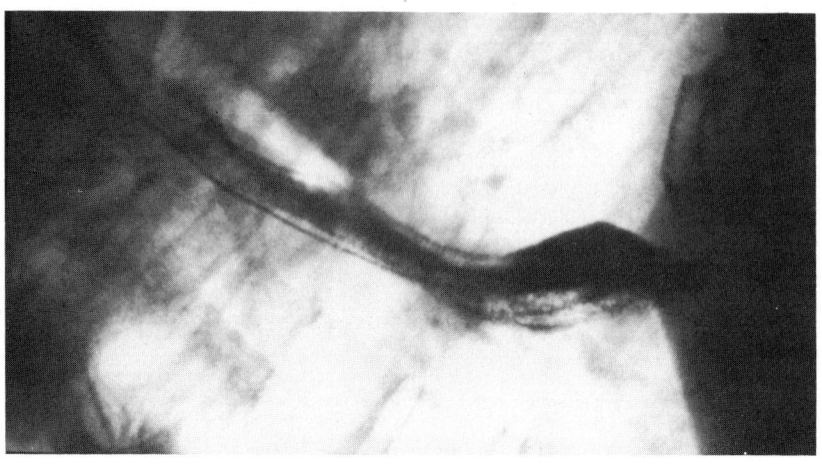

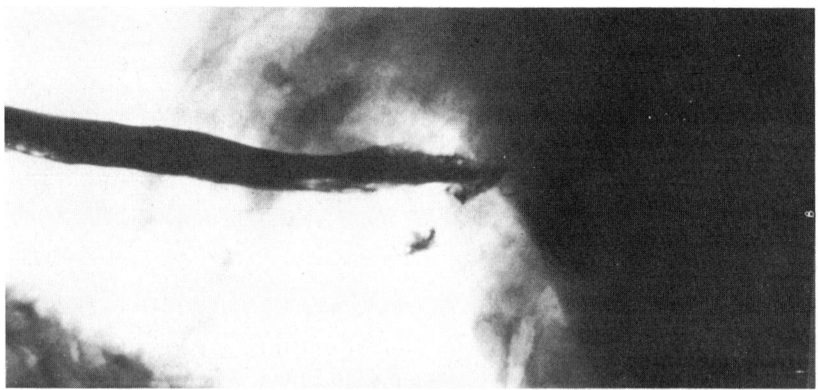

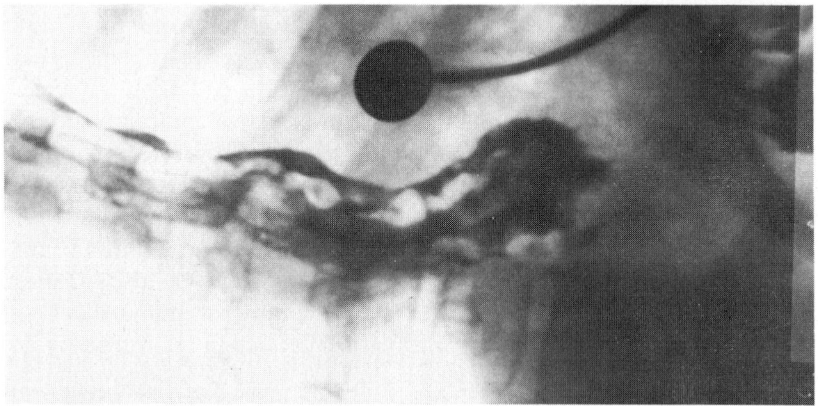

FIGURE 11. Barium swallow in an 8 year old boy with portal thrombosis, demonstrating incomplete necrosis of the esophageal wall (B) after paravariceal sclerotherapy (A and C) for acute massive hemorrhage. (From Paquet, K. J., and Lindecken, K. D., *Ztschr. Kinderchir.*, 23, 269, 1978. With Permission.)

Table 13
EFFECT OF OPERATIVE PROCEDURES PERFORMED IN 30 PEDIATRIC PATIENTS BEFORE SCHLEROTHERAPY WAS DONE

Number of patients	Type of operation	Months free of hemorrhage	Shunts	
			Patent	Clotted
1	Fundectomy	23 months	—	—
9	Mesocaval shunt	3—12 months	0	9
8	Splenectomy	1—6 months	—	—
8	Splenectomy and splenorenal shunt	6—14 months	0	8
4	Transthoracic Ligation of varices	4—12 months	—	—
30	Total	1—23 months	0	16

has restricted this procedure to patients not responding to any conservative or semiinvasive means.

Laser photocoagulation is a powerful method in treating gastrointestinal hemorrhage. Kiefhaber[64] effectively controlled more than 90% of variceal bleedings by means of a high-power Neodymium-Yag laser device. Argon lasers are not suitable to the management of such massive hemorrhage because of insufficient energy emission. As the effect of laser treatment is restricted to the coagulated bleeding site, recurrence of hemorrhage is inevitable when no other definitive treatment is initiated.

The disappointing results of emergency shunts delineated above need no further comment.

In summary, transhepatic obliteration is not sufficiently hemostatic and bears the risk of portal thrombosis. Photocoagulation by means of a Neodymium-Yag laser effectively controls acute bleeding in expert hands, but long-term effects cannot be expected. Paravariceal sclerotherapy appears to be somewhat superior to the intravariceal technique concerning recurrence and complication rate, whereas no significant differences can be detected in terms of hemostatic efficacy and in-hospital mortality. Both techniques appear as the desirable treatment of variceal hemorrhage. To finally prove superiority of this method, we have designed a prospective controlled randomized trial of emergency paravariceal sclerotherapy which is presently being performed.

Which procedure provides reasonable reliability in preventing further bleed?

Elective treatment has been performed by us in 540 adult patients with an in-hospital mortality of 11% and recurrence and complication rates as mentioned above. In this group, 84% were categorized as Child C patients. Denck[17,42] reported an admission mortality of 16.5% in 511 patients; 15% had rebled with fatal outcome within 0 to 17 years after primary treatment. Wodak[28] delineates similar data.

Intravariceal injection sclerotherapy has been tested recently in a controlled trial by Terblanche et al.[24] In his chronic injection treatment group of 11 patients, 7 recurrent bleeds occurred within 2 years (64%) compared to 34 rebleeds observed in 13 patients on control medical treatment. Mortality rates were similar in both groups (5/13 in the medical and 5/11 in chronic injection group). Lewis and co-workers lost two of their nine electively treated patients within one year (22%). One fatal recurrent hemorrhage occurred in a patient whose varices never could be eradicated.

From these considerations, paravariceal sclerotherapy may be superior to intravariceal injection concerning prevention of recurrent hemorrhage. Data on long-term survival, which is more than 50% after five years in our patients, are not sufficient to judge chronic intravariceal sclerotherapy. Since patent portal-systemic shunts performed in patients elected according to Child's criteria diminish the risk of rebleeding to about 25%,[49] the aim of long-term sclerotherapy must be equal to or stay within this rate. Retrospective data of Paquet[26] and Denck[42] encourage controlled trials to solve the question whether sclerotherapy might be able to replace portal-systemic shunt operations in patients considered fit for shunting.

No data from outside our group are published on sclerotherapy in pediatric patients. Our experience in 52 children demonstrates this method to be much more effective than any surgical method previously applied to these patients. Seventeen children had clotted shunts with no chance of repeated operation for anatomical reasons. Since any portal-systemic shunt performed under 10 years of age is hampered by a high risk of shunt thrombosis within several months, surgery should be postponed until the children are at least 10 to 14 years old. Therefore, endoscopic paravariceal sclerotherapy serves to definitely control the varices until shunt operations can be successfully done.

The question, if prophylactic endoscopic sclerotherapy might be effective in patients who are not considered suitable to shunt surgery and who have not bled previously, is approached by a prospective controlled trial presently carried on by us. Preliminary data are encouraging, but they need further clarification and consolidation by greater numbers of patients and longer follow-up periods.

Which special technique should be used?

The answer to the question, which particular technique of sclerotherapy one should perform, might be simply to use the technique in which an individual physician is most skilled. This procedure will be probably the most effective in his hands.

To definitely compare intravariceal and paravariceal injection, a controlled trial would be necessary. We favor paravariceal injection, as we feel that this technique will more effectively prevent hemorrhage by not obliterating, but preserving, the portal-systemic collaterals under a fibrous layer. Therefore, pressure at the gastric level is unlikely to increase. This might become a problem of intravariceal injection. Recently, preliminary results of a prospective controlled study on elective intravariceal sclerotherapy was presented by Clark et al.[65] with rebleeds from gastric varices as frequent as 55%. No such results have been reported by other groups.

The flexible instrument in our hands is used to treat nonbleeding grade 1 to 3 varices and to perform acute injections when seeping variceal hemorrhage is seen at emergency endoscopy. Since grade 4 esophageal varices are difficult to control by the flexible fiberscope and view is insufficient in massive hemorrhage, the rigid esophagoscope is preferred. In addition, there is considerable danger of pulmonary aspiration in massively bleeding patients. Thus, the rigid instrument is used in these situations. We have not seen any significant problems arising from a cautious general anesthesia.

Despite frequent criticism during the last 40 years, sclerotherapy of esophageal varices is now widely accepted for the indications shown in Table 14.

VI. SUMMARY

Endoscopic sclerotherapy of bleeding esophageal varices has been performed for more than 40 years. In uncontrolled studies, it has been effective in controlling acute hemorrhage and in preventing recurrent bleeds. Controlled trials of acute and elective treatment are necessary to finally assess the value of this method.

Table 14
INDICATIONS OF ESOPHAGOSCOPIC PARAVARICEAL SCLEROTHERAPY

1. Acute massive hemorrhage from esophageal varices
2. Prophylaxis of recurrent hemorrhage after one or more previous bleeds in all patients not suitable to shunt surgery
3. Prophylaxis of recurrent hemorrhage in babies and children up to 10—14 years old
4. Prophylaxis of first hemorrhage in grade III and IV esophageal varices?
5. Prophylaxis of recurrent hemorrhage as alternative to shunt operations?

Two different techniques of injection sclerotherapy have been developed: (1) the intravariceal method that obliterates the varices and, in addition, induces submucous fibrogenesis, and (2)para-variceal method that preserves important collateral channels by covering them by a fibrous layer. To date, we have treated more than 1000 patients by the latter technique. Both methods provide definitive hemostatis in 90% of acute variceal bleedings and prevent further bleeds. Preliminary results on a controlled study of prophylactic sclerotherapy in 24 patients suggests prevention of first variceal hemorrhage. In pediatric patients, effective control of varices is achieved until shunt surgery can be performed. The following indications for sclerotherapy are suggested:

1. Acute massive variceal hemorrhage
2. Previous variceal bleeding in patients not suitable to shunt surgery and all patients refusing shunt operation
3. Bleeding varices in babies and children up to 10 to 14 years old.

REFERENCES

1. **Crafoord, C. and Frenckner, P.,** Nonsurgical treatment of varicose veins of the oesophagus, *Acta. Otolaryngol. (Stockholm),* 27, 422, 1939.
2. **Moersch, H. J.,** The treatment of esophageal varices by injection of a sclerosing solution, *J. Thorac. Surg.,* 10, 300, 1940.
3. **Moersch, H. J.,** Further studies on the treatment of esophageal varices by injection of a sclerosing solution, *Ann. Otolaryngol. Rhinol. Laryngol.,* 50, 1233, 1941.
4. **Moersch, H. J.,** Treatment of esophageal varices by injection of a sclerosing solution, *JAMA,* 135, 754, 1947.
5. **Patterson, C. O. and Rouse, M. O.,** The injection treatment of esophageal varices, *JAMA,* 130, 384, 1951.
6. **Kempe, S. G. and Koch, H.,** Injection of sclerosing solutions in the treatment of esophageal varices, *Acta Otolaryngol. (Stockholm) Suppl.,* 118, 120, 1954.
7. **Jackson, F. C., Perrin, E. B., de Gradi, A. E., Smith, A. G., and Lee, L. E.,** Clinical investigation of the portocaval shunt. I. Study design and preliminary survival analysis, *Arch. Surg.,* 91, 43, 1965.
8. **Resnick, R. H., Chalmers, T. C., Ishihara, A. M., Garceau, A. J., Callow, A. D., Schimmel, E. M., and O'Hara, E. T.,** A controlled study of the prophylactic portocaval shunt; a final report., *Ann. Intern. Med.,* 70, 675, 1969.
9. **Mikkelsen, W. P. and Pattison, A. C.,** Emergency portocaval shunt, *Am. J. Surg.,* 96, 183, 1958.
10. **Guetgemann, A. and Esser, G.,** Portal hypertension varicose vein bleeding and shunt operation, *Minn. Med.,* 51, 1517, 1968.
11. **Wantz, G. E. and Payne, M. A.,** Experience with portocaval shunt for portal hypertension, *N. Engl. J. Med.,* 265, 721, 1961.
12. **Macbeth, R.,** Treatment of esophageal varices in portal hypertension by means of sclerosing injections, *Br. Med. J.,* 2, 877, 1955.
13. **Hunt, P. S., Johnston, G. W., and Rodgers, H. W.,** The emergency management of bleeding esophageal varices with sclerosing injections, *Br. J. Surg,* 56, 305, 1969.

14. **Johnston, G. W. and Rodgers, H. W.,** A review of 15 years experience in the use of sclerotherapy in the control of acute hemorrhage from esophageal varices, *Br. J. Surg.*, 60, 797, 1973.
15. **Wodak, E.,** Ösophagusvarizenblutung bei portaler Hypertension: ihre Therapie und Prophylaxe, *Wien. Med. Wochenschr.*, 110, 581, 1960.
16. **Denck, H.,** Zur Frage der zweckmäβigen Behandlung blutender Ösophagusvarizen, *Wien. Klin. Z.*, 16, 274, 1963.
17. **Denck, H.,** Endooesophageal sclerotherapy of bleeding oesophageal varices, *J. Cardiovasc. Surg.*, 12, 146, 1971.
18. **Paquet, K. J.,** Indikationen und Ergebnisse der Sklerosierungstherapie von Ösophagusvarizen, *Therapiewoche,* 22, 262, 1972.
19. **Raschke, E. and Paquet, K. J.,** Management of hemorrhage from esophageal varices using endoscopic method, *Ann. Surg.*, 177, 99, 1973.
20. **Paquet, K. J. and Oberhammer, E.,** Sclerotherapy of bleeding oesophageal varices by means of endoscopy, *Endoscopy,* 10, 7, 1978.
21. **Fleig, W. E., Rüttenauer, K., Stange, E. F.,** and **Ditschuneit, H.,** Endoscopic sclerotherapy controls acute bleeding from esophageal varices, *Gastroenterology,* 78, 1165, 1980.
22. **Fleig, W. E., Rüttenauer, K., and Strange, E. F.,** Endoscopic sclerotherapy for bleeding esophageal varices: a prospective trial in patients not responding to balloon tamponade, *Gastrointestinal Endoscopy,* in press.
23. **Stange, E. F. and Fleig, W. E.,** The visible vessel land gastrointestinal hemorrhage, (Letter), *N. Engl. J. Med.*, 301, 892, 1979.
24. **Terblanche, J., Northover, J. M. A., Bornman, P., Kahn, D., Siller, W., Barbezat, G. O., Sillais, S., Campbell, J. A. H., and Saunders, S. F.,** A prospective controlled trial of sclerotherapy in the long term management of patients after esophageal variceal bleeding, *Surg. Gynecol. Obstet.*, 148, 323, 1979.
25. **Johnson, L. S., Kinnear, D. G., Brown, R. A., and Mulder, D. S.,** "Downhill" esophageal varices, *Arch. Surg.*, 113, 1463, 1978.
26. **Paquet, K. J., Albrecht, M., and Kliems, G.,** Wandsklerosierung bei Ösophagusvarizen: prophylaktisch—bei akuter Blutung—im Intervall?, in *Operative Endoskopie,* Demling, L, and Rösch, W., Eds., Acron Verlag, Berlin, 1979, 33.
27. **Stelzner, F. and Lierse, W.,** Der angiomuskuläre Verschluβ der Speiseröhre, *Arch. Klin. Chir.*, 321, 35, 1968.
28. **Wodak, E.,** Akute gastrointestinale Blutung; Resultate der endoskopischen Sklerosierung von Ösophagusvarizen, *Schweiz. Med. Wochenschr.*, 109, 591, 1979.
29. **Liebowitz, H. R.,** Pathogenesis of esophageal varix rupture, *JAMA,* 175, 874, 1961.
30. **Orloff, N. J. and Thomas, H. S.,** Pathogenesis of esophageal varix rupture. A study based on gross and microscopic examination of the esophagus at the time of bleeding, *Arch. Surg.*, 87, 301, 1963.
31. **Mörl, M., Wannagat, L., and Gehring, D.,** Laparoscopic manometry of the liver circulatory system—comparative examinations of the different stages of portal hypertension in cirrhosis of the liver, in IV World Congress of Digestive Endoscopy, Madrid, June 1 to 3, 1978, 88.
32. **Terblanche, J., Northover, J. M. A., Bornman, P., Kahn, D., Barbezat, G. O., Sellais, S. L., and Saunders, S. F.,** A prospective evaluation of injection sclerotherapy in the treatment of acute bleeding from esophageal varices, *Surgery,* 85, 239, 1979.

32a. **Eckhardt, V. F., Grace, N. D., and Kantrowitz, P. A.,** Does lower esophageal sphincter incompetency contribute to esophageal variceal bleeding? *Gastroenterology,* 71, 185, 1976.

32b. **Eckhardt, V. F., and Grace, N. D.,** Gastroesophageal reflux and bleeding esophageal varices, *Gastroenterology,* 76, 39, 1979.

33. **Lewis, J., Chung, R. S., and Allison, J.,** Sclerotherapy of esophageal varices, *Ann. Surg.*, 115, 476, 1980.
34. **Johnson, A. G.,** Injection sclerotherapy in the emergency and elective treatment of oesophageal varices, *Ann. R. Coll. Surg. Engl.*, 59, 497, 1977.
35. **Williams, K. G. D. and Dawson, J. L.,** Fibreoptic injection of oesophageal varices, *Br. Med. J.*, 2, 766, 1979.
36. **Soehendra, N., Reynders-Frederix, V., Doehn, M., Bützow, G. H., and Erbe, W.,** Fiberendoskopische Ösophagusvarizenverödung, *Dtsch. Med. Wochenschr.*, 104, 161, 1979.
37. **Barsoum, M. S., Khattar, N. Y., and Risk-Allah, M. A.,** Technical aspects of injection sclerotherapy of acute oesophageal variceal haemorrhage as seen by radiography, *Br. J. Surg.*, 65, 588, 1978.
38. **Sugawa, C., Okumura, Y., Lucas, C. E., and Walt, A. J.,** Endoscopic sclerosis of experimental esophageal varices in dogs, *Gastrointest. Endosc.*, 24, 114, 1978.
39. **Soehendra, N.,** Behandlung der ösophagusvarizenblutung durch Verödung (intravasale Injektion), 1st German-Austrian-Swiss Symposium on Portal Hypertension, Zell a.S., Austria, March 21 to 23, 1980.

40. **Paquet, K. J., Büsing, V., and Kliems, G.,** Wandsklerosierung der Speiseröhre wegen akuter, konservativ unstillbarer und drohender Varizenblutung, *Dtsch. Med., Wochenschr.,* 102, 59, 1977.
41. **Fleig, W. E., Rüttenauer, K., Stange, E. F., and Ditschuneit, H.,** Treatment of bleeding esophageal varices by endoscopic sclerotherapy, in *Portal Hypertension,* Paquet, K.J. and Denck, H., Eds., S. Karger, Munich, 1981, in press.
42. **Denck, H.,** Indikation, Technik und Ergebnisse der endoskopischen Behandlung von Ösophagusvarizen, *Zentralbl, Chir.,* 103, 213, 1978.
43. **Haslhofer, L.,** Pathologisch-anatomische Beobachtungen zur Wandsklerosierung, *Wien. Z. Inn. Med.,* 51, 118, 1970.
44. **Bailey, M. E. and Dawson, J. L.,** Modified oesophagoscope for injecting oesophageal varices, *Br. Med. J.,* 2, 540, 1975.
45. **Paquet, K. J.,** Ein neues Instrument zur Wandsklerosierung der Speiseröhre in der Behandlung der akuten Ösophagusvarizenblutung bzw. von Varizen im blutungsfreien Intervall, *Akt. Gastrol.,* 4, 441, 1975.
46. **Kapp, F. and Buess, H.,** Ösophaguswandsklerosierung als Therapie blutender Ösophagusvarizen bei inoperablen Patienten, *Dtsch. Med. Wochenschr.,* 98, 2465, 1973.
47. **Brunner, G.,** Intravasale und submuköse ösophagusvarizensklerosierung mit einem neuen flexiblen Gerät, *Z. Gastroenterol.,* 18, 443, 1980.
48. **Brooks, W. S., Jr.,** Adapting flexible endoscopes for sclerosis of oesophageal varices, (letter), *Lancet,* 1, 266, 1980.
49. **Galambos, J. T.,** Cirrhosis, in *Major problems in Internal Medicine,* Vol. XVII, Smith, L.H., Jr., Ed., W. B. Saunders Philadelphia, 1979.
50. **Brooks, W. S., Jr., Galambos, J. T., Warren, N. D., and Millikan, W. J., Jr.,** Modification of the flexible endoscope for endoscopic sclerosis of esophageal varices, Digestive Disease Week, Salt Lake City, May 19 to 21, 1980, A-53, No. 211.
51. **Johanson, C. A. and Shapiro, H. A.,** Transfiberscope sclerotherapy in the control of esophageal variceal hemorrhage, Digestive Disease Week, Salt Lake City, May 19 to 21, 1980, A-53, No. 209.
52. **Sivak, M. V., Jr., Stout, D., and Skipper, G.,** Injection sclerosis of esophageal varices using a fiberoptic endoscope, Digestive Disease Week, Salt Lake City, May 19 to 21, 1980.
53. **Conn, H. O., Leavy, C. M., Vlahcevic, Z. R., Rodgers, J. B., Maddrey, W. C., Seeff, L., and Levy, L. L.,** Comparison of lactulose and neomycin in the treatment of chronic portal-systemic encephalopathy. A double blind controlled trial, *Gastroenterology,* 72, 573, 1977.
54. **Reiter, H. J., and Bode, J. Ch.,** Parenteral application of a special amino acid solution in the treatment of severe hepatic encephalopathy, *Z. Gastroenterol.,* 7, 457, 1978.
55. **Pugh, R. N. H., Murray-Lyon, I. M., Dawson, J. L., Pretroni, M. C., and Williams, R.,** Transsection of the oesophagus for bleeding esophageal varices, *Br. J. Surg.,* 60, 646, 1973.
56. **Vosmik, J., Jedlicka, K., Mulder, J. L., and Cort, J. H.,** Action of the triglycyl hormogen of vasopressin (glypressin) in patients with liver cirrhosis and bleeding esophageal varices, *Gastroenterology,* 72, 605, 1977.
57. **Chojkier, M., Groszmann, R. J., Atterbury, C. E., Bar-Meir, S., Blei, A. T., Frankel, F., Glickman, M. G., Kniaz, J. L., Schode, R., Taggart, G. F., and Conn, H. O.,** A controlled comparison of continuous intraarterial and intravenous infusions of vasopressin in hemorrhage from esophageal varices, *Gastroenterology,* 77, 540, 1979.
58. **Conn, H. O. and Simpson, J. A.,** Excessive mortality associated with balloon tamponade of bleeding varices, *JAMA,* 202, 587, 1967.
59. **Pitcher, J. L.,** Safety and effectiveness of the modified Sengstaken-Blakemore tube: a prospective study, *Gastroenterology,* 61, 291, 1971.
60. **Novis, B. H., Duys, P., Barbezat, G. O., Clain, F., Bank, S., and Terblanche, J.,** Fibreoptic endoscopy and the use of the Sengstaken tube in acute gastrointestinal hemorrhage in patients with portal hypertension and varices, *GUT,* 17, 258, 1976.
61. **Soehendra, N.,** Fiberendoskopische Ösophagusvarizenverödung, in *Operative Endoskopie,* Demling, L., and Rösch, W., Eds., Acron-Verlag, Berlin, 1979, 47.
62. **Lunderquist, A. and Vang, J.,** Transhepatic catheterization and obliteration of the coronary vein in patients with portal hypertension and esophageal varices, *N. Engl. J., Med.,* 291, 46, 1974.
63. **Bengmark, S., Börjesson, B., Hoevels, B., Joelsson, B., Lunderquist, A., and Owman, T.,** Obliteration of esophageal varices by PTP. A follow-up of 43 patients, *Ann. Surg.,* 190, 549, 1979.
64. **Kiefhaber. P., Moritz, K., and Heldwein, W.,** Endoscopische Blutstillung blutender ösophagus—und Magenvarizen mit einem Hochleistungs-Neodym-Yag-Laser, in *Operative Endoskopie,* Demling, L., and Rösch, W., Eds, Acron-Verlag, Berlin, 1979, 19.
65. **Clark, A. W., Mitchell, J. K., McDougall, B., et al.,** A prospective controlled clinical trial of injection sclerotherapy in cirrhotic patients with recent hemorrhage, 14th Meeting European Association Study of the Liver, Düsseldorf, 1979.

Chapter 5

LASER PHOTOCOAGULATION PRINCIPLES

David C. Auth

TABLE OF CONTENTS

I. INTRODUCTION

The objective of laser photocoagulation (endoscopic or otherwise) is the conversion of light energy into thermal energy with a subsequent temperature rise leading to thermal denaturation or "coagulation". As such, the use of a laser might be regarded as a rather expensive "heater" or "cautery". There is no proven evidence that laser light improves the normal biochemical coagulation cascade. Thus, if laser cautery is justified as an expensive clinical technique, it should provide improved efficacy and/or safety over other available thermal cautery devices.

There has been a good deal of fanfare about lasers in the contemporary press as being "death rays" or "miracle cures" or insidious carriers of mysterious energy. While it is possible with great effort and expense to construct lasers which can vaporize targets as big or bigger than a breadbox, most lasers which are sold are deemed useful because of two fundamental physical characteristics: (1) Laser light is highly directional and can be focused to small spots; and (2) laser light is usually confined to one or more narrow regions of the optical spectrum.

These fundamental physical characteristics will be discussed below in so far as they are important to endoscopic coagulation.

II. LASER UTILITY IN ENDOSCOPY

A. Fiberoptic Transmission

The use of optical fibers for flexibly conveying an optical image is familiar to endoscopists. Ordered arrays of small optical channels of 10-μm diameter cylinders enable excellent visualization of internal anatomical cavities. Disordered arrays are used for conveying light for illumination of dark cavities. The ability of a glass cylinder to trap and transport an optical wave is a result of a phenomenon referred to as "critical internal reflection". This means that a light ray which intercepts a boundary between two dissimilar transparent materials can be perfectly (= to 100%) reflected if the angle of intercept is greater than or equal to the critical angle. This angle is shown in Figure 1 as ϕ_c. The defining equation is:

$$\phi_c = \tan^{-1} n_2/n_1 , \tag{1}$$

where n_2 and n_1 are the respective indices of refraction for the dissimilar materials. This means that total internal reflection can only be obtained when n_2 is greater than n_1. Thus, a cylinder of glass with an optical index of 1.5 can easily provide trapping of an optical ray when the cylinder is immersed in air or water. The problem with optical fibers consisting of a single cylinder of glass when used as a conveyor of light is that of loss. That is, light is scattered by impurities which may come in contact with the light at the boundary layer of the cylinder and the external medium. In order to reduce this loss and provide an efficient conveyor of light, a cladding[1] is normally used as shown in Figure 1. This cladding is made of material whose index of refraction is less than the core cylinder. The function of the cladding is to provide isolation of impurities from the core cylinder and to provide a consistent reflector of light for the core cylinder. Cladded fibers have now been developed which possess such low loss that the telephone companies have begun installing them in communications service instead of conventional copper cables. This new generation of low-loss optical fiber waveguides has enabled the passage of high-power beams of laser light through the biopsy channel of conventional endoscopes. Without low loss characteristics, an optical fiber would selfdestruct if high-power laser light were confined. When a fiber possesses significant

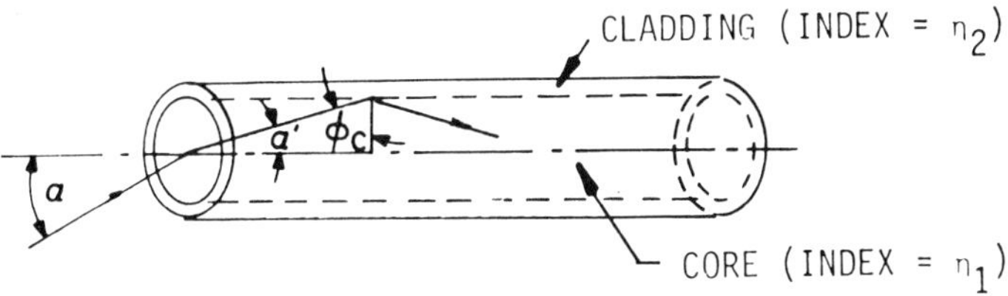

FIGURE 1. The cladded optical waveguide. Note the trapping of optical radiation by the transparent cylindrical core. (From Gilbert, D. A., Silverstein, F. E., Auth, D. C., and Rubin, C. E., Progress in Hemostasis and Thrombosis, 1978, 349. With permission.)

loss because of optical absorption, it heats up in the presence of intense optical radiation. Eventually, the fiber melts and it is destroyed. A similar form of destruction has been experienced by endoscopists when blood collects on a fiber during laser endoscopy which can lead to absorption and heating with eventual destruction of the fiber.

The maximum angle for trapping of light in a fiber is shown in Figure 1 as α. Rays which exceed this angle are lost, since they imply a value for ϕ which is less than the critical angle for internal reflection. A typical value for α for useful endoscopic laser fibers is 12°. Of course, smaller angles of incident radiation can easily be confined. In order to provide flexibility, optical fibers are drawn from a hot melt to a thin filiamentary structure with diameters ranging from 5 to 1000 μm (1 mm). Fibers of 1000 μm are quite stiff and are normally rejected for flexible endoscopy. Fibers of 400 to 600 μm are most commonly used for laser endoscopy at the present time, since they combine flexibility with a sufficiently large diameter as to enable easy projection of a laser light spot onto the input end of the fiber. This is shown in Figure 2a. Although the argon laser can be focused to a spot of less than 5-μm diameter, larger diameter fibers provide easy alignment of the spot with the fiber's entrance pupil. The ready availability of larger diameter (several hundred microns diameter) low-loss fibers has made it possible to transmit Nd:YAG laser radiation of high power, even though this laser can have minimal focal spot sizes exceeding 200 μm.

One may be inclined to ask why it is not possible to use a conventional light bulb for coagulation. In fact, it is. However, if one attempts to transport the radiation of a light bulb through an optical fiber that is small enough to be flexible, one finds out rather quickly that only a small portion of the light can be trapped within the optical fiber. This is graphically depicted in Figure 2b where the classical incandescent candle is focused on the entrance pupil of an optical fiber. It is easy to see that only a very small fraction of the candlelight reaches the focusing lens and an even smaller amount is presented to the fiber. Thus, a key parameter in favor of lasers for flexible fiber photocoagulation is "focusability".

B. Radiant Transfer and Selective Absorptivity

Figure 3 illustrates the impact of the three most important surgical laser beams upon a specimen of tissue. The carbon dioxide laser operates at 10.6 μm wavelength in the middle infrared region of the electromagnetic spectrum. This wavelength is such that the water molecule strikes up a sympathetic vibration. When this happens, energy is extracted from a laser beam and converted to heat. Since tissue contains water, the CO_2 laser beam is rapidly absorbed by tissue. Thus, as shown in Figure 3, its penetration is shallow. When the radiation from a CO_2 laser is focused on tissue at high-power levels, it causes rapid evaporation of cell water, which in turn forms a crater. A series of side-by-side craters forms an incision. The CO_2 laser is a popular laser scalpel.

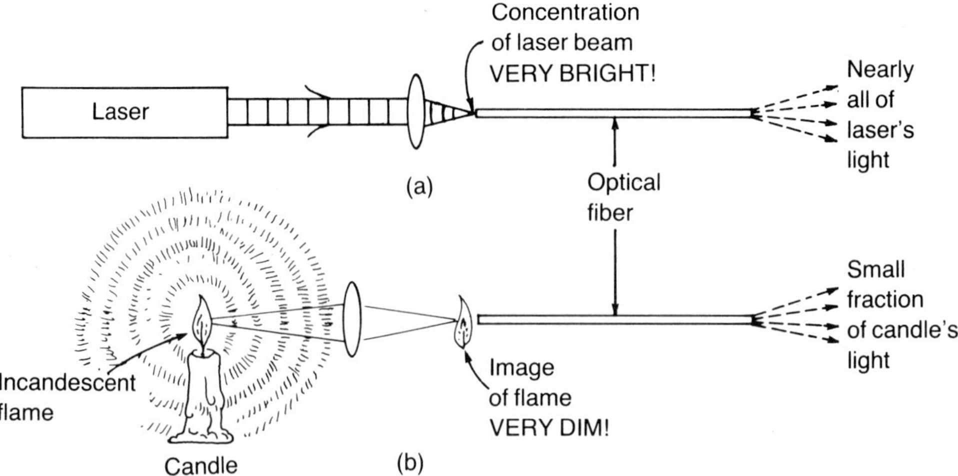

FIGURE 2. Coupling of light into an optical fiber waveguide. (a) Efficient coupling of laser light having high directivity into fiber; (b) inefficient coupling of light from an incandescent source having poor directivity.

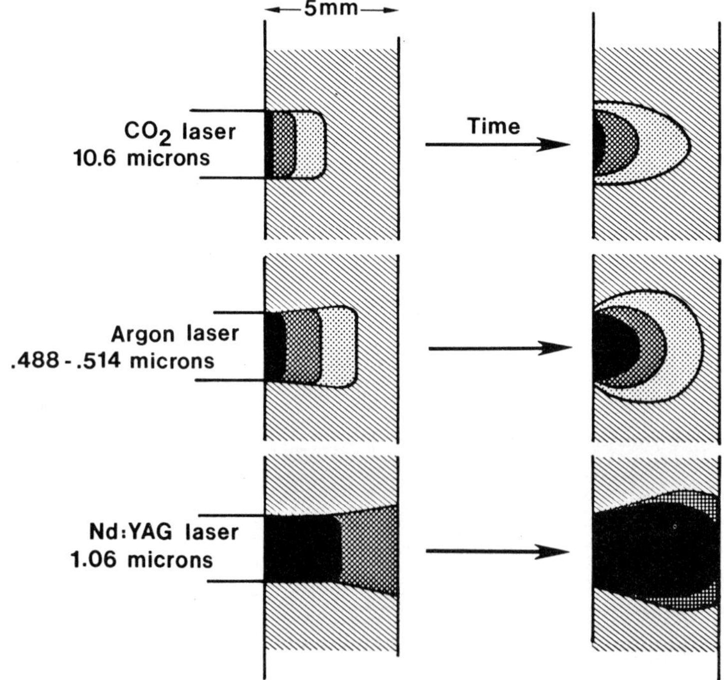

FIGURE 3. Laser radiation incident upon tissue. Penetration depth is a function of laser wavelength. After passage of time, thermal diffusion in the tissue causes additional dispersal of heat.

The second laser illustrated in Figure 3 is the argon laser. This laser emits two strong wavelengths in the blue-green region of the spectrum visible to the human eye. Its color is well absorbed by the hemoglobin molecule, but not by water. Thus, the argon laser is well absorbed by blood, but not by white tissue. Perfused pink tissue is a good absorber of argon laser radiation, although not as good as whole blood. An argon laser beam will penetrate about 1 mm in normal stomach tissue before its intensity has dropped to 5%

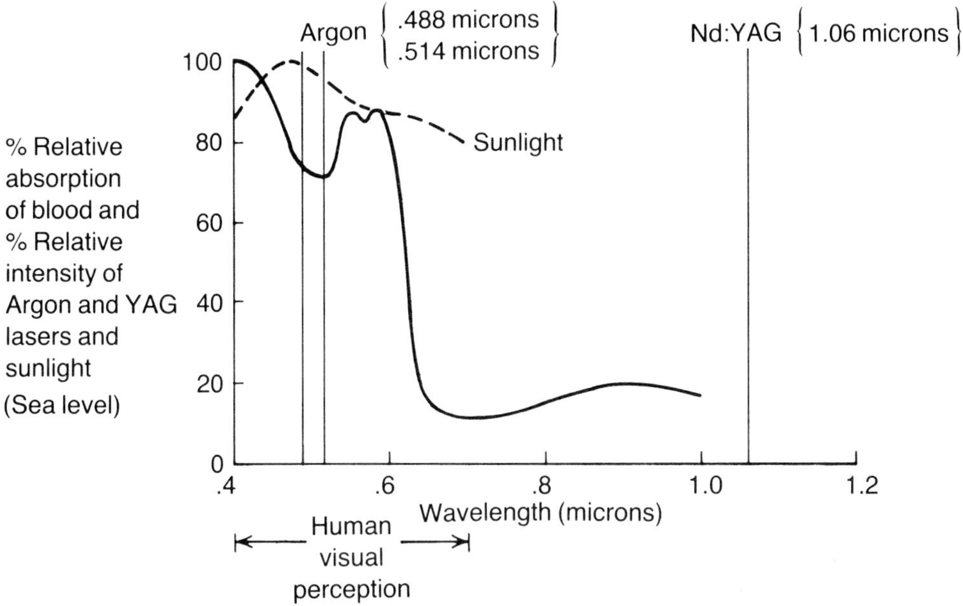

FIGURE 4. Spectral absorption of whole blood with overlay of spectral emission of sunlight and the argon and Nd:YAG lasers.

of its initial value at the surface. Obviously, variations in the number of red blood cells per cubic centimeter will affect the actual absorption in a clinical application.

The third laser depicted in Figure 3 is the Nd:YAG laser which reads as the neodymium doped yttrium aluminum garnet laser. This laser operates in the near infrared region of the electromagnetic spectrum at 1.06μm. At this wavelength, absorption by water is nearly insignificant, but absorption by whole blood is substantial although much less than with the argon laser. This laser is able to penetrate more deeply into whole blood or into blood perfused pink tissue. Whereas the argon laser is able to penetrate to a level of about 1 mm in normal gastric tissue, the YAG laser is able to penetrate to approximately 4 mm. Deeper penetration enables deeper coagulation which can be argued to be necessary for hemostasis of large vessels. Several authors[2-5] have experimented on relative efficacies of the deep penetrating YAG laser vs. the shallow penetrating argon laser.

Figure 3 illustrates another important consideration of photocoagulation which is "instant penetration". This means that light penetrates at the speed of light into the tissue and begins heating the tissue in the depth immediately. A hot iron applied to the surface of the tissue will rely on the slow diffusion of heat to raise the temperature of tissue at a depth of several millimeters. Heat diffusion also accompanies laser coagulation leading to a change of the thermal profile as time progresses. Figure 3 depicts this time evolution (somewhat arbitrarily) as the right-hand column of pictures proceeding from the left-hand column. Comparisons can be made to electrosurgery and electrocautery.[6]

Figure 4 illustrates the relative spectral absorption of blood as a function of wavelength. The argon laser emits its primary energy in a local "valley" in the hemoglobin absorption curve. Thus, a 100-μm thick specimen of whole human blood would absorb about 72% of the incident argon laser light which impinges upon it. If a high-power laser were available at 0.58 μm, it would experience nearly 90% absorption in a similar thickness of whole blood. It is apparent that the hemoglobin absorption is much reduced above 0.7 μm. The dashed curve showing the relative *emission* by our sun is provided to demonstrate the utter overlap of the argon laser emission and normal sunlight. A prime difference in the character of sunlight and laser light is the diffuse emission of sunlight over a wide band of wavelengths in contrast with the laser which concentrates its energy in a very narrow band of the electromagnetic spectrum. Since sunlight emits in a spectral range which overlaps a high absorption range for hemoglobin, it would cause thermal coagulation if it were focused onto a bleeding area. However, if it were focused onto a fiberoptic waveguide, a situation similar to that depicted in Figure 2b would be obtained—namely, poor (inefficient) coupling of the light into the fiber.

C. Power and Energy Control

The laser provides very precise adjustment of power and energy that can be injected into a flexible fiberoptic waveguide. Commercial lasers of high-power output (greater than 1 W) routinely offer power adjustment. With straightforward ancillary apparatus, a pulse timer can be attached to a conventional laser to provide a precisely adjustable timed pulse of energy. Since energy equals power times time, i.e.,

$$E = P \times \text{Time}\ , \qquad (2)$$

it follows that energy is well controlled if power and time are controlled. In order to establish a range of useful benefit/risk ratio, control of energy is essential and the laser does this well. A laser/fiberoptic system can easily provide an aiming beam so that exact targeting of coagulating doses can be accomplished. Indeed, laser "designators" are used as "spotters" for nonlaser missiles in modern weapons. Control of laser energy density is also important in obtaining effective and safe coagulation. This is a much more difficult parameter to control. Figure 5 depicts laser light emanating from the distal end of a flexible endoscope. The divergence of light as it travels away from the fiber tip is one of the primary characteristics of laser coagulation. Various researchers[7] have indicated preferences regarding the divergence angle. The primary consideration is twofold:

1. The angle should be sufficiently acute to assure adequate energy density when the beam intersects the tissue that is to be coagulated when used at a normal and convenient operating distance.
2. The beam angle should be sufficiently obtuse so as not to cause excessive energy density when operated at a normal and convenient operating range. From a practical viewpoint, a range of 4 to 16 degrees is manageable, provided the endoscopist takes the individual case into account when adjusting the "stand-off" distance prior to coagulation. In practice, endoscopists either adjust the stand-off distance by measured displacement of the proximal end of the catheter with respect to the entrace port of the endoscope or use a small divergence angle (4°) and back away from the bleeding site a distance which is "sure" to be enough.

D. Trade-offs of Laser Coagulation

Table 1 presents a series of pro and con arguments for the use of lasers in coagulation. Without discussing Table 1 point by point, the fact remains that lasers are generally considered to be effective for stopping bleeding, but at a very high monetary price. Some proponents have argued the installation of multipurpose laser suites to distribute the cost over a larger number of procedures.

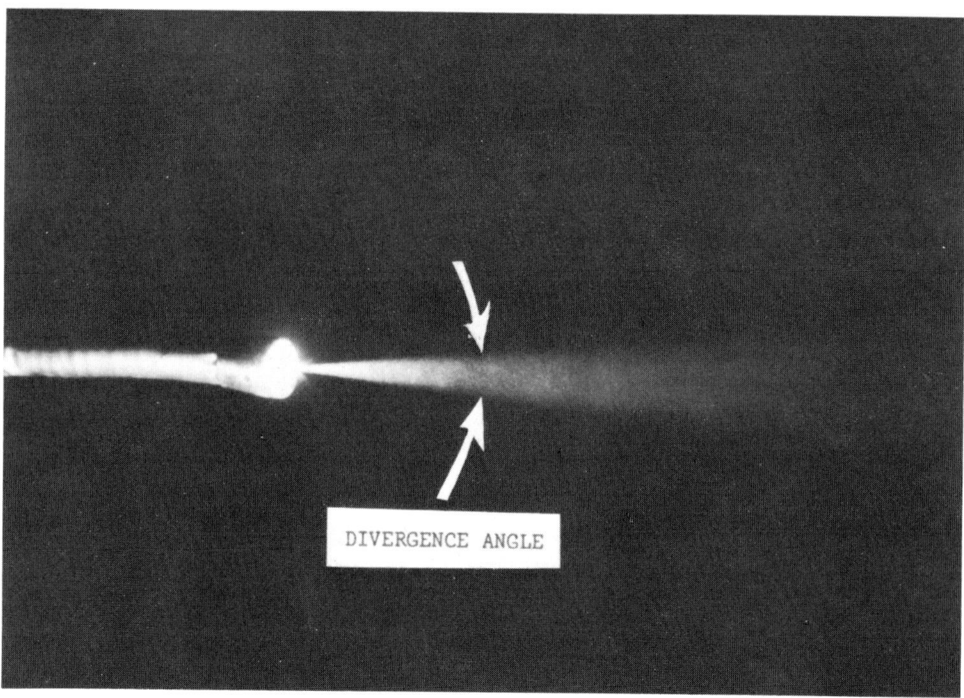

FIGURE 5. Argon laser light issuing from a flexible endoscope. Divergence angle equal to approximately 12°.

Table 1
TRADE-OFFS WITH ENDOSCOPIC LASER COAGULATION

Pro	Con
Noncontacting (no sticking)	High Initial cost
Adjustable penetration	Special installation
Argon—shallow penetration	Argon requires gas assist and fail-safe Recirculation system
YAG—Deep penetration	Optical hazard
YAG—Short high energy pulses	YAG—risk of deep injury
Selective absorption by blood	No coaptation of vessels
Adjustable area of coverage	Nontrivial training required
Easily aimed	High maintenance
Instant penetration to a predetermined depth	Not portable
Excellent power control	Buildup of surface char with argon lasers
	Subject to motional perturbations

III. LASER PHYSICS

A. Historical Roots and Atomic Energy Levels

Laser is an acronym for *L*ight *A*mplification by *S*timulated *E*mission of *R*adiation. In a simplified model, the atom (no longer an indivisible natural entity) consists of electrons circling about a dense nucleus of protons and neutrons. As the electrons gain speed, and hence energy, they increase the size of their orbit. If they gain enough speed, they will leave the nuclear core altogether which then becomes "ionized". One of the fundamental tenants of the quantum theory of nature (and hence atoms) is that electrons will in general not be able to increase their orbital energies in a continuous fashion, but rather in "jumps" or "quanta". These characteristic energy jumps are the very parameter that spectroscopic chemists utilize to label atoms based on the wavelengths which they absorb. According to Planck,[8] the relationship between the wavelength of light and its energy per photon is given as:

$$E_p = hc/\lambda \ , \tag{3}$$

where h is Plack's constant, c is the speed of light, and λ is the wavelength. Thus, light of a particular wavelength may be viewed as a collection of photons of equal energy. By carefully noting (using absorption spectroscopy) which energy of photons are absorbed by a particular atom, the chemist is able to identify the atom under scrutiny because its "signature" is known. Likewise, the photons which an atom is capable of emitting are energetically related to its own particular quantum levels or energies. Spectroscopy which uses the emission signature of an atom is referred to as emission spectroscopy. Sometimes the emission is forced using a spark or flame in an atmosphere of the atom being tested. The emission of light by an atom can occur at any time provided it has a lower energy state which nature allows for it. The fact that the emission can occur at any time means that the scientist must use a statistical estimate of the likelihood of emission, rather than an absolute prediction of the occurrence. This kind of statistical emission is referred to as "spontaneous emission".

"Stimulated emission" implies a form of energy change in an atom which is encouraged by the presence of an external ambiance of electromagnetic energy whose frequency of oscillation is equal to that which the atom would give off if it were to emit. This "encouragement" or "stimulation" of emission is the fundamental property of lasers and the reason for their acronym. The characterization and explanation of stimulated emission was first provided by Einstein.[9]

Since the emission must be between two energy states of a particular atom, the frequency or color of the light which is emitted is well defined depending upon the atom involved. An example is the color of the argon laser as seen in Figure 4. A further advantage of stimulated emission is the ability of a laser oscillator to predispose the atoms to radiate their energy in a particular and well-defined direction. This is seen in Figure 6 where a trapped beam of radiation is shown reflecting back and forth between two mirrors. The trapped beam has very well-defined direction, since it must be perpendicular to the point of contact with the mirrors. The trapped beam can "stimulate" other atoms to radiate in the same direction, which means that new radiation is also aligned with the mirrors. By allowing some of the radiation to "leak out" of one of the mirrors (using semitransparent mirrors), a beam is extracted which exactly replicates the beam as it reflects from the mirror. Since a portion of the beam reflects back into the space between the mirrors (the optical cavity), the process may continue without being selfextinguished.

B. Typical Laser Configurations

Several methods for raising the energy of atoms in preparation for a "stimulating experience" have been devised. The two most common are illustrated in Figure 6a and 6b. In Figure 6a, atoms are forced to carry an electric current by undergoing ionization and becoming electrical charge carriers. As they accelerate under the influence of an applied electric field, their energy increases. When they collide with other atoms, they can cause orbital electrons to jump up in energy. If the energy jump is to the proper level, laser action can then proceed. This type of energy excitation is easily

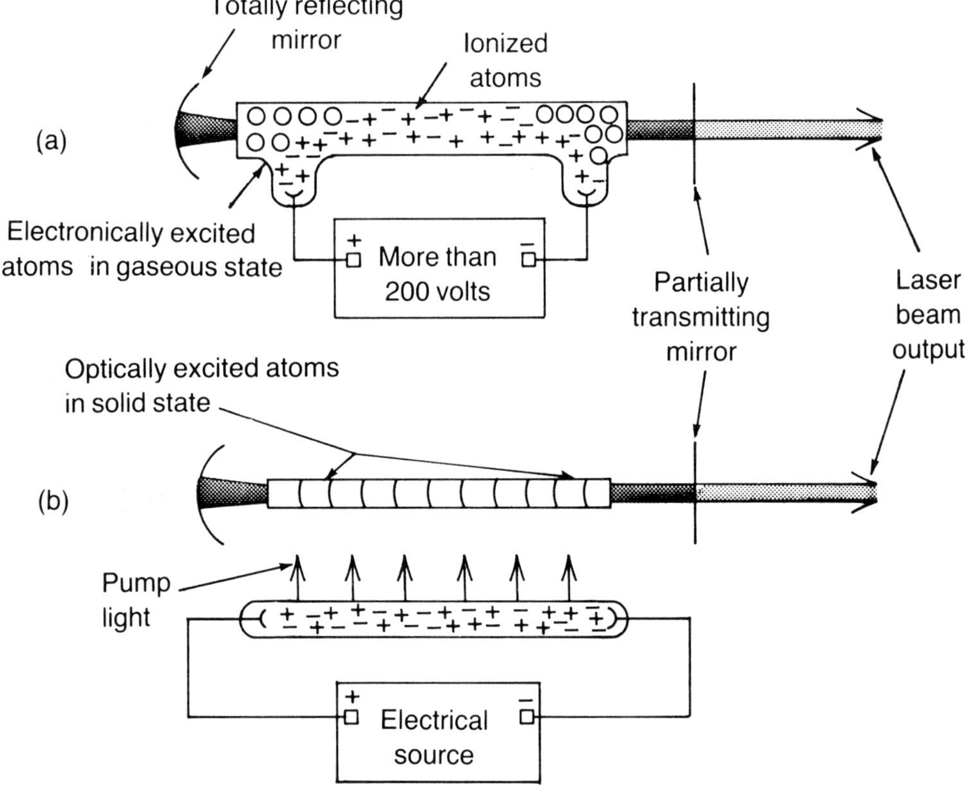

FIGURE 6. Two common laser systems. (a) Electrical discharge pumped gas laser representative of the argon and CO_2 lasers; (b) optically pumped solid-state laser representative of the Nd: YAG and ruby lasers.

accomplished in a gaseous laser such as the argon laser. In Figure 6b, the lasing material is excited by an external source of light of very high (similar to the most powerful used in photography). This type of excitation is useful for solid laser materials such as the Nd: YAG laser. Normal YAG material is a gemstone quality crystal which, without the presence of Nd impurity, is water-white and widely used as a fake diamond material.

C. Important Physical Parameters for the Clinic

In addition to the specification of wavelength, the output power and power consumption of a laser are relevant considerations for the clinician. For argon laser coagulation, a range of 1 to 20 W is most frequently encountered with 1 to 3 W being used for ophthalmology and 5 to 10 W for GI bleeding. Due to its deep penetration, the YAG laser is not used in ophthalmology, but for GI bleeding its useful power range is 50 to 100 W. In order to supply 10 W of argon laser power, an electrical power input to the machine of approximately 25 kW is typical. By contrast, to supply 100 W of YAG laser radiation, the electrical power input to the machine is typically 14 kW. Thus, we might say that the YAG laser is more energy efficient. The cost of kilowatt hours of electrical energy is insignificant in these applications. What is more significant is the cost of the electrical "hook-up" and the inconvenience of not being able to portably transport the laser from place to place. The argon laser may require up to 440 V if very high power is desired (greater than 10 W). A 440-V electrical service is not commonplace, although some large X-ray machines do require it. Most YAG lasers used for coagulation operate with single or three-phase current at 220 to 240 V. This electrical service is more readily available in hospitals and clinics. For purposes of comparison, a modern electrosurgery generator (Bovie®) can deliver 300 W of radio frequency power with 1100 W of input power at 120 V (normal room outlet).

IV. TISSUE INTERACTION AND SAFETY

A. Scattering vs. Absorption

Propagation of light through fog is a commonplace example of the physical phenomenon known as scattering. Light bounces from water droplet to water droplet in an irregular manner. Some of the light reflects back from whence it came. In general, if a well-directed beam of light impinges upon a fog bank, it rapidly becomes a plume. Thus, the illustration of light propagating in tissue as shown in Figure 3 is naive. The actual shape of radiation in the tissue tends to fan out sideways due to scattering. If the beam intersecting the tissue is large at the surface, the effects of scattering are relatively minor since they cause a further broadening which is only a few percent more than the initial beam diameter. However, if the beam is small to start with, the effects of scattering can cause a very large percentage change in beam diameter as it propagates within the tissue. The analogy between the water droplets of fog and the fibrous structure of tissue is close except that the droplets are spheroidal in shape and tissue fibers are linear filaments. In general, scattering is an advantage for coagulation, since it diffuses light and reduces the probability for deep damage or damage to organs adjacent to the serosa if endoscopic coagulation is performed.

A fundamental difference between absorption and scattering is that scattering deflects energy into another direction in a random manner whereas absorption changes energy into another form such as transformation of light into heat.

B. Thermal and Nonthermal Effects

The dominant mechanism for therapy and destruction as laser light interacts with tissue is *heat.* Laser energy is transformed via absorption into thermal energy manifested as vibrational agitation of the constituent molecules. This thermal agitation is measurable as temperature. The more vigorous it becomes, the hotter is the substance. If it becomes sufficiently hot, denaturation of protein ensues or in other words, thermal coagulation. This is normally associated with tissue death. This tissue death can be therapeutic if it results in cessation of bleeding and regeneration of viable tissue. Thermal coagulation begins in a range from 50°C to 80°C. If thermal energy is further deposited beyond that which is necessary to cause therapeutic coagulation, the temperature will continue to rise to 100°C and remain there until the water *in situ* is evaporated. After the entrained water is evaporated, the temperature will continue to rise, eventually forming a carbon residue. Since the carbon is a good absorber of laser radiation, it can rise to thousands of degrees centigrade causing an incandescent glow. Evaporation of water can lead to the development of steam vesicles which explode within the depth of the tissue. This has been referred to as the "popcorn effect" which is sometimes observed with the YAG laser. This type of microexplosion is illustrative of a mechanical effect brought on by a thermal interaction. Some of the "bad press" associated with the early experiments using lasers for destruction of cancers involved the dissemination of metastases following an explosive impact of a short-pulsed laser beam upon tissue. When a large amount of energy is released within tissue in a time which is so short as to not allow perfusion of steam through the microstructure, mechanical rupture and explosion can occur.

When laser light is able to directly stimulate a chemical reaction in tissue such as in photosynthesis, we refer to the process as nonthermal, since conversion to thermal

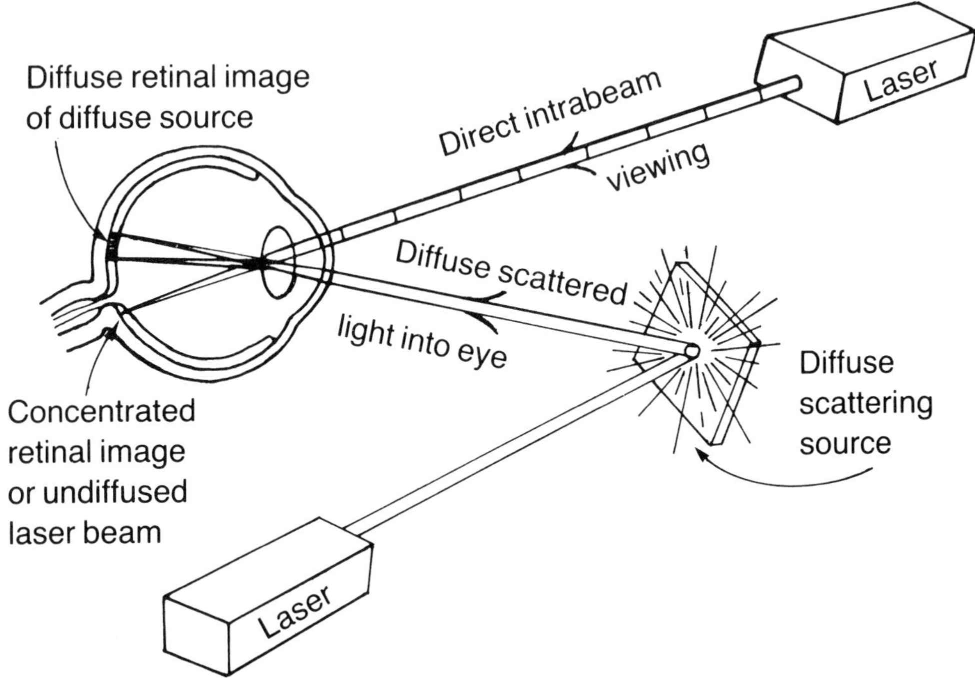

FIGURE 7. Two principal forms of laser hazard to the human eye. Direct laser beam interception by the cornea and secondary scattering by intermediate objects.

energy is not necessary to initiate the event. Bronchoscopic use of lasers for stimulation of tumor specific fluorescence is an example of a nonthermal application of lasers.[10]

C. Ophthalmic Hazards

Figure 7 depicts the two important cases of laser light entering the human eye. When a laser beam travels directly from its source into the eye, it is focused to a very tiny spot on the retinal surface. This concentration of energy can cause thermal and/or mechanical damage. It is used to advantage by the ophthalmologist to perform microcoagulation of retinal vessels. Direct intrabeam viewing of greater than 10 mW of laser radiation can be damaging to the retina. Laser coagulation of 100 W implies 10,000 times the power of this threshold level. Once the laser radiation is inserted into an optical fiber, its hazard level drops significantly. For this reason, clinical systems should not be designed with open beams issuing directly from the laser generator source. They should be coupled into the fiber cables before being available to the clinical staff in order to avoid inadvertent retinal damage.

The other example of laser exposure of the human eye is depicted in the lower portion of Figure 7. Laser light is incident upon an object such as a piece of paper and is simultaneously reflected and scattered into the space in front of the object. Scattering of light from objects is what makes normal vision possible. When the incident light is intense, the scattered light can be uncomfortably bright. The light which reaches the cornea of the eye is apertured by the pupil and then partially focused of the retina. If the eye attempts to focus on the scattering object, it will image the object on the retina of the eye. This means that the size of the focal spot of laser light will be proportionate to the size of the spot which is illuminated on the object. A 2-mm spot on the object will be imaged in proportion to the amount of visual field which is encompassed by the eye. As the observer moves closer to the object, the 2–mm spot appears to grow in size as a fraction of the visual field subtended. To a good approximation, the power density within the image on the retina does not change as the observer draws closer to the scattering object, but the total power intercepted by the pupil increases markedly. This is an example of "diffuse reflection". Laser light which undergoes diffuse reflection can still be hazardous, but the hazard is drastically reduced when compared to the intrabeam viewing case discussed above for the following reasons:

1. The light is no longer well collimated and cannot be focused to as small a spot on the retina.
2. The light is being scattered throughout a hemisphere of space, and the amount that reaches the eye is a very small fraction of the total.
3. Since the light is scattered throughout the half-space, it provides its own secondary prewarning system. In other words, a surprise overexposure is unlikely because the ambiance of bright light within the room raises caution.

During the process of endoscopic laser photocoagulation, the scattered light which returns to the viewing optics of the endoscope can cause discomfort to the endoscopist because of its brightness. In some cases,[11] the light which leaves from the eyepiece of the endoscope can be in excess of safe levels if a special intervening filter is not in place.

D. Clinical Parameters

1. Spot Size

The diameter of the coagulating beam of radiation as it intercepts the tissue is referred to as the spot size. Typical useful values range from 1.5 mm to 4 mm for endoscopic coagulation. If the spot size is too small, the beam is likely to cavitate the tissue because of its high-power density. This follows since the power per unit volume is sufficient to rapidly evaporate tissue before heat is conducted away. If the spot size is too large, the process of coagulation is slow to occur because of inadequate power density. The distance of separation between the tip of the laser fiber and the tissue should be adjusted for the desired spot size. If one is using a 14° divergence angle and desires a 2.5-mm spot on the tissue, the distance should be approximately

$$(57/14) \times 2.5 \text{ mm} = 10.1 \text{ mm} \doteq 1 \text{ cm}. \quad (4)$$

Maintaining a distance of 1- to 2 cm is possible, but not always easy in endoscopy. Some practitioners have stated a preference for a laser which operates at high power so that a quick dose of laser energy may be deposited before motion disrupts target alignment and distance. YAG laser coagulationists have been using short bursts of 0.5 to 1.0 sec with power outputs of approximatey 75 W. Argon laser coagulation is performed at power levels of 5 to 10 W and time durations of 1 to 10 sec.

2. Energy Density and Power Density

These parameters are frequently a source of much discussion and confusion. Part of the confusion is due to the fact that a well defined, all encompassing rule of operation is not practical. Energy density is specified as joules per square centimeter. Power density is specified as watts per square centimeter. Since power times time equals energy, it follows that a certain power density applied for a certain time duration will result in a certain energy density. If one attempts to develop strict guidelines for the endoscopist which state that "thus and so" joules per square centimeter should be deposited without regard to the duration of application, then one is neglecting the effects of vascular cooling and thermal conduction (which evacuate the local heat) during the coagulation

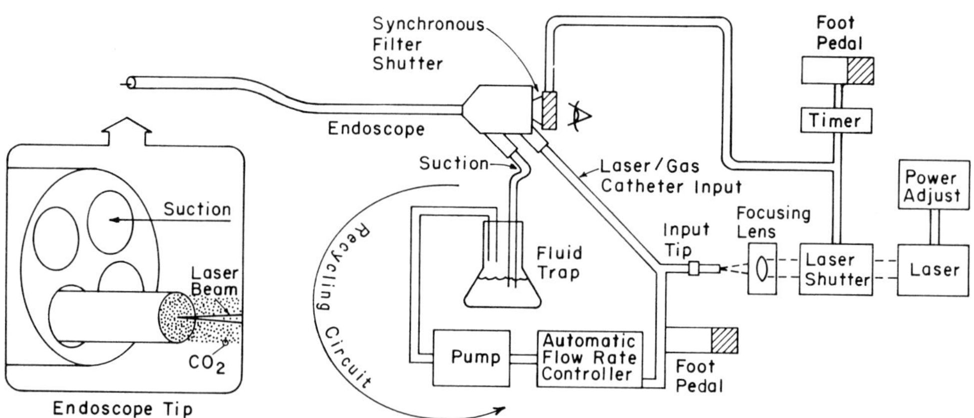

FIGURE 8. A comprehensive endoscopic laser photocoagulation system with fail-safe eye shutter, gas-assist recycling, and ancillary automatic control modules.

process. It is more meaningful to state the power density, the time of application, the spot size, and the wavelength, when attempting to communicate the true coagulation potential and risk of deep injury.

V. CLINICAL INSTRUMENTATION

A. Optical Source

For endoscopic coagulation, the laser is flexibly connected via a thin cable (= 2.5 mm) to the endoscope with intervening controls for power, and time duration (see Figure 8). Aiming light is inserted to provide the endoscopist with a preview of the coagulation zone. With the argon laser, the preview beam is most conveniently supplied by inserting a filter into the main laser beam[12] which allows a harmless but visible amount of light through the system, thereby delineating the coagulation zone. The spot size of the aiming beam is the same as the coagulation beam when the system is configured in this way. The Nd: YAG laser is not visible to the human eye and another aiming beam must be inserted for targeting. The lower power (approximately 5 mW) helium-neon laser is most commonly used to provide this aiming function for the YAG coagulation systems. The helium-neon laser operates at 0.6328 μm which is in the visible red region of the spectrum. This color is disconcerting to some practitioners since it does not provide good contrast with a red background. When an auxiliary laser is used for aiming, its spot size is not necessarily the same as the coagulating laser.

B. Optical Safety

When an argon laser is used for coagulation, a synchronous filter is convenient in order to protect the endoscopist's eyes during coagulation. Since it is synchronous, it does not distort color perception before and after coagulation. This synchronous filter should be "fail-safe", meaning that the laser cannot be fired at a high power unless the filter is directly in front of he endoscopist's eye. An electromechanical interlock can provide this feature. The synchronous orange filter reduces the amount of argon laser light which reaches the endoscopist during coagulation and, although the color balance is distorted, the process of coagulation can still be observed. In YAG laser coagulation, a permanent filter may be inserted on the endoscope, since it is possible to make a filter which will block the 1.06 μm infrared radiation without significantly affecting the intensity or color balance in the visible region of the spectrum.

C. Washing and Gas Assist

Visualization of the precise bleeding point is an important factor in safe and effective control of bleeding. Deposited energy which misses the target not only fails to stop the bleeding but increases unnecessary tissue necrosis. Sprays of water or gas are useful to delineate the precise bleeding vessel. Coaxial gas jet assist[13,14] has been found to be very important for successful argon laser coagulation of actively bleeding vessels. Since the argon laser light is heavily absorbed in the surface layer of red blood, it is unable to accomplish coagulation when a pool of blood is overlying the vascular source. By blowing the overlying blood away, the laser light can penetrate to the vessel and cause it to shrink and coagulate. In order to provide adequate gas flushing of serious bleeders, flow rates of approximately 75 cc/sec are used. This amount of gas flow can rapidly overdistend a patient if an evacuation channel is accidentally obstructed. For this reason, a fail-safe gas recycling system has been developed[15] which automatically discontinues gas jet assistance if the return channel is obstructed. A further feature of this system is its ability to automatically correct the gas flow rate after laser catheters of varying pneumatic resistance are interchanged.

REFERENCES

1. **Hirschowitz, B. I., Curtiss, L. E., Peters, C. W., and Pollard, H. M.,** *Gastroenterology,* 35, 50, 1958.
2. **Silverstein, F. E., Protell, R. L., Gilbert, D. A., Gulacsik, C., Auth, D. C., Dennis, M. B., and Rubin, C. E.,** Argon vs. neodymium YAG laser photocoagulation of experimental canine gastric ulcers, *Gastroenterology*, 77, 491, 1979.
3. **Kiefhaber, P., Nath, G., and Moritz, K.,** Endoscopic control of massive gastrointestinal hemorrhage by irradiation with a high power neodymium-YAG laser, *Prog. Surg.*, 15, 140, 1977.
4. **Dwyer, R. M. and Bass, M.,** Laser phototherapy in man using argon and Nd:YAG lasers (abstract), *Gastrointest. Endoscop.,* 24, 195, 1978.
5. **Dixon, J. A., Berenson, M. M., and McCloskey, D. W.,** Neodymium-YAG laser treatment of experimental canine gastric bleeding, acute and chronic studies of photocoagulation, penetration and perforation, *Gastro enterology,* 77, 647, 1979.
6. **Gilbert, D. A., Silverstein, F. E., Auth, D. C., and Rubin, C. E.,** Nonsurgical management of acute nonvariceal upper gastrointestinal bleeding, in *Progress in Hemostasis and Thrombosis*, Vol. 4, Spaet, T. H., Ed., Grune & Stratton, New York, 1978, 349.
7. **Silverstein, F. E., Auth, D. C., Rubin, C. E., and Protell, R. L.,** High power argon laser treatment via standard endoscopes: I. A. preliminary study of efficacy in control of experimental erosive bleeding, *Gastroenterology*, 71, 558, 1976.
8. **Halliday, D. and Resnick, R.,** *Physics,* John Wiley & Sons, New York, 1960, 1178.
9. **Einstein, A.,** Zur quantentheorie der strahlung, *Phys. Z.,* 18, 121, 1917.
10. **Doiron, D. R., Profio, E., Vincent, R. G., and Dougherty, T. J.,** *Chest,* 76, 27, 1979.
11. **Gulacsik, C., Auth, D. C., and Silverstein, F. E.,** Ophthalmic hazards associated with laser endoscopy, *Appl. Opt.*, 18, 1816, 1979.
12. **Auth, D. C., Lam, V. T. Y., Mohr, R. W., Silverstein, F. E., and Rubin, C. E.,** A high-power gastric photocoagulator for fiberoptic endoscopy, *IEEE Trans. Biomed. Eng.,* 32, 129, 1976.
13. **Silverstein, F. E., Protell, R. L., Gulacsik, C. Auth, D. C., Deltenre, M., Dennis, Piercey, J., and Rubin, C.,** Endoscopic laser treatment: III. Development and testing of a gas-jet-assisted argon laser waveguide in control of bleeding experimental ulcers, *Gastroenterology*, 74, 232, 1978.
14. **Kimura, W. D., Gulacsik, C., Auth, D. C., Silverstein, F. E., and Protell, R. L.,** Use of gas jet appositional pressurization in endoscopic laser photocoagulation, *IEEE Trans. Biomed. Eng.*, 25, 218, 1978.
15. **Opie, E. A.,** A Fail-Safe Servo-Controlled Recycling System for Laser Endoscopy, Digest: Conference on Laser and Electrooptical Systems, San Diego, 1980, 82.

Chapter 6

LASER PHOTOCOAGULATION: EXPERIMENTAL AND CLINICAL STUDIES

Fred E. Silverstein, David A. Gilbert, Andrew D. Feld, and Robert L. Protell

TABLE OF CONTENTS

I. INTRODUCTION

Upper gastrointestinal bleeding is a commonly encountered problem in clinical medicine and gastroenterology. There are approximately 100 admissions for gastrointestinal bleeding per 100,000 population per year.[1] The care of patients with upper gastrointestinal bleeding has improved in the past ten years with the use of central intravascular pressure monitoring and intensive care units. However, despite advances in the care of critically bleeding patients, the mortality from upper gastrointestinal bleeding has remained constant at 10% for several decades.[2] This lack of improved survival has been attributed to the increasing age of bleeding patients and the associated, often life-threatening, underlying illnesses. In the past ten years, there have been dramatic advances in the technology of fiberoptic endoscopy. Many investigators have sought to find a method to control upper gastrointestinal bleeding using endoscopic access to the gastrointestinal tract.[3] Techniques investigated include laser photocoagulation, direct thermal coagulation,[4,5] electrocoagulation,[6,7,8] and the application of topical hemostatic agents such as cyanoacrylate glues[9,10] and clotting factors.[11,12] In his Chapter, Dr. Auth has presented the physics of lasers and engineering aspects of tissue interaction. In this Chapter, we will discuss the role of laser photocoagulation in upper gastrointestinal bleeding. We will discuss some of the technical and biologic aspects of the lasers being studied, the animal work reported, and the American clinical experience. Cotton and Vallon will present the status of the nonAmerican clinical trials in the next Chapter. We will comment on the biologic effects of lasers, the medical aspects of laser delivery systems, the necessity for gas-jet assistance, removal of insufflated gas, laser safety, and some of the problems with laser photocoagulation that are yet to be solved.

II. LASER SYSTEMS

The word *laser* is an acronym for *L*ight *A*mplication by *S*timulated *E*mission of *R*adiation. The intense monochromatic light energy of a laser can be directed at a tissue which absorbs the energy, generating heat which can coagulate proteins in the blood and tissue. For the treatment of upper gastrointestinal bleeding, the laser's energy must be absorbed by red blood and tissue. If the target is a bleeding blood vessel, the laser's energy may be able to coagulate the blood and surrounding tissue proteins and stop the hemorrhage. To be effective and safe, the laser's energy must stop the bleeding without injuring the underlying tissue too severely. Excessive injury could result in a perforation or injury to adjacent organs. The laser beam must also be passable via a flexible waveguide inserted into the biopsy channel of a modern fiberendoscope.

A. Carbon Dioxide Laser

The carbon dioxide laser was the first laser to be used for the endoscopic control of bleeding. This laser has a wave length of 10.2 μm and is invisible. Goodale reported that this laser when directed into a dog stomach via a rigid, open gastroscope could slow experimental gastric bleeding.[13] However, the carbon dioxide laser beam cannot be passed down an available flexible waveguide and, therefore, is not a practical method for use with fiberoptic endoscopes at the present time. A flexible delivery waveguide may soon be available, but no studies with this system have yet been reported. A second problem with the CO_2 laser is that its energy is absorbed so superficially that it may not be able to stop significant bleeding.

There are two lasers which are currently being studied for endoscopic use—the argon laser and the neodymium-YAG (Nd:YAG) laser.

B. Argon Laser

The argon laser emits a visible blue-green light which is highly absorbed by red surfaces including red blood. The light is absorbed by a thin layer of blood 100 μm thick. The light is coherent (wavelength 0.44 to 0.52 μm) and can be focused onto the tip of flexible quartz fibers varying from 100 to 600 μm in diameter. These quartz fibers can be encased in a Teflon® or polyethylene catheter which protects the fiber. There is space for a coaxial jet of CO_2 gas or water to pass around the quartz fiber to be directed at the bleeding lesion. These catheters can be passed down the biopsy channel of a standard fiberendoscope. The divergence angle at the tip of the catheter can be varied from 7 to 20 degrees. The most commonly reported full angles of divergence range from 8 to 12 degrees. Available lasers put out up to 23 W of power. The argon laser is generally used with powers exiting from the tip of the catheter of 5 to 10 W. The coaxial jet of CO_2 has been found to enhance the laser's efficacy by blowing blood off of the surface of the target lesion so that the laser's energy can be deposited on the bleeding vessels.[14,15]

C. Neodymium-YAG Laser

The Nd:YAG laser has a longer wavelength (1.06 μm) in the near infrared range. This laser's energy is well absorbed by red surfaces, but less so than is the argon laser's energy. The Nd: YAG laser is not well absorbed until it passes through a layer of blood 300 μm thick. The neodymium-YAG laser penetrates three to five times more deeply into tissue than does the argon laser; therefore, higher powers are required to adequately heat and coagulate tissue proteins. Available lasers have output powers of up to 120 W.

There are two types of delivery systems for the Nd:YAG laser. The first system is a triconical quartz waveguide developed by Nath and Kiefhaber.[16] The laser exits from this fiber with a divergence angle of 4 degrees. The fiber must be enclosed in one channel of a two-channel upper endoscope which must be specially modified to accommodate the fiber and protective quartz lens at the endoscope tip. Recently, several investigators have evaluated delivery of the neodymium-YAG laser via quartz fiber waveguides similar to those used for the argon laser. The neodymium-YAG laser can be focused onto the tip of a 400 to 600 μm quartz fiber exiting the fiber with divergence angles of from 8 to 28 degrees.[17] This system does not focus the beam as narrowly as does the triconical fiber. A distinct advantage of the quartz waveguide is that the fiber and its protective catheter can be passed down the biopsy channel of a standard fiberoptic instrument without special modification. A coaxial gas jet can be passed around the fiber and through the catheter. This contrasts with the triconical fiber for which a noncoaxial jet must be built into the modified endoscope.

Overall, the single fiber delivery system would seem to be preferable to the triconical fiber. A standard two-channel or large one-channel endoscope can be used. If a gas jet is not needed, the waveguide can be passed down the biopsy channel of a standard endoscope. This allows a variety of endoscopes to be used for laser phototherapy depending on the clinical circumstances. The fiber and waveguide are cheaper and the waveguide is reportedly less fragile. With this system, the gas jet is truly coaxial. Finally, the fiber waveguide can be advanced from the tip of the instrument towards the target without moving the endoscope.

III. ENDOSCOPES

The type of fiberendoscope required for laser photocoagulation varies with the type of waveguide. To use the quartz fiber encapsulated waveguide, any standard fiberendoscope is adequate. This includes the newer 28-30 French circumference instruments which are being used with increasing frequency in clinical gastrointestinal endoscopy. The quartz fiber is so small that even with the polyethylene or Teflon® covering tube, it still can be passed down the biopsy channel of these smaller instruments. These types of quartz catheters can be used with either argon or neodymium-YAG lasers. If one uses the triconical fiber system or a fixed fiber which requires a distal lens to focus the beam at the tip, a two-channel endoscope must be obtained. One channel would be occupied by the laser delivery system.

When gas recycling is used, one needs a vent to remove insufflated gas. This can be a second channel, a single large channel with the space around the laser gas waveguide used to remove gas, or an N/G tube passed next to the endoscope. Most of the reported experience has been with standard-sized (36 to 39 French) endoscopes which are end-viewing. For the patient with a gastric ulcer which is high on the lesser curvature, a side-viewing endoscope might be preferable. A prototype side-viewing endoscope with two channels is available. The retroflexion (>180°) of the newest models of endoscopes makes visualization of the bleeding lesion somewhat less difficult, although this is still a significant problem in a patient with active bleeding and a stomach full of blood.

IV. COAXIAL GAS JET

If a coaxial jet of gas is used with either the neodymium-YAG or argon laser, the endoscopist must have a system to remove this gas to prevent overdistention of the stomach. Johnston, et al.[18] demonstrated that overdistention and thinning of the stomach wall may be associated with deeper wall injury during argon laser photocoagulation. There are several systems to remove gas from the stomach during gas-assisted photocoagulation. We have developed a fail–safe recycling system which removes the gas, filters it, and recompresses it for reuse as the coaxial gas jet, thereby theoretically preventing overdistention because the same volume of gas is recycled.[19,20] Other alternatives are to vent the channel to room pressure or to attach a suction pump to the venting channel running at approximately the same flow as is the insufflation system. In several experimental studies, gas flow rates have been 75 cc/sec.[21] Johnston has studied the effect of the gas jet and feels that the direct back-pressure on the target measured in centimeters of water is a better parameter to follow than is gas flow.[18]

V. LASER SAFETY

Safety considerations are very important with laser photocoagulation. In addition to potential adverse effects of the laser on the intestinal wall, there are other dangers to the patient and operators using laser photocoagulation. Both the argon and the neodymium-YAG laser can injure the eye. Therefore, it is essential that the patient and all other people present in the room wear appropriate protective filter goggles. These should be clearly marked as to which type of laser energy is filtered. We have demonstrated in a series of studies that both argon laser and Nd:YAG laser energy can be highly transmitted up the visual bundle of a standard fiberoptic endoscope during laser photocoagulation.[22] The laser beam can exit from the waveguide in the stomach, reflect off of the mucosal surface, and come back up the fiberendoscope visual bundle. There is a clear potential hazard for the operator during photocoagulation unless some type of filter is placed between this visual bundle and the endoscopist's eye. This type of filter shutter is available and should be included in any photocoagulation system with either the argon or Nd:YAG laser. The argon filter attenuates the endoscopist's vision, and therefore, should move into position just before the laser fires at full power. It should move out of position after the laser firing is completed. The Nd:YAG filter is clear to the eye, does not attenuate the endoscopist's view, and therefore, can be installed on the endoscopist's eyepiece at the beginning of the endoscopy. It remains in place throughout the procedure.

VI. EXPERIMENTAL ANIMAL STUDIES

A. Argon Laser Photocoagulation in Animals

The first argon laser endoscopic photocoagulation was reported by Nath, et al. in 1973.[23] Frühmorgen, et al. reported their endoscopic argon laser system shortly thereafter, including their studies of argon laser photocoagulation in the esophagus, stomach, duodenum, and colon of experimental animals.[24] Waitman, et. al[25] and Dwyer, et al.[26] then reported the use of argon photocoagulation to stop bleeding from experimental lesions using low power (less than 1 W). At the University of Washington, we reported the experimental use of argon photocoagulation in an animal model of erosive gastric bleeding.[27] At this point, our group in Seattle developed a model of an acute standard-sized mucosal defect using a modification of the multipurpose intestinal biopsy tube.[28] These standard ulcers are approximately 1.0 cm in diameter and 0.15 cm deep. The bleeding which results is moderately brisk and long-lasting when dogs are heparinized. The ulcers extend into the vascular submucosa without injuring the muscularis externa. This model is not an accurate physiologic model of a bleeding chronic gastric ulcer in man. However, there is no such model available at this time. The ulcer maker does provide rapid, standard-sized acute ulcers which can be readily reproduced so that different investigators can compare their results and different techniques can be compared to each other. After acute studies of hemostatic efficacy, the dogs recover and are sacrificed at approximately seven days. The ulcers are then removed and processed for histologic examination. At seven days, the maximal depth of tissue injured can be clearly seen.

A study on argon photocoagulation in this standard acute ulcer model in heparinized dogs found that higher powers (5 to 7 W) were required to stop bleeding and that low power (1 W) was not hemostatically effective.[29] However, the argon laser is so well absorbed by blood that its hemostatic efficacy is impaired in rapidly bleeding lesions. The flowing blood absorbs the laser's energy and prevents the laser beam from coagulating the bleeding vessels in the base of the ulcer. To overcome this problem, our group and that of Frühmorgen simultaneously developed and reported the gas jet system.[14,15] The jet of gas exits from the tip of the laser waveguide coaxially to the beam and clears blood off of the surface of the bleeding lesion, transiently back-pressurizing the bleeding vessels. The vessels are then exposed directly to the argon laser beam and photocoagulation is more rapid and more effective. We compared argon laser photocoagulation with coaxial CO_2 to the argon laser without coaxial CO_2 in the standard bleeding ulcer model in heparinized dogs.[21] Our results were as follows:

	7 W with CO_2	**7 W without CO_2**
Stopped bleeding/total ulcers	16/16	12/14
Number of 5-sec exposures (range)	3 (1—6)	11 (2—33)

Therefore, with coaxial CO_2, we were able to stop all bleeding ulcers with fewer 5-sec laser applications.

The many factors which may influence the hemostatic efficacy and resulting depth of tissue injury during argon laser photocoagulation have been studied. The photocoagulation variables include: laser power (watts), laser energy (joules), duration of application (seconds), power density (watts/cm^2), energy density (J/cm^2), spot size, angle of divergence of the laser, angle of divergence of the coaxial gas, gas flow rate, back-pressurization by the gas, and catheter-to-target distance. Obviously, many of these factors are interrelated. Several groups have examined these variables to determine a method to maximize hemostatic efficacy with minimal injury to the tissue. This work is summarized below.

1. Laser Power and Spot Size

Johnston et al. reported a study of argon laser photocoagulation with coaxial gas in acute standard ulcers in dogs using three different distances from the tip of the laser catheter to the target (0.5 cm, 1.0 cm, and 2.0 cm) with three different laser powers (6 W, 9 W, and 12 W).[30] All nine combinations resulted in hemostatic efficacy in more than 90% of treated ulcers. When examined at seven days, the incidence of full-thickness injury was reported as follows:

	Distance		
Power	**2.0 cm**	**1.0 cm**	**0.5 cm**
6 W	8%	8%	14%
9 W	4%	8%	32%
12 W	19%	15%	50%

(% = incidence of full-thickness injury to the gastric wall)

During some ulcer treatments, an erosive effect of the argon laser was noted, which resulted in increased arterial bleeding or rebleeding in 5% of the ulcers treated at 6 W, 9% of ulcers treated at 9W, and 23% of ulcers treated at 12 W. This erosive effect was only noted when the catheter was held very close (0.5 cm) to the tissue. They concluded that in this standard experimental model the argon laser was effective, but caused deeper tissue injury at 12 W than at 9 W or at 6 W, and that there was a risk of tissue erosion resulting in arterial bleeding when the laser catheter was held very close to the target.

2. Gas Pressure, Laser Power, and Treatment Distance

Several groups have now found that a jet of carbon dioxide gas exiting coaxially to the laser beam increases the hemostatic efficacy of the argon laser and reduces the depth of injury.[14,15] Johnston et al. performed a study to determine the relationship of gas back-pressurization and laser power.[18] In standard acute bleeding ulcers using a spot size of 3 mm, they found that lower power argon (6 W) required a higher gas back-pressure ($\geq$ 8 cm of water) than higher laser power (10 W) which required only 4 cm of water back-pressure. Using a gas flow of 7.3 *l*/min, they also found that a pressure of $>$ 8 cm of water could be obtained with a treatment distance of $<$ 1.75 cm. A gas pressure of 4 cm of water at the same flow rate was produced at a treatment distance of $\leq$ 2.5 cm. Therefore, with the same flow rate of gas, the catheter had to be held closer to the target to generate the higher gas back-pressure necessary for lower power photocoagulation. Treatment distances of 1.5 to 2.5 cm yielded adequate gas back-pressure.

The degree of gastric distention was found to correlate with resulting depth of injury at endoscopic photocoagulation. With normal distention of the canine stomach, only 1 of 22 treated ulcers had full-thickness injury to the muscularis externa when examined at seven days. However, when ulcers were treated during gastric overdistention, 16 of

22 ulcers had full-thickness injury. Thus, increased depth of injury with gastric overdistention and its consequent wall thinning was observed.

3. Total Energy and Depth of Injury

Bown et al. have suggested that the depth of tissue injury resulting from photocoagulation on normal dog mucosa correlates well with the total energy delivered.[31] This group found that a full-thickness injury was rare if the total injury delivered to normal mucosa was less than 50 J. The energy density (J/mm^2) did not correlate as well with depth of injury as did the total energy. This group performed a study of hemostatic efficacy of the argon laser in experimental bleeding lesions in dogs using three laser power ranges: 2 to 5 W, 7 to 9 W, and 12 W. Standard acute ulcers and nonstandard ulcers were used. They found:

Power	Stopped bleeding/total ulcers
2—5 W	2/6 (33%)
7—9 W	22/23 (96%)
12 W	2/5 (40%)

They concluded that the laser's hemostatic efficacy depended on the power delivered and that in these animal models, 9 W seemed to be most effective. The failures at 12 W were reported with the nonstandard lift-and-cut acute ulcerations.

4. Argon Laser Photocoagulation in the Esophagus and Duodenum

The effects of argon laser photocoagulation have been studied extensively in the stomach. Yet bleeding ulcers in patients occur with the greatest frequency in the duodenum. Machicado et al. compared the effect of argon laser photocoagulation and bipolar electrocoagulation in esophageal and duodenal mucosa.[32] They evaluated the hemostatic efficacy and resulting depth of injury using standard acute ulcers in the duodenum treated at laparotomy, as well as in the esophagus treated at thoracotomy. The ulcers were resected one week later for histologic evaluation. They reported:

		Argon laser			
	Bipolar	4 W	5.5 W	6 W	10 W
Duodenum					
Stopped bleeding/ total ulcers	21/21	16/20	21/24	21/24	23/23
Full-thickness injury	20%	35%	30%	55%	60%
Esophagus					
Stopped bleeding/ total ulcers	20/20	19/19	20/20	19/19	19/19
Full-thickness injury	15%	31%	35%	47%	74%

They concluded that bipolar electrocoagulation and the argon laser both stopped bleeding from standard ulcers in the esophagus and duodenum, but that deeper tissue injury resulted in these organs than was reported in the stomach. They also concluded that high-power argon resulted in deeper damage than was found with either lower-power argon or bipolar electrocoagulation.

5. The Argon Laser in Primates

Experimental argon laser photocoagulation in primates was reported by Butler, et al.[33] This group treated bleeding mucosal biopsies in six rhesus monkeys with a 3-W argon laser. Two monkeys were heparinized and four monkeys were not heparinized.

Of six lesions in the stomach, the laser stopped five with an average coagulation time of 38.2 sec. In the duodenum, the laser stopped four of four lesions with an average coagulation time of 28.5 sec.

Several groups have studied the argon laser through a variety of application parameters in different animal models. In general, the argon laser in these models has been found to be hemostatically effective with minimal injury to the underlying gastrointestinal tissue.

B. Nd:YAG Laser Photocoagulation in Animals

Our group has performed several studies of ND:YAG photocoagulation. In our first study, we evaluated the hemostatic efficacy and resulting depth of injury of a ND:YAG laser with a 4° divergence angle in our standard acute bleeding ulcer model.[34] In each experiment, treated ulcers were removed after seven days for evaluation of depth of injury. Three experiments were performed.

1. Varying Pulse Duration

In the first experiment, we used 55 W of power with coaxial CO_2 gas, varying the laser pulse duration—0.5 sec with 5-sec cooling intervals between pulses, 1.0 sec pulses without obligate cooling intervals, or continuous laser exposure to achieve hemostasis. In these studies we found:

	Duration		
	0.5 sec with interval cooling	**1.0 sec**	**Continuous**
Stopped bleeding/ total ulcers	10/10	9/9	11/11
Full-thickness injury	50%	66%	55%

Therefore, in this experiment, the pulse interval did not significantly reduce the depth of tissue injury.

2. Coaxial Gas Jet

In the second experiment, we used the Nd:YAG laser at 55 W with 1.0 sec pulses with or without coaxial CO_2. The results were:

	With CO_2	**Without CO_2**
Stopped bleeding/total ulcers	12/12	11/12
Full-thickness injury	66%	66%

Coaxial CO_2 in this model did not reduce the depth of injury.

3. Laser Power

In the third experiment, we used the Nd:YAG laser with 1.0-sec pulses with coaxial CO_2, but at three laser powers. We found:

	15 W	**30 W**	**55 W**
Stopped bleeding/total ulcers	6/12	12/12	12/12
Full-thickness injury	17%	75%	66%

Therefore, the laser was not effective at 15 W, but was effective at 30 and 55 W. However, both 30 W and 55 W resulted in deep tissue injury.

We are now evaluating the Nd:YAG laser at higher powers (30 to 75 W), varying the pulse duration (0.5 to 1.0 sec), and with wider divergence angles of 14 and 25 degrees.[17] We hope to determine whether changing to higher power with short durations and wider divergence angles will result in less tissue injury with maintenance of hemostatic efficacy.

Other investigators have evaluated the histologic effects of the Nd:YAG laser in animals.

4. Penetration and Perforation Times

Dixon et al. studied the 55 W Nd:YAG laser in acute standard bleeding ulcers.[35] He found that he could stop the bleeding in 51 of 51 ulcers with a mean time of photocoagulation of 3.56 ± 1.65 sec (range 1 to 8.5 sec). In 19 treated ulcers, a free perforation was produced with a mean of 9.6 ± 1.5 sec (range 6.33 to 12.28 sec). When examined histologically after 9 to 14 days, 13 of 22 treated lesions had greater than 80% damage to the muscularis externa. Nineteen ulcers were photocoagulated until the bleeding stopped and then treated with 4 to 15 sec of additional laser exposure. Fourteen of these 19 ulcers had greater than 80% injury to the muscularis externa when examined after several days. In their final study, a free perforation was produced in nine dogs using the Nd:YAG laser. The perforation in the gastric wall was not sutured closed. All of these dogs survived without clinical peritonitis. This study lends a note of caution indicating that one cannot extrapolate from the results in animal models to the anticipated clinical results in patients. Not only does the dog tolerate a full-thickness wall injury without developing clinical peritonitis, but this experiment demonstrated that the dog will also survive a free perforation without developing peritonitis. Therefore, conclusions regarding the consequences of a full–thickness injury in dogs should not be directly extrapolated to patients.

5. Nd:YAG Compared to Monopolar Electrocoagulation

Escourrou et al. performed a study of the hemostatic efficacy and resulting depth of injury of an 80 W Nd:YAG laser compared to monopolar electrocoagulation in acute standard bleeding ulcers.[36] Their results were:

	Nd:YAG	**Monopolar Electrocoagulation**
Stopped bleeding/total ulcers	30/30	28/30
>50% injury to muscularis externa	5/60	24/60
Average time (sec)	5.4 ± 2	28.7 ± 22

They concluded that both methods were hemostatically effective, but that the Nd:YAG laser stopped the bleeding faster than did monopolar electrocoagulation with a significantly lower incidence of deep injury to the muscularis externa. This group is now involved in a controlled clinical trial of Nd:YAG photocoagulation in patients with gastrointestinal bleeding. It is possible that in their animal experiments the high laser power with short exposure times accounts for the reduced depth of tissue injury.

6. Nd:YAG Pulse Durations and Power

Bown et al. reported a series of studies of Nd:YAG laser photocoagulation in experimental canine ulcers performed to evaluate the optimal pulse energy.[37] They found that effective hemostasis required a pulse energy of greater than 20 J. Thirty J was optimal except with pumping arteries, which required 40 J pulses. The pulse duration was also evaluated and the optimum range was found to be 300 to 500 msec.

Thirty J pulses at shorter durations (50 or 100 msec) or longer durations (1 sec) were not as effective. Stopping the bleeding point with one pulse seemed to be better than multiple pulses. They then used the Nd:YAG laser with 75 W of power using 30 J pulses and a pulse duration of 400 msec to treat experimental acute bleeding ulcers and found that they were able to stay within their safe limit for full-thickness injury. This group plans to use the Nd:YAG laser with these application parameters in a clinical trial in patients with upper gastrointestinal bleeding.

7. The Nd:YAG Laser in Pigs

Sluis et al. reported studies of Nd:YAG photocoagulation in gastric ulcers in pigs.[38] The Nd:YAG laser was studied with 0.5 to 5.0 sec total exposure times, powers of 50 to 80 W, pulse durations of 0.5, 1.0, 1.5 and 2.0 sec on both normal mucosa and experimental bleeding ulcers. In this report, the investigators noted that the histologic depth of injury correlated with total laser energy, but that intermittent bursts produced less damage. They made an interesting observation that the pig antrum resisted the photocoagulative damage of the Nd:YAG laser better than did other gastric areas, perhaps related to the wall thickness. The hemostatic efficacy correlated with laser power. Low laser power was not effective hemostatically and actually increased bleeding in some instances. This group concluded that 82 W of power was most effective. In their bleeding model, 12, 1-sec applications at 82 W were effective hemostatically and produced the least tissue injury. These are the parameters they plan to use in a controlled clinical trial in patients.

Thus, several groups have found the Nd:YAG laser to be rapidly hemostatically effective, but with a high incidence of full-thickness injury to the gastric wall. However, animals tolerate this deep injury without apparent adverse sequelae.

C. Comparisons of Argon in Experimental Models

Several investigators have compared the hemostatic efficacy and resulting tissue injury for the argon and Nd:YAG lasers in animal models.

Our group compared a 55 W Nd:YAG laser with 4 degree divergence, 1 sec applications with coaxial CO_2 gas to a 7 W argon laser with a 14° divergence, 5-sec application durations, and coaxial CO_2.[34] These lasers were compared at laparotomy in heparinized dogs using standard acute bleeding ulcers. We found:

	55 W Nd:YAG	**7 W Argon**
Stopped bleeding/total ulcers	15/15	15/15
Full-thickness injury	79%	0

The difference in depth of injury was highly significant statistically. In this experiment using this model, both lasers stopped bleeding, but the Nd:YAG laser caused deeper injury to the muscularis externa.

Three other groups have recently compared the argon laser to the Nd:YAG laser in animals. Dixon et al. compared the argon laser at 6 W to the Nd:YAG laser at 55 W in standard acute bleeding ulcers.[39] He found:

	55 W Nd:YAG	**6 W Argon**
Stopped bleeding/total ulcers	51/51	35/39
Full-thickness injury	80—90%	Minimal
Sec required for treatment	3.6 ± 1.6	25 ± 8.2
Sec required to perforate	9.4 ± 1.2	54 ± 8.5

This group concluded that these lasers might complement each other in terms of hemostatic efficacy. They suggested that the argon laser could be used for superficial or multiple bleeding arteries and veins, whereas the more deeply penetrating and perhaps more hemostatically effective Nd:YAG laser could be used for single site, massive, arterial, and large venous bleedings. As will be reported below, this group has used both lasers in clinical trials in patients.

Waitman reported comparative evaluation of argon and Nd:YAG lasers in bleeding acute ulcers.[40] He concluded that the argon laser could staunch ulcer bleeding with or without coaxial CO_2 without perforating the gastric wall or causing full-thickness injury if the power was less than 7.5 W. This group reported the Nd:YAG laser's hemostatic efficacy was similar to argon, but the resulting depth of injury was higher with the Nd:YAG laser. More than 50% of ulcers treated with the Nd:YAG laser had injury through the full thickness of the muscularis externa. Based on these experiments, they are now engaged in a controlled clinical trial of the argon laser in patients with upper gastrointestinal bleeding.

The laser research group at UCLA and the Wadsworth VA Hospital have reported two studies comparing argon and Nd:YAG laser photocoagulation.[41,42] In the first study, Johnston et al. reported an endoscopic comparison of the argon laser at 8 W and 10 W to the Nd:YAG laser at 70 W, bipolar electrocoagulation, and monopolar electrocoagulation in the treatment of acute standard bleeding gastric ulcers in dogs.[41] They found:

	Argon		**Nd:YAG**		
	8 W	**10 W**	**70 W**	**Bipolar**	**Monopolar**
Bleeding stopped/ total ulcers	28/30	30/30	30/30	29/20	30/30
Full-thickness injury	10%	10%	43%	17%	53%

They concluded that each technique studied was hemostatically effective at endoscopy, but that the Nd:YAG laser and monopolar electrocoagulation damaged more deeply than did the argon laser at 8 or 10 W, or the bipolar electrode.

In the second study, Jensen et al. reported similar endoscopic data but also reported a series of experiments at laparotomy.[42] In these studies, the argon laser at three power levels was compared to the Nd:YAG laser at five power levels in the photocoagulation of acute standard bleeding ulcers in dogs. They found:

	Argon			**Nd:YAG**				
	6 W	**10 W**	**12 W**	**40 W**	**50 W**	**60 W**	**70 W**	**90 W**
Stopped bleeding/ total ulcers	22/31	30/33	32/32	30/30	30/30	29/30	28/29	27/30
Full-thickness injury	16%	15%	18%	77%	97%	80%	76%	83%

They concluded that at laparotomy in this model, both lasers stopped bleeding effectively, but that the Nd:YAG photocoagulation caused more damage at powers of 6 to 12 W.

In conclusion, a number of carefully controlled studies have been performed in animals with the argon laser and the Nd:YAG laser photocoagulation systems. Several groups have compared results prospectively with these two lasers. In most of these animal studies, both lasers stopped bleeding. The high-power Nd:YAG laser coagulates more rapidly than does the argon laser, but the Nd:YAG laser causes significantly deeper injury to the gastrointestinal wall. The significance of this full-thickness injury in animals is not yet clear. In these experiments, no dogs developed free perforation or peritonitis despite significant full-thickness injury extending to the serosa.

VII. CLINICAL STUDIES OF LASER PHOTOCOAGULATION

Most of the nonrandomized and controlled clinical trials of laser photocoagulation have been reported from outside the U.S. and will be subsequently described in detail by Dr. Cotton. In the U.S., there are several clinical trials of the argon laser and the Nd:YAG laser in massive upper gastrointestinal bleeding now in progress. Several of these are using a controlled clinical trial protocol which was developed by a committee consisting of members of the American Gastroenterological Association, the American Society for Gastrointestinal Endoscopy, and other experts in the field. The results of these trials have not yet been reported. A multicenter trial to compare laser photocoagulation with electrocoagulation is planned.

A. Argon Clinical Trials in the U.S.

Waitman et al. reported treating a series of bleeding patients considered to be exceptionally high-risk for surgery.[43] The lesions bleeding included gastric ulcer, stress ulcer, duodenal ulcer, hemorrhagic gastritis, gastric cancer, and telangiectasia. The exact number of patients was not reported. An argon laser was used to photocoagulate these lesions using 4 W of power. Bleeding stopped in all patients, but two patients rebled within 24 hr. There were no complications.

Jensen et al. reported using argon laser and bipolar electrocoagulation to treat intestinal telangiectasia.[44] They treated four patients with a total of 145 lesions in the stomach and 5 lesions in the colon. Ten lesions were treated with a bipolar electrode and 140 with the argon laser using 7 to 10 W. In some treated lesions the coagulation induced bleeding. This occurred with all ten lesions treated with bipolar electrocoagulation and in some lesions ($>$ 10 mm diameter) treated with the argon laser. No other complications occurred. On follow-up, small, new, vascular lesions were noted in two patients within two months. The clinical course after treatment was compared to the period before treatment. In these patients, they found a reduction in the need for emergency admissions, transfusions, anemia, and surgery after treatment when compared to the 13-month period before treatment.

This same group has also reported treating four patients with acutely bleeding ulcers with an argon laser.[45] These ulcers included three duodenal ulcers and one gastric ulcer. Power output was 8 to 11.5 W. CO_2 back-pressure was 8 cm of water. Bleeding stopped in all patients, but one duodenal ulcer with a large bleeding gastroduodenal artery rebled and required emergency surgery. There were no complications. This group suggested that patients with severe active bleeding gastroduodenal arteries be considered for primary surgical therapy rather than argon laser photocoagulation.

B. Nd:YAG Clinical Trials in the U.S.

Most of the American clinical experience of Nd:YAG has been reported by Dwyer.[46] A total of 58 patients with a variety of bleeding lesions have been treated using a 60 W Nd:YAG laser with 2 to 12 seconds of exposure. He reports the laser treatment to be 90% effective. In two patients, variceal bleeding could not be controlled. In one instance, the patient was too unstable clinically to continue with photocoagulation, and in one instance, the laser output fell below 50 W. One perforation occurred in this series.

C. Combined Laser Trials in the U.S.

Dixon has reported treating nine patients with acute upper gastrointestinal bleeding who were considered to be poor surgical risks.[39] These patients were treated with either the argon laser or the Nd:YAG laser. Bleeding was controlled in seven of nine patients. The two failures were caused by inadequate visualization. There were no complications. The exact type of bleeding lesions and treatment parameters have not yet been reported.

VIII. CONCLUSION

Laser photocoagulation using the argon and Nd:YAG lasers has been studied fairly extensively in animal models of gastrointestinal bleeding. Controlled clinical trials are now underway in patients with upper gastrointestinal bleeding. Hopefully, these trials will define the exact benefit of laser photocoagulation for bleeding patients in terms of a reduction in morbidity, mortality, transfusions, and duration of hospitalization, as well as the risk of laser treatment. These studies of the argon and Nd:YAG lasers should be completed prior to the widespread clinical use of these expensive and potentially hazardous techniques.

There remain some questions regarding laser photocoagulation. Which laser is preferable? What delivery parameters for the selected laser are ideal regarding power, total energy, spot size, and CO_2 flow rate? What type of endoscope should be used? Is a gas recycling system necessary or can the gas simply be vented to the outside? Can portable lasers be developed that can be taken to the bedside? How do these techniques compare to endoscopic hemostatic techniques now being studied which are much less expensive and can be taken to the bleeding patient's bedside? Is the cost and technical difficulty of installing a laser justified? How many patients would be eligible for laser photocoagulation of upper gastrointestinal bleeding lesions?[47] We hope that many of these questions will be answered in the controlled clinical trials currently underway throughout the world to determine the role of laser photocoagulation in the therapy of upper gastrointestinal bleeding.

ACKNOWLEDGMENT

This study was supported by contract NO1-AM-52211 from the U.S. Public Health Service and by NIH Gastroenterology Research Training Grant 5T32 AM 07113.

REFERENCES

1. **Morgan, A. G., McAdam, W. A. F., Walmsley, G. L., Jessop, A., Horrocks, J. C., and de Dombal, F. T.,** Clinical findings, early endoscopy, and multivariate analysis in patients bleeding from the upper gastrointestinal tract, *Br. Med. J.*, 2, 237, 1977.
2. **Allan, R. and Dykes, P.,** A study of the factors influencing mortality rates from gastrointestinal haemorrhage, *Q. J. Med. New Series 45,* 180, 533, 1976.
3. **Gilbert, D. A., Silverstein, F. E., Auth, D. C., and Rubin, C. E.,** "The nonsurgical management of acute nonvariceal upper gastrointestinal bleeding," in *Progress in Hemostasis and Thrombosis,* Vol. 4, Spaet, T.H., Ed., Grune & Stratton, New York, 1978.
4. **Protell, R. L., Rubin, C. E., Auth, D. C., Silverstein, F. E., Terou, F., Dennis, M., and Piercey, J. R. A.,** The heater probe: a new endoscopic method for stopping massive gastrointestinal bleeding, *Gastroenterology,* 74, 257, 1978.

5. **Protell, R. L., Lawrence, D. M., Peoples, J. E., Majoch, T. R., and Auth, D. C.,** A new endoscopic thermal cautery which stops experimental bleeding safely, *Gastroenteroloy,* 78 (Abstr.), 1239, 1980.
6. **Piercey, J. R. A., Auth, D. C., Silverstein, F. E., Willard, H. R., Dennis, M. B., Ellefson, D. M., Davis, D. M., Protell, R. L., and Rubin, C. E.,** Electrosurgical treatment of experimental bleeding canine gastric ulcers: development and testing of a computer control and a better electrode, *Gastroenterology,* 74, 527, 1978.
7. **Papp, J. P.,** Endoscopic electrocoagulation of upper gastrointestinal hemorrhage, *JAMA*, 236, 2076, 1976.
8. **Gaisford, W. D.,** A new prototype 2-channel upper gastrointestinal operating fiberscope, *Gastrointest. Endosc.,* 22, 148, 1976.
9. **Protell, R. L., Silverstein, F. E., Gulacsik, C., Martin, T. R., Dennis, M. B., Auth, D. C., and Rubin, C. E.,** Failure of cyanoacrylate tissue glue (Flucrylate, MBR 4197) to stop bleeding from experimental canine gastric ulcers, *Am. J. Dig. Dis.*, 23, 903, 1978.
10. **Martin, T. R., Onstad, G. R., and Silvis, S. E.,** Endoscopic control of upper gastrointestinal bleeding with a tissue adhesive (MBR 4197), *Gastrointest. Endosc.,* 24, 73, 1977.
11. **Linscheer, W. G. and Fazio, T. L.,** Control of upper gastrointestinal hemorrhage by endoscopic spraying of clotting factors, *Gastroenterology,* 77, 642, 1979.
12. **Jensen, D. M., Machicado G., Tapia J., and Mautner, W.,** Clotting factors fail to control bleeding from standard ulcers or gastric erosions, *Gastroenterology,* 78 (Abstr.), 1187, 1980.
13. **Goodale, R. L., Okada, A., and Gonzales, R.,** Rapid endoscopic control of bleeding gastric erosions by laser radiations, *Arch. Surg.,* 101, 211, 1970.
14. **Silverstein, F., Protell, R., Auth D., Dennis M., Piercey J., and Rubin C.,** Comparison of high-power and low-power argon laser photocoagulation using an animal model of acute bleeding ulcer, *Gastroenterology,* 70 (Abstr.), 938, 1976.
15. **Frühmorgen, P., Bodem, F., Reidenbach, H. D., Kaduk, B., and Demling, L.,** The first successful endoscopic laser coagulations of bleeding and potential bleeding lesions in the human gastrointestinal tract, *Gastrointest. Endosc.* 22 (Abstr.), 224, 1976.
16. **Kiefhaber, P., Nath, G., and Noritz, K.,** Endoscopical control of massive gastrointestinal hemorrhage by irradiation with a high-power neodymium–YAG laser, *Prog. Surg.,* 15, 140, 1977.
17. **Gilbert, D. A., Gulascik, C., Auth, D. C., Silverstein, F. E., and Dennis, M. B.,** Nd-YAG laser photocoagulation at wider beam divergence angles produces deep tissue injury, *Gastroenterology,* 78 (Abstr.), 1272, 1980.
18. **Johnston, J. H., Jensen, D. M., and Mautner, W.,** Limitations of endoscopic argon laser with coaxial CO_2, *Gastroenterology,* 76 (Abstr.), 1161, 1979.
19. **Gilbert, D. A., Silverstein, F. E., Protell, R. L., Auth, D. C., Gulacsik, C., and Dennis, M. B.,** Animal endoscopic studies of CO_2 assisted argon laser photocoagulation preparatory to controlled trials in man, *Gastroenterology,* 74 (Abstr.), 1037, 1978.
20. **Opie, E. A.,** A fail safe servo-controlled recycling system for laser endoscopy, in Conference Digest: The Conference on Laser and Electrooptical Systems, San Diego, 1980, 82.
21. **Silverstein, F. E., Protell, R. L., Gulacsik, D., Auth, D. C., Deltenre M., Dennis, M., Piercey J., and Rubin, C. E.,** Endoscopic laser treatment III: the development and testing of a gas-jet-assisted argon laser waveguide in control of bleeding experimental ulcers, *Gastroenterology,* 74, 232, 1978.
22. **Gulacsik, C., Auth, D. C., and Silverstein, F. E.,** Ophthalmic hazards associated with laser endoscopy, *Appl. Opt.,* 18, 1816, 1979.
23. **Nath, G., Gorisch, W., and Kiefhaber, P.,** First laser endoscopy via a fiberoptic transmission system, *Endoscopy,* 5, 208, 1973.
24. **Frühmorgen, P., Kaduk, B., Reidenbach, H. D., Bodem, F., Demling, L., and Brand, H.,** Long-term observations in endoscopic laser coagulations in the gastrointestinal tract, *Endoscopy,* 7, 189, 1975.
25. **Waitman, A. M., Spira I., Chryssanthou, C. P., and Steng, A. J.,** Fiberoptic–coupled argon laser in the control on experimentally produced gastric bleeding, *Gastrointest. Endosc.,* 22, 78, 1975.
26. **Dwyer, R. M., Haberback, B. J., Bass, J., Chenow, J.,** Laser-induced hemostasis in the canine stomach. Use of a flexible fiberoptic delivery system, *JAMA*, 231, 486, 1975.
27. **Silverstein, F. E., Auth, D. C., Rubin, C. E., and Protell, R. L.,** High power argon laser treatment via standard endoscopes, I. A preliminary study of efficacy in control of experimental erosive bleeding, *Gastroenterology,* 71, 558, 1976.
28. **Protell, R. L., Silverstein, F. E., Piercey, J., Dennis M., Sprake W., and Rubin, C. E.,** A reproducible animal model of acute bleeding ulcer—The "Ulcer Maker," *Gastroenterology,* 71, 961, 1976.
29. **Silverstein, F. E., Protell, R. L., Piercey, J., Rubin, C. E., Auth, D. C., and Dennis M.,** Endoscopic laser treatment III: comparison of the efficacy of high and low power photocoagulation in control of severely bleeding experimental ulcers in dogs, *Gastroenterology,* 73, 481, 1977.

30. **Johnston, J. H., Jensen, D. M., and Mautner, W.,** Is argon laser safe at close treatment distance or high powers?, *Gastroenterology,* 76 (Abstr.), 1161, 1980.
31. **Bown, S. G., Salmon, P. R., Kelly, D. F., Galder, B. M., Pearson, H., Weaver, B. M. Q., and Read, A. E.,** Argon laser photocoagulation in the dog stomach, *Gut,* 20, 680, 1979.
32. **Machicado, G. A., Jensen, D. M., Tapia, J. I., and Mautner, W.,** Argon laser photocoagulation and bipolar electrocoagulation in the treatment of bleeding duodenal and esophageal ulcers, *Gastroenterology,* 76 (Abstr.) 1191, 1979.
33. **Butler, M. L. and Morris, W.,** Use of argon laser in the treatment of experimentally induced upper gastrointestinal bleeding in primates, *Gastrointest. Endosc.,* 24, 117, 1978.
34. **Silverstein, F. E., Protell, R. L., Gilbert, D. A., Gulacsik, C., Auth, D. C., Dennis, M. B., and Rubin, C. E.,** Argon vs. neodymium YAG laser photocoagulation of experimental canine gastric ulcers, *Gastroenterology,* 77, 491, 1979.
35. **Dixon, J. A., Berenson, M. M., and McCloskey, D. W.,** Neodymium-YAG laser treatment of experimental canine gastric bleeding, acute and chronic studies of photocoagulation, penetration and perforation, *Gastroenterology,* 77, 647, 1979.
36. **Escourrou, J., Frexinos, J., Balas, D., Monrozies, X., Ribet A., and de Rangueil, C. H. U.,** Comparison of a new method of electrocoagulation and YAG laser photocoagulation in the treatment of bleeding canine gastric ulcers, *Gastroenterology,* 76 (Abstr.), 1128, 1979.
37. **Bown, S. G., Adams, N. L., Storey, D., Salmon, P. R., and Brunetaud, J. M.,** "Pulsed Nd:YAG laser photocoagulation in the dog stomach," in Abstracts of the IV European Congress of Gastrointestinal Endoscopy, George Thieme Verlag, Stuttgart, Germany, 1980, 25.
38. **Sluis, R. F. v.d., Holland, R., and Yap, S. H.,** "Experience with neodymium–YAG laser photocoagulation in experimental gastric ulcers in pig," in Abstracts of the IV European Congress of Gastrointestinal Endoscopy, George Thieme Verlag, Stuttgart, Germany, 1980, 115.
39. **Dixon, J., Berenson, M.,** "Experimental and clinical observations in application of argon and Nd:YAG lasers in upper gastrointestinal bleeding lesions," presented at Int. Med. Laser Symp., Detroit, March 29 to 31, 1979.
40. **Waitman, A. M.,** "Clinical and experimental argon laser therapy of the UGI tract," presented at Int. Laser Symp., Detroit, March 29, 1979.
41. **Johnston, J. H., Jensen, D. M., and Mautner, W.,** Comparison of laser photocoagulation and electrocoagulation in endoscopic treatment of UGI bleeding, *Gastroenterology,* 76 (Abstr.), 1162, 1979.
42. **Jensen, D. M., Johnston, J. H., and Mautner, W.,** "Comparisons of laser photocoagulation and electrocoagulation in control of experimental GI bleeding," presented at Int. Med. Laser Symp., Detroit, March 29 to 31, 1979.
43. **Waitman, A. M., Grant, D. Z., DeBeer, R., and Chryssanthou, C.,** Endoscopic argon laser photocoagulation in upper gastrointestinal hemorrhage, *Gastroenterology,* 76 (Abstr.), 1265, 1979.
44. **Jensen, D. M., Machicado, G., Tapia, J., Mautner, W., and Franco, P.,** Endoscopic treatment of telangiectasia with argon laser photocoagulation and bipolar electrocoagulation in patients with chronic gastrointestinal bleeding, *Gastrointest, Endosc.,* 26 (Abstr.), 69, 1980.
45. **Jensen, D. M., Machicado, G., Mautner, W., Tapia, J., and Franco, P.,** Endoscopic argon laser photocoagulation of patients with severe gastrointestinal bleeding, *Gastroenterology,* 78 (Abstr.), 1188, 1980.
46. **Dwyer, R. M.,** Safe and effective laser phototherapy in man using the Nd:YAG laser, *Gastroenterology,* 76 (Abstr.), 1126, 1979.
47. **Overholt, B. F. and Mahan, G.,** GI bleeding in a metropolitan hospital—or is there a need for laser coagulation in upper GI bleeding?, *Gastrointest. Endosc.,* 26 (Abstr.), 73, 1980.

Chapter 7

EUROPEAN CLINICAL EXPERIENCE IN LASER PHOTOCOAGULATION IN UPPER GASTROINTESTINAL TRACT

P. B. Cotton and A. G. Vallon

TABLE OF CONTENTS

I. INTRODUCTION

Endoscopic laser photocoagulation has been in clinical use in Europe since 1975. Frühmorgen and his colleagues[1] in Erlangen—Nurenburg introduced the Argon laser while Kiefhaber and colleagues[2] used the Neodymium-Yag laser in Munich. Their preliminary results encouraged others to follow so that laser machines are now being used in at least 50 European centers. Despite its widespread use, the clinical contribution of laser photocoagulation remains in some doubt. Most reported studies do not include control data.[3-9] Evaluation is difficult because many lesions stop bleeding spontaneously and both clinical practice and patient selection varies considerably between units. Substantial controversy remains first, as to which type of laser is preferable and second, whether either makes a clinical contribution sufficient to justify its cost. We believe that these and other related questions can only be answered through randomized controlled trials. Preliminary results from such trials are not immediately convincing, but several others are in progress.

We have attempted to summarize current European practice based on published results and a survey of users.

II. CENTERS AND PATIENT MATERIAL

Information has been received from 50 centers; 40 of these (30 in Germany and Austria) were using Neodymium-Yag lasers supplied by M.B.B.-AT (MediLas), Molectron Medical, or Barr and Stroud. The remainder were using the Spectra-Physics Argon ion laser. At the time of this writing, many centers were only just beginning to use their equipment.

Only six of these centers admitted more than 250 patients with acute upper gastrointestinal bleeding each year. Three admitted over 700. There was considerable variation in the type of patients encountered and in the spectrum of responsible lesions (Table 1). Twenty centers provided data on the timing of endoscopy and the percentage of patients seen to be actively bleeding at endoscopy. Not surprisingly, the percentage of active bleeders was higher in those centers practicing emergency endoscopy within two hours of admission. The majority (11 centers) saw active bleeding in less that 20% (Table 2). This has considerable implications for all methods of endoscopic hemostasis.

Most centers were not performing or planning to do controlled trials. The vast majority of those using Neodymium-Yag lasers, but very few of those using Argon lasers, were treating patients with varices as well as those with ulcers. Approximately half of all centers were only treating ulcers which were actively bleeding at the time of endoscopy. The remainder were also treating nonbleeding ulcers with visible vessels or clot attached. As a result of these factors, more than half of the centers were treating less than 20% of their patients judged to have bled from ulcers.

Most groups were using standard forward-viewing fiberscopes. A few used double-channeled instruments or those with a single-larger channel. Many types of laser fiber were in use. Estimates of their durability varied enormously. Most centers used coaxial gas. Information was not obtained about venting systems. Most centers with Neodymium-Yag lasers used a power output of 70 to 90 W—those with Argon lasers, 6 to 8 W, measured at the fiber tip. The reported length of laser shot varied considerably, from ½ to 4 sec. Most centers did not have any fixed maximum duration for laser exposure. In the treatment of ulcer vessels, most users aimed both at the tip and at the base of any exposed vessel.

Table 1
VARIABILITY IN PROPORTIONS OF ULCERS AND VARICES

	Ulcers	Varices
81—100%	4	0
61—80%	7	1
41—60%	8	0
21—40%	2	4
0—20%	1	11

Note: Figures indicate numbers of centers.

Table 2
URGENCY OF ENDOSCOPY AND RELATIONSHIP TO THE PERCENTAGE OF ULCERS ACTIVELY BLEEDING AT ENDOSCOPY

Timing of endoscopy (hr)		0—2	2—6	6—12	12—24	Total
Ulcers actively bleeding at endoscopy (%)	40+	3	0	0	1	4
	20—40	3	1	1	0	5
	10—20	3	2	5	1	11
Total centers		9	3	6	2	20

III. RESULTS

More than 1000 patients have now been treated in Europe. The majority were treated with Neodymium-Yag lasers in uncontrolled studies. The results are summarized in Tables 3 to 8. While giving interesting information, the data do not permit firm conclusions. Techniques, definitions, indications for surgery, and particularly the selection of patients for endoscopic treatment, all differ between centers.

IV. BLEEDING PEPTIC ULCERS

A. Uncontrolled studies (Tables 3 and 4)

Both Neodymium-Yag and Argon lasers can provide immediate hemostasis in a high proportion of patients with actively bleeding peptic ulcers. The overall success rate appears to be greater for the Neodymium-Yag laser (90% against 81%), but the incidence of early rebleeding is also higher (14% against 11%), so that the results for hemostasis at one week are quite similar (76% against 71%). The data for surgical intervention and death are difficult to evaluate. The mortality rate is dependent upon the population of patients selected. Many deaths are not related to surgery or bleeding.

B. Controlled Studies (Tables 5 and 6)

Two controlled studies have been completed[10,11] (one each with the Argon and Neodymium-Yag lasers) and at least five others are known to be in progress.[12] Presently, available results are insufficient for any final conclusions. Perhaps the most interesting fact is that a significant proportion (40 to 60%) of ulcers in the control groups stopped bleeding spontaneously—a much higher figure than had been assumed by those advocating emergency treatment and from other reported studies. Both Neodymium-Yag and Argon lasers provided immediate hemostasis significantly more often (77%).

Table 3
NONRANDOMIZED STUDIES WITH ARGON-ION LASER IN PATIENTS WITH ACTIVELY BLEEDING ULCERS

		Le Bodic[19] et al.	Brunetaud[9] et al.	Laurence[3] et al.	Others	Total
Total attempts		46	67	60	15	188
Immediate hemostasis	%	83	83	80	80	81
Rebleed within 1 wk	%	17	9	8	7	11
Hemostasis > 1 wk	%	65	74	72	73	71
Surgery for bleeding	%	0	?	22	7	16
Deaths overall	%	26	?	7	0	13

Table 4
NONRANDOMIZED STUDIES WITH NEODYMIUM—YAG LASER IN PATIENTS WITH ACTIVELY BLEEDING ULCERS

		Kiefhaber[20] et al.	Shonekas[21] et al.	Sander[22] et al.	Eight others	Total
Total attempts		273	256	64	142	735
Immediate hemostasis	%	93	99	83	73	90
Rebleed within 1 wk	%	15	11	17	17	14
Hemostasis > 1 wk	%	78	88	66	57	76
Surgery for bleeding	%	10	5	2	8	7
Deaths overall	%	27	1	16	15	15

This figure is lower than that seen in the uncontrolled studies (Tables 3 and 4) and the incidence of rebleeding is also higher. While rebleeding appeared to be more frequent with the Neodymium-Yag laser than with the Argon laser (32% against 13%), the numbers are too small for serious analysis. The most important fact is that the present data for surgical intervention and death do not show any convincing benefit for laser therapy when compared with controls.

Similar conclusions were drawn from another study in which the results of Neodymium-Yag laser photocoagulation in 62 patients were compared with those in 43 patients in whom coagulation was impossible for technical reasons.[13] Continuing or recurrent hemorrhage was equally common in both groups. Although emergency surgery was performed more frequently in controls (41% against 13%), the overall mortality rates were similar (27% and 24%).

V. BLEEDING ESOPHAGEAL VARICES

The Neodymium-Yag laser appears to give excellent results in patients with bleeding esophageal varices (Table 7). Immediate hemostasis was achieved in 90% of 298 patients, with a 19% incidence of early rebleeding. Mortality data were not included. The preliminary results of Argon laser treatment in this context are less encouraging (Table 7).

VI. NONBLEEDING PEPTIC ULCERS

In most centers, the majority of ulcers were not actively bleeding at the time of emergency endoscopy. It has recently been emphasized that the appearance of visible vessels[14] and stigmata of recent hemorrhage[15] can give some indication as to the risk of

Table 5
RANDOMIZED CONTROLLED TRIALS WITH ARGON-ION LASER IN PATIENTS WITH ACTIVELY BLEEDING PEPTIC ULCERS

	LeBodic et al.[19]		Vallon et. al[10]		Totals (%)	
	L[a]	C[b]	L	C	L (%)	C (%)
Total patients	15	10	15	13	30 (100)	23 (100)
Immediate hemostasis	13	5	10	4	23 (77)	9 (39)
Rebleed within 1 wk	2	1	2	2	4 (13)	3 (13)
Hemostasis > 1 wk	11	4	8	2	10 (64)	6 (26)
Surgery for bleeding	0	0	7	9	7 (23)	9 (39)
Deaths	3	1	2	3	5 (17)	4 (17)

[a] L = laser group.
[b] C = controls.

Table 6
RANDOMIZED CONTROLLED TRIALS WITH ND-YAG LASER IN PATIENTS WITH ACTIVELY BLEEDING PEPTIC ULCERS

	Ihre el al.[11]		Van Trappen[a23]		Escourrou[24]		Totals	
	L	C	L	C	L	C	L (%)	C (%)
Total patients	19	13	27	27	31	30	77 (100)	70 (100)
Immediate hemostasis	11	8	27	20	21	14	59 (77)	42 (60)
Rebleed within 1 wk	4	4	2	3	16	4	22 (37)	11 (26)
Haemostasis > 1 wk	7	4	25	17	5	10	37 (48)	31 (44)
Surgery for bleeding	9	9	1	4	7	6	17 (22)	19 (27)
Deaths	1	2	1	2	2	2	4 (5)	6 (9)

[a]Van Trappen's series excludes ulcers with *arterial* bleeding.

rebleeding and provides a justification for the prophylactic use of endoscopic hemostatic methods. Relatively few centers have reported their results in such patients (Table 8). The apparently impressive results in uncontrolled data fall into perspective in the reported controlled studies, which show no benefit in terms of rebleeding, surgical intervention, or death (Table 8).

VII. COMPLICATIONS

No complications to the endoscopist or other staff during laser treatment have yet been reported. The assessment of hazard to the patient is complex. Emergency endoscopy carries its own risks in actively bleeding and sick patients. Laser photocoagulation may contribute to these risks simply by the inherent prolongation of the procedure, or by the necessary use of a larger instrument, or by the fact that the suction channel of a single-channeled instrument is necessarily blocked.

Laser perforation of the gastric or duodenal wall has been reported by Kiefhaber in approximately 1% of treatments, particularly in patients with acute ulcers.[6] One patient in the Barcelona trial developed an exacerbation of pain during Argon laser treatment and was found to have a covered perforation of a duodenal ulcer at surgery. Rapid gas distension of the stomach is believed to have aggravated a problem present prior to hospital admission.[10] Over-distension of the stomach and intestines with gas may give

Table 7
NONRANDOMIZED STUDIES IN PATIENTS WITH BLEEDING ESOPHAGEAL VARICES

		ND-YAG				ARGON
		Kiefhaber[20] et al.	Shonekas[21] et al.	Five others	Total	LeBodic[19] et al.
Total attempts		103	128	67	298	18
Immediate hemostasis	%	91	85	97	90	61
Rebleed within 1 wk	%	14	19	24	19	30
Hemostasis > 1 wk	%	77	66	73	71	31

Table 8
STUDIES IN PATIENTS WITH NONBLEEDING PEPTIC ULCERS

	Nonrandomized	Controlled studies			
	Nd-Yag 4 groups	Nd-Yag Ihre[11]/Van trappen[12] et al.		Argon Vallon et al.[10]	
	L (%)	L (%)	C (%)	L (%)	C (%)
Total patients	113 (100)	21 (100)	31 (100)	53 (100)	55 (100)
Rebleed within 1 wk	9 (8)	3 (14)	6 (19)	13 (25)	12 (22)
Surgery for bleeding	3 (3)	3 (14)	4 (13)	9 (15)	9 (16)
Deaths	3 (3)	1 (5)	0 (0)	3 (6)	7 (13)

rise to other problems. Exacerbation of bleeding by laser photocoagulation has been reported by several groups. One patient is known to have developed esophageal stenosis after Neodymium-Yag laser treatment of esophageal varices.

Overall, laser photocoagulation appears to be reasonably safe, but further precise data are certainly required.

VIII. DISCUSSION

Endoscopic laser photocoagulation is already being used widely in European patients. This popularity, despite the considerable costs involved, suggests that the technique is valuable, but proof of this is still lacking. The spread of laser photocoagulation, particularly with the Neodymium-Yag instrument in Germany, is largely due to the enthusiasm of Kiefhaber and his group in Munich. They have reported a reduction in mortality in high-risk patients with bleeding ulcers by comparison with earlier years,[6] but such data are difficult to evaluate in a center with a changing referral base. We believe that controlled trials constitute the only method for arriving at an independent assessment. The history of the technique of gastric freezing provides a salutory warning.

Many controlled studies have been started in patients with ulcers, but few are yet complete. Present results do not indicate any major clinical superiority for laser techniques. The results of Escourrou and colleagues are particularly instructive (Table 6). Their treated patients stopped bleeding more quickly than controls, but there was no difference between the two groups after one week. Patients bleed from a spectrum of lesions and vessels. Large clinical trials, or a collection of smaller trials, will be necessary to ensure adequate numbers in all subsets. It is particularly disappointing that present studies have shown no benefit for laser photocoagulation performed prophylactically to prevent rebleeding once initial hemorrhage has ceased; since this is the largest group of patients seen at emergency endoscopy.

The reported results for Neodymium-Yag laser treatment of patients with bleeding esophageal varices are surprisingly good (Table 7) and compare well with those achieved by other emergency procedures.[16-18] It will take many years to establish the precise role of laser photocoagulation in this context.

There are many potential reasons for failure of laser treatment in any individual patient and for failure of particular trials to show a benefit. In the individual patient, laser photocoagulation may fail through lack of adequate access to the bleeding point, because of excess bleeding, or because of anatomical distortion. This has been particularly apparent in the duodenal bulb, where scarring may prevent an accurate aim. The personal skill of the endoscopist concerned is important. It is apparent that the best results have been reported from those centers with the most experience (Table 4); a factor rarely stated, but often important. The size and number of bleeding vessels in a particular ulcer will also affect the results. In this context, it is important to note that the Argon laser has less penetration than the Neodymium-Yag. In the Barcelona study, there are two failures of hemostasis shown later to be due to the size of the vessels—2 and 3 mm in diameter.[10]

A controlled trial may fail to show an existing benefit if its size or protocol is inadequate. There was a trend towards clinical benefit in our own small study in Barcelona. Larger numbers might have reached conventional statistical significance. Most protocols have assessed the value of a single laser treatment. It would be equally logical to repeat laser photocoagulation if rebleeding occurs.

Laser photocoagulation appears to be relatively safe. Although a few perforations have occurred with the Neodymium-Yag equipment, it should be emphasized that other and less obvious hazards must be taken into account in any cost-benefit analysis. Mere prolongation of emergency endoscopy carries hazards to the patient. The time may be better spent in the operating room. These procedures require considerable technical expertise. It is probable that the risks will increase, when and as laser equipment is more widely used outside the developing centers.

The whole concept of emergency endoscopic treatment has considerable implications. The provision of expert teams on very short stand-by call is difficult and expensive. If laser photocoagulation is definitely shown to be of benefit, it is likely to result in the aggregation of bleeding patients into a smaller number of large hospitals. Indeed, it seems probable that the development of "bleeding centers" would improve the prognosis by better application of simple conventional techniques even without expensive new technology.

The high costs of laser equipment is a major disincentive to the uncommitted and has provided a major stimulus to the development and reevaluation of alternative endoscopic techniques. Laser photocoagulation was welcomed because treatment could be provided without touching the lesion and because direct diathermy was considered to be inherently dangerous. This latter disadvantage has not been proven. New diathermy and thermal probes appear to have considerable potential. Several centers initially involved actively in laser photocoagulation are now turning their attention to simpler techniques. However, their lower cost does not reduce the need for stringent clinical evaluation.

REFERENCES

1. **Frühmorgen, P., Bodem, F., Reidenbach, H. D., Kaduk, B., Demling, L., and Brand, H.,** The first endoscopic laser coagulation in the human gi-tract, *Endoscopy,* 7, 156, 1975.
2. **Kiefhaber, P., Nath, G., and Moritz, K.,** Endoscopical control of massive gastrointestinal haemorrhage by irradiation with a higher power Neodymium-Yag laser, *Proc. Surg.,* 15, 140, 1977.
3. **Laurence, B. H., Vallon, A. G., Cotton, P. B.,** Armengol Miro, J. R., Salord-Oses, J. C., LeBodic, L., Sudry, P., Fruhmorgen, P., and Bodem, F., Endoscopic laser photocoagulation for bleeding peptic ulcers, *Lancet,* i, 124, 1980.
4. **Brunetaud, J. M., Enger, A., Flament, J. B., Petit, J., Bergot, M., and Moschetto, Y.,** Utilisation d'un laser a argon ionise en endoscopie digestive: photocoagulation des lesions hemorragiques, *Rev. Phys. Appl.,* 14, 385, 1979.
5. **Frühmorgen, P., Bodem, F., Reidenbach, H. D., and Demling, L.,** Was ist gesichert in der Lasercoagulation zur Stillung gastrointestinaler Blutugen, *Internist,* 19, 707, 1978.
6. **Kiefhaber, P., Moritz, K., Schildberg, F. W., Feifel, G., and Herfarth, C.,** Endoscopic Neodymium-Yag lazer irradiation for control of bleeding acute and chronic ulcers, *Langenbecks Arch. Chir.,* 347, 567, 1978.
7. **Stauber, R. and Schandalik, R.,** Indikationen und Tecknik der endoscopischen laser therapie, *Chirurgica,* 51, 99, 1980.
8. **Stange, E. F., Fleig, W. E., Junge, Y., Merkle, N., and Dirschunert, H.,** Neodymium-Yag laser treatment of upper gastrointestinal bleeding in man: safe and effective, *Gastroenterology,* 78, 1268A, 1980.
9. **Brunetaud, J. M., Brown, S. G., Houche, P., Storey, D., Paris, J. C., and Salmon, P. R.,** Argon laser photocoagulation. The current situation, 4th European Congress Gastrointestinal Endoscopy, Hamburg, 1980.
10. **Vallon, A. G., Cotton, P. B., Laurence, B. H., Armengol Miro, J. R., Salord–Oses, J. C.,** Randomized trial of endoscopic argon laser photocoagulation bleeding peptic ulcers, *Gut,* 1981, in press.
11. **Ihre, T., Johansson, C., Seligson, U., and Torngren, S.,** Endoscopic Yag-laser treatment in massive gastrointestinal bleeding, 1981, in press.
12. **Van Trappen, G., Rutgeerts, P., Broeckaert, L., Janssens, J., and Coremans, G.,** Is treatment of upper gastrointestinal haemorrhage by Nd-Yag laser useful? *Gastroenterology,* 78, 1283A, 1980.
13. **Rohde, H., Thon, K., Fischer, M., Ohmann, C., and Lorenz, W.,** Early endoscopy combined with endoscopic Nd-Yag laser therapy in patients with actively bleeding lesions, IV European Congress Gastrointestinal Endoscopy, Hamburg, 1980.
14. **Griffiths, W. J., Neumann, D. A., and Welsh, J. D.,** The visible vessel as an indicator of uncontrolled or recurrent gastrointestinal haemorrhage, *N. Engl. J. Med.,* 300, 1411, 1979.
15. **Foster, D. N., Miloszewski, K. J. A., and Losowsky, M. S.,** Stigmata of recent haemorrhage in diagnosis and prognosis of upper gastrointestinal bleeding, *Br. Med. J.,* i, 1173, 1978.
16. Editorial. Injection sclerotherapy for oesophageal varices, *Lancet,* ii, 233, 1979.
17. **Scott, J. Long, R. G., Dick, R., and Sherlock, S.,** Percutaneous transhapetic obliteration of gastro-oesophageal varices, *Lancet,* ii, 53, 1976.
18. **Orloff, M. J., Charters, A. C., Chandler, J. G., Condon, J. K., Gramborl, D. E., Modafferi, T. R., Levin, S. E., Brown, N. B., Sviokla, S. C., and Knox, D. G.,** Portacaval shunt as emergency procedure in unselected patients with alcoholic cirrhosis, *Surg. Gynecol. Obstet.,* 141, 59, 1975.
19. **LeBodic, L. and Sudry, P.,** Survey data, 1980.
20. **Kiefhaber, P.,** Survey data, 1980.
21. **Shonekas, H.,** Survey data, 1980.
22. **Sander, R., Posl, H., Spuhler, A., Hitzler, H.,** Der Neodym-Yag-Laser: Ein effecktives instrument fur die Stillung der lebensbedrohlichen. Gastrointestinal blutung, *Leber Magen Darm,* in press, 1980.
23. **Van Trappen, G.,** Survey data, 1980.
24. **Escourrou, J.,** Survey data, 1980.

Chapter 8

TOPICAL THERAPY: CYANOACRYLATES AND OTHER MODALITIES

Stephen E. Silvis

TABLE OF CONTENTS

I. INTRODUCTION

Gastrointestinal endoscopes allow direct visualization of the entire gastrointestinal (GI) tract. In routine clinical medicine, this is generally limited to the mucosa from the mouth to the third portion of the duodenum, and from the anus to the ileo-cecal valve. Examination of the small bowel continues to be rather difficult and bleeding lesions in that area are uncommon; therefore, this procedure is not commonly used. With fiberoptic endoscopes, clear visualization is obtained, and the single or multiple biopsy channels allow the introduction of various instrumentation for treatment. This has allowed consideration of a number of potential agents for the control of GI bleeding.

There are rather strict limitations on the size of the biopsy channel. Whenever the biopsy channel is increased or a second channel added, a compromise must be made between enlarging the total diameter of the instrument or reducing the visual and light-carrying bundles. These limitations exclude the attractive technique of controlling bleeding using conventional surgical methods, i.e., mechanically occluding the vessel with hemostat clips or sutures. Some attempts have been made to produce clips that can be inserted through the endoscope. It has not been feasible to obtain large enough clips to control bleeding and which could be passed through the channel of an endoscope. It is particularly difficult to close a clip on a bleeding vessel. To my knowledge, no one has attempted to use suture material through an endoscope; for this does not seem to be feasible with present instruments. There remains the possibility of modified clips being used through a large-channel endoscope.

The previous Chapters have reviewed the ancient and well-established method of closing bleeding vessels, that is, the application of heat (i.e., direct heat, laser photocoagulation, and electro-coagulation). All of these methods have the disadvantage of producing additional tissue destruction at the site of the bleeding lesion. The modalities considered in this Chapter have major advantages: the relative or complete absence of any additional tissue damage, not having to touch the bleeding lesion with the applicating tube, and the ability to treat wide areas.

Gastrointestinal bleeding remains a major problem. It accounts for approximately 150,000 hospital admissions per year within the U.S. with a median duration of hospitalization of 7.5 days.[1] The average cost per day approximates $300 to $400. A conservative estimate of the national cost of upper GI hemorrhage is between $300 to $450 million per year. Obviously, the economic impact of this problem is immense. In spite of the improvement of diagnostic techniques, the mortality for upper GI bleeding remains approximately 10% which is the same figure noted 30 years ago.[2-22] The reasons for this constant mortality rate are subject to varying influences. For example, the population at risk has changed over the years, particularly with respect to an increasing age. Many of the patients die from causes unrelated to their upper GI hemorrhage. There are numerous etiologies for GI bleeding. However, in all series peptic ulcer disease, diffuse erosive gastritis (or stress ulceration) and esophageal varices make up the majority of cases (generally in the range of 90%).[23-30] The other 10% represents a long list of miscellaneous problems. It is obvious that the treatment of the three major categories of bleeding must be distinctly different. Treatment of esophageal varices requires some effect on either the venous pressure or occlusion of the vein. Peptic ulcer disease responds to local therapy but necessitates the ability to stop sizeable arterial bleeding.

Diffuse hemorrhagic gastritis is a much less clearly defined entity. It may bleed massively and require surgical procedures. In addition, the only effective surgical procedure is either a vagotomy and pyloroplasty or total gastrectomy. This group would be very difficult to study. It requires the treatment of large areas of the gastrointestinal tract without further significant tissue destruction. Mallory-Weiss tears are localized and more easily defined. These lesions can be treated by electrocoagulation or surgery if necessary, but the majority stop bleeding.

A recent ASGE National Prospective Survey demonstrated that the risk of recurrent bleeding was considerably higher in gastric, duodenal, and stomal ulcers.[31-32] Age, associated disease, orthostatic hypotension, hematemesis, and severe anemia on admission are all high-risk factors. From these data, a group of patients can be defined in whom 30% require urgent surgery to stop continued or recurrent bleeding. The surgical mortality in this group was over 20% in contrast with surgical mortality of under 1% in elective gastric surgery. This emphasizes the significant advantage of endoscopy to control bleeding.

In designing a control study of the treatment of GI bleeding, a number of factors must be considered. One of the major problems is that a high percentage of the bleeding lesions will stop spontaneously. If the study includes a large number of patients who spontaneously stop bleeding, then: (1) A very large number of patients need to be included in the study; and (2) the spontaneous rate of cessation is likely to cloud any effect of the therapeutic modality. Another significant problem is: How effective must the therapy be for it to be of interest to the practicing medical community, the endoscopist, and particularly the patient? A modality that would influence the need for surgery in 40 to 50% of the patients would certainly be welcome by all groups. A lower success rate would be of interest if the modality did not produce destruction of normal tissue and was without significant systemic complications. We must bear in mind that even if the group of ulcer patients in whom 30% required urgent surgery, only 30 out of each 100 patients are significant in the results of the study. If effectiveness rates of less than 40 to 50% are of interest, then large groups (over 200) are necessary. An effectiveness rate of 20% would require huge groups of patients (over 800) even when studying the severe group. This amounts to a truly massive endeavor.

It is advisable that patients who rebleed be considered separately from those who continue to bleed for the first 24 hr. A number of patients need to be excluded from any study. If patients with catastrophic associated illnesses are to be included, this would obviously skew the results of the studies. They would need to have another stratification of the randomization process and, under any circumstances, this would complicate evaluation of results.

There are also ethical considerations. Upper GI endoscopy has a low but real morbidity.[33-37] It is probably higher in the actively bleeding patient.[31-32] This brings up the question of whether sham therapy can be justified, i.e., where the patient is endoscoped and the therapy is either given or not given by randomization. If sham therapy is not given, the question of whether the therapy is injurious or not remains unanswered. In addition, the study becomes a single, rather than a double-blind study.

From the previously mentioned problems, it is obvious that no hospital in this country has adequate numbers of patients for a control clinical trial. This makes a multicentered study imperative. There are numerous advantages and disadvantages to multicentered studies. The obvious advantage is that sufficient numbers of cases to obtain data can be studied in a reasonable period of time. The disadvantages are—the complexity of the administration of the study, the difficulty in assuring that the patient populations are similar, and that the operators are using identical criterion to admit and treat the patients. There probably needs to be a separate randomization within the hospitals, so that like numbers of patients from each institution fall into each therapeutic group. In a number of control studies, flaws in design or execution can cloud the final results and can lead to an ongoing debate after the study is completed. Examples of this phenomenon would be the control study on hypoglycemia agents in diabetes[38-40] and the coronary bypass control studies.[41-44] While these studies were carefully planned, problems with the execution cause a continuing debate as to whether their findings are valid for many reasons.[39,40,43,44] The discussion of these debates is inappropriate to the current Chapter. Notwithstanding these disadvantages, it is obvious that control studies of the endoscopic treatment of upper GI bleeding should be done early, carefully, and with sufficient numbers to make an intelligent scientific decision. In any disease entity that is so variable, both in its etiology and course, as upper GI bleeding, uncontrolled studies no matter how large are not going to give a convincing answer. We have all studied the reports of enthusiastic investigators with a new modality showing an improvement over historical controls only to see the effect disappear with controlled studies. The reasons for this phenomenon are multiple relating to other therapeutic agents being used, differences in technique, and difference in patient selection for entry into the study. The fact that we generally accept a probability of less than 5% as effective, and the probability of positive studies being published over negative, is at least in a ratio of 20:1 or greater. Therefore, the negative studies will probably not be published in medical journals until after the positive ones have already been printed.

It is questionable if a decrease in mortality from gastrointestinal bleeding has been realized with modern endoscopic techniques.[45-54] This suggests the urgent need for improvements in therapy. One of these potential improvements would be a satisfactory endoscopic method.[55] The techniques of applying heat are not applicable in an extensive lesion such as a hemorrhagic gastritis and the topical agent may not be effective in the localized lesions with brisk bleeding. It may be that a combination of a local treatment such as coagulation of a bleeding vessel followed by protecting the area with a coating agent will be the ultimate method of controlling bleeding, that is, (a suture and a band-aid).

II. TISSUE ADHESIVES

Considerable interest in clinical and experimental medicine has been raised by tissue adhesives since the synthesis of cyanoacrylate analogs.[56-58] The structural formula of these compounds is shown below:

$$\begin{array}{ccccccc} & & C \equiv N & & & & \\ & & 1 & & & & \\ CH_2 & = & C & - & C = O & - & R \end{array}$$

Cyanoacrylates

$$\begin{array}{ccccccccccccc} & & & & C \equiv N & & & & & & \\ & & & & 1 & & & & & & CH_3 \\ CH_2 & = & C & - & C = O & - & O & - & C & - & C\,F_3\text{—}R \\ & & & & & & & & 1 & & \\ & & & & & & & & H & & \end{array}$$

Trifluoroisopropyl—cyanoacrylate MBR 4197 (flucrylate)

They differ in the side-chain substitution (R) onto the cyanoacrylate nucleus. The compounds that have been studied in clinical or experimental medicine have been methyl, ethyl, butyl, N-butyl, isobutyl, propyl, isopropyl, and trifluoroisopropyl cyanoacrylate.[59-71] Rather extensive literature has developed in using these agents to occlude blood vessels to control bleeding in seriously contused areas, in treatment of dental socket bleeding, and more recently, in treating upper GI bleeding both topically and by the occlusion of vessels.[72-100]

The various cyanoacrylates differ primarily in the speed with which they polymerize, the degree of tissue irritation they produce, and their biodegradability. For example, methyl-cyanoacrylate (the super glue) polymerizes extremely rapidly, is relatively rapidly biodegradable, and produces an intense tissue irritation. At the other extreme, the isopropyl-cyanoacrylate is slowly biodegradable, produces minimum tissue reaction, and polymerizes more slowly. The trifluoroisopropyl (MBR 4197) is intermediate in these reactions, as is the ethyl-cyanoacrylate. Cyanoacrylate polymerization is triggered by the exposure to moisture; the polymer is resistent to both acid and alkaline pH. There does not appear to be systemic toxicity from the cyanoacrylates.[72-100]

The only other resin which has been suggested for control of GI bleeding is carboset reported by Keller and Logan.[101] This compound, however, is not resistant to alkaline digestion (personal observation).

MBR 4197 (flucrylate) has been extensively studied by both Minnesota Mining and Manufacturing Company and other investigators. In studies by Nelson et al.,[89] this compound was shown to have significantly less tissue irritation than the methyl-cyanoacrylate and to have a high bonding strength essentially equal to methyl and butyl cyanoacrylates. It is slowly biodegradable. Bonding strength was studied in comparison to the isobutyl compound by Dellevigne et al.[90] He found the tensil strength of bonds between tissue and various substrates to be about equal in the two polymers. The agent was studied in dogs by Payne et al.[91] who concluded that it gave a rapid satisfactory bond when properly applied. He used it in intestinal anastomosis, skin grafts, and to obtain hemostasis in hepatic lobectomy. The biological reactivity of the compound in his model was rather low.

The story of the development and investigation of the cyanoacrylates illustrates many of the pitfalls of clinical research and development. These compounds were originally believed to have their potential role as an adjunct to suturing during operations. There are at least two reasons most investigators have abandoned this as a role: (1) If any of the material comes between the cut edges of tissue, it tends to interfere with healing, and (2) the automatic stapling devices have come into use in the time-consuming intestinal anastomoses. In addition, it has been shown that at least some suture material is necessary to hold tissues together to approximate the edges when a polymer is being used. The agents have been rather extensively used in the Viet Nam conflict to control bleeding from contused lesions.[80,82,87] It is somewhat difficult to evaluate this literature because these patients were very severely injured and had multiple therapies, including treatment with the cyanoacrylate.

It became apparent that the methyl-cyanoacrylate was probably too irritating to tissues to be useful. In addition, it polymerized extremely rapidly which was probably neither necessary nor desirable. Additional compounds were synthesized with different characteristics. Toxicology studies were performed failing to show systemic toxicity of the compounds.[63,77,93] Due to the very long biological half—life of these compounds, a concern about carcinogenesis was raised. There were two studies of MBR 4197 by Mesrobian and Sklar[92,93] which failed to demonstrate a carcinogenic effect of the compound when painted for long periods on hamster pouches. They concluded that the compound was not carcinogenic.

Tissue adhesives have been shown to be of value in the closing of spinal fluid fistula leaks,[94] vascular aneurysms,[95] large wounds of vascular organs such as the kidney, liver, spleen, or retroperitoneal space,[91,96] in the clotting of varices,[97] and in supplying a dressing that could not otherwise be applied.[88] They produce rapid and complete hemostasis in dental surgery[59-63,98] and more recently have been used for the injection of esophageal varices.[99,100]

Two animal studies of MBR 4197 have been conducted. The first by Martin and

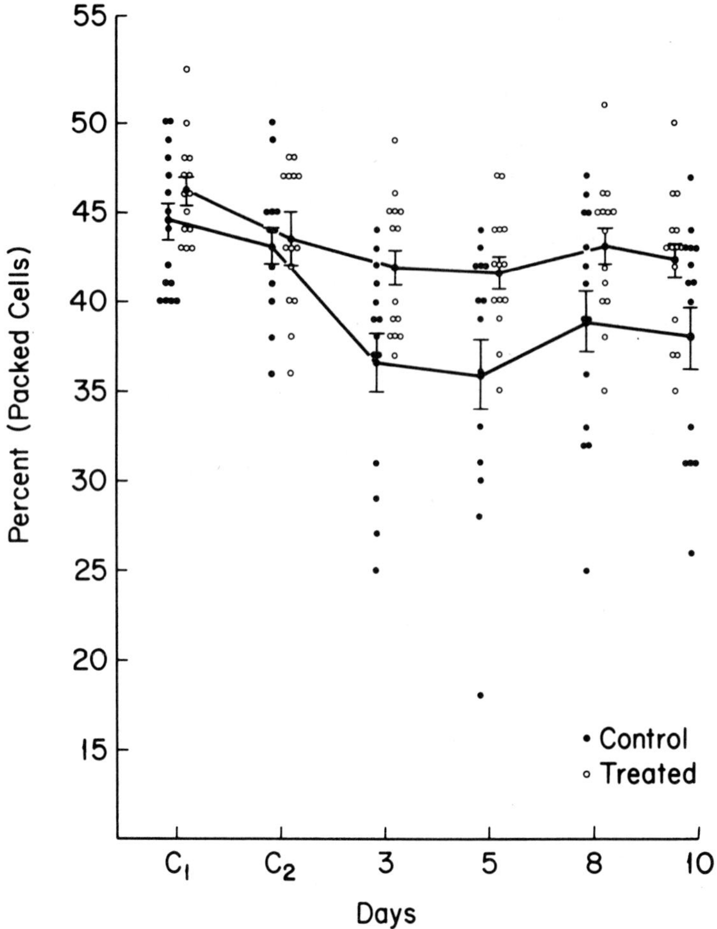

FIGURE 1. The hematocrits of the control dogs are shown in the black circles and the hematocrits of the treated dogs are shown in the open circles. The brackets show two standard errors of the mean (2 SEM) and the lines connect the means. C_1 represents the hematocrits done at the time the ulcers were made and C_2, the hematocrits at the time that the first therapy or placebo was given. The slight decrease in the mean hematocrit between C_1 and C_2 represents bleeding from the ulcer production. Significantly different hematocrits were found on days three, five, and ten ($p < 0.05$). In addition, it can be seen that five of the 14 control dogs, but none of the treated animals, had hematocrits below 35%.

Silvis[102] showed a significant decrease in the degree of bleeding from chronic ulcer model in dogs. This model consisted of removing a loop of gastric mucosa with a snare and minimum cutting current, waiting three days, anticoagulating the dog, and measuring the degree of hematocrit fall. Figure 1 shows the individual hematocrits of the dogs treated with MBR 4197. It illustrates that all of the severe bleeding demonstrated by a marked fall in hematocrits, was eliminated by the treatment.

In addition, these studies answered the questions: Could MBR 4197 be delivered through an endoscope, did it adhere to the tissue, did it reduce bleeding in the chronic model, and did it affect the rate of healing? All of these questions were answered in an affirmative manner. The agent would adhere for 2 to 6 days to abnormal tissue. It adhered very briefly to normal gastric mucosal tissue. The polymer is aerosolized down a plastic delivery tube. Figure 2 shows the equipment to wash the lesion and to blow CO_2

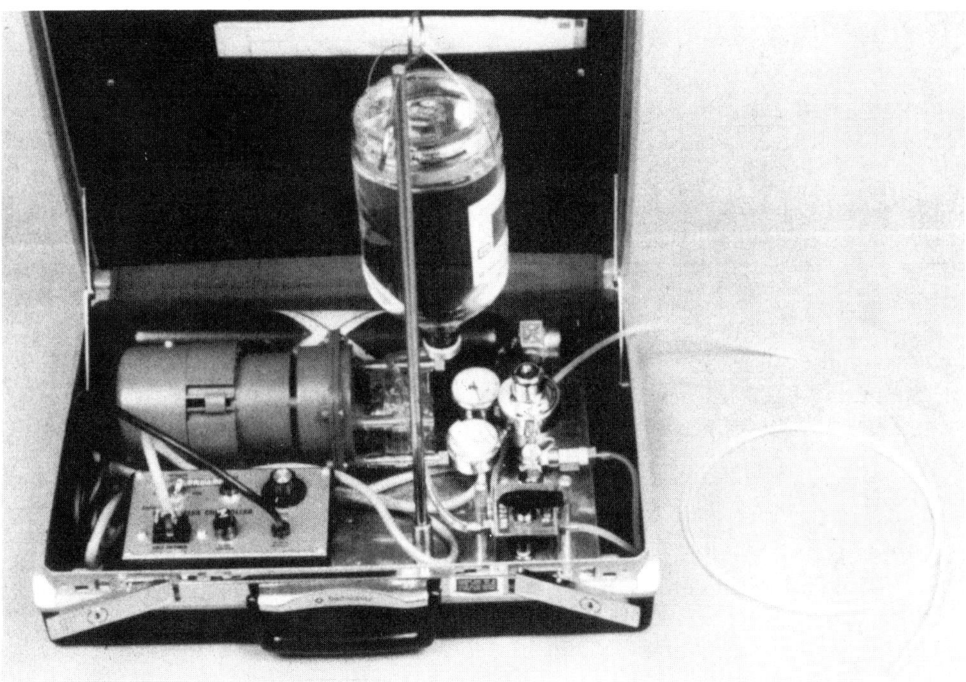

FIGURE 2. This machine was developed to wash and "dry" lesions. Normal saline is used to wash the lesion and a short burst of CO_2 (30 psi) is delivered through the same catheter to dry the lesion.

Table 1
SUMMARY OF PATIENTS, TREATED WITH MBR 4197

Diagnosis	Success
Bleeding ulcers	5/6
Varices	0/1
Esophagitis	6/6
Cancer	1/1
Technical failures (4)	
Success: treated	12/14
Total	12/18

to dry the lesion preceding the delivery of the polymer. The second study was done by Protell et al.[103] with the standard ulcer model.[104] In this study, they could not demonstrate a significant effect of the polymer in a brisk bleeding model.

Clinical experience was obtained and reported by Martin et al.[105] He reported on six patients in whom bleeding was controlled in five of the six and was felt to be life-saving in three patients. These same investigators have now treated a total of 14 patients and have demonstrated control of the bleeding in 12 of the 14.

Table 1 shows a summary of the patients treated with MBR 4197.

On the basis of these encouraging animal and clinical studies, notwithstanding the one negative animal study, a controlled clinical trial was designed and undertaken. The reason for going ahead even with a negative animal study was that the ulcer maker produces an acute lesion with a loose area between the mucosa and submucosa. This is not present in chronic ulcer disease where it is bound down by inflammatory tissue. In addition, very brisk arterial bleeding is produced with this model with bleeding at the rate of up to 2 to 3 cc/min. This type of bleeding in clinical medicine is seldomly observed (3 cc/min. would result in 180 cc an hour or over 4000 cc in 24 hr). This is higher than the rate of bleeding usually seen or that one would be willing to temporize with for any length of time prior to surgical intervention.

Design of the controlled protocol was as follows—patients with peptic ulcer (gastric or duodenal), significant bleeding defined as a hemoglobin under 10, supine or postural hypotension, and recent bleeding from the ulcer. Active bleeding—defined as active bleeding at endoscopy or evidence of recent blood loss with the presence of a clot in the ulcer base. Exclusions were as follows:

1. Hereditary clotting defects
2. Bleeding from multiple sites
3. The presence of more than two peptic ulcers
4. Previous ulcer surgery
5. Coma, delerium tremers, psychosis
6. Hepatic, cardiac, renal, or respiratory failure

In summary, the group of cases selected were those with peptic ulcers who had bled recently and would be candidates for surgery if they continued to bleed and did not have extremely severe associated diseases.

The design was to randomize between conventional therapy, which would include blood transfusions, antacids, or cimetidine and nasogastric suction for 24 to 48 hr, and MBR 4197 therapy, which was given at the time of admission and repeated in 2 to 3 days. Observations were:

1. Hemoglobin, hematocrit changes
2. Blood transfusion requirements
3. Need for surgery
4. Overall mortality

This study was designed to determine if direct endoscopic application of trifluoroisopropyl cyanoacrylate (MBR 4197) would effectively stop bleeding from gastric and duodenal ulcers and prevent rebleeding from these lesions. Active and recent active bleeders with gastric and duodenal ulcers were randomized to receive conventional therapy alone (controls) or conventional therapy plus MBR 4197 (treatment) applied immediately and reapplied in 48 hr. Cessation of bleeding, evidence of rebleeding, number of units of blood transfused, and requirements for surgery were then assessed. Fifty-two patients, 24 treatment and 28 controls, were evaluated. Six of the 24 patients continued to bleed or rebled in spite of MBR 4197 application, and all required surgery. Four of 28 controls continued bleeding and 3 of 4 required surgery. Total number of units transfused in the treatment group before and after application of polymer were 56/56 compared to 33/55 for the controls before and after entrance into the study.[106]

A somewhat more severe group was assigned by randomization into the treatment group. There were considerable problems with the delivery system in this multicentered study. On analysis of this data, it was apparent that a very large study would be necessary to show efficacy. There was difficulty in obtaining material and the sponsoring company elected to terminate the study in August of 1979. This compound has not been entirely abandoned, but is not actively being investigated at the present time. The lessons learned from this study are multiple. It is essential to pick out a group of patients that will have a high incidence of rebleeding. It is necessary to stratify randomization so the treated and control group distribute equal risk factors. As previously discussed, unless an agent is almost 100% effective, a rather sizeable group will be necessary to show efficacy. Any technical problems will seriously interfere with the evaluation of the study.

This author feels that the cyanoacrylates may have potential as a method of controlling GI bleeding and should not be abandoned.

From the above study, a number of questions remain:

1. Was the wrong group of patients studied? This agent may be effective against diffuse mucosal bleeding, but not arterial bleeding.
2. Stratified randomization may have given more equal groups and may have shown a positive effect.
3. Washing and drying may have increased bleeding while mechanical problems may have obliterated the effect of the polymer.
4. The polymer may not be effective.

Attempts to aerosol some of the other polymers would be worthwhile. When properly applied in patients, brisk arterial spurting was very impressively and immediately controlled.[105] Its great advantages are the lack of tissue destruction, the ability to use standard equipment, and the relatively inexpensive agent and delivery system. Although no polymers are currently available for investigation, this modality may yield a positive method for treating bleeding patients which would allow treatment of all bleeding lesions.

III. THE USE OF ENDOSCOPIC CLOTTING AGENTS

The addition of clotting agents to irrigation solutions was used rather extensively in the past with generally disappointing results. This technique produced massive clotting of blood within the stomach, but did not affect the bleeding lesion.

Recently, special endoscopic delivery equipment has been devised by Linscheer and Fazio.[107] With the combination of fibrinogen thrombin with saline and Co_2 wash, they have shown the ability to control the bleeding from an artificial ulcer model. This technique should produce no tissue damage. It produces a clot which could be autodigested by the enzymes in the stomach and may require some protection of the clot while healing occurs. There are only the minimal risks of the endoscopy and hepatitis from the fibrinogen used in this therapeutic procedure. The risk of hepatitis upon topical application may be less than with intravenous administration, but this is not established. The authors who have developed the method feel that it is ready for controlled clinical trial. It has the advantages of the other topical methods, the delivery equipment is portable, relatively inexpensive, and can be used through standard equipment and the technique can probably be mastered in a short time.

In Figure 3, reprinted from the article by Linscheer and Fazio,[107] the delivery system is shown consisting of a molded four-lumen catheter which allows separate delivery of saline and compressed CO_2 to wash and cleanse the lesion and two channels for delivering the thrombin and fibrinogen. In Figure 4,[107] the result of these studies is shown. The technique reduces bleeding both with and without heparinization. Saline irrigation increases the bleeding which was not entirely stopped by the therapy. This suggests that brisk arterial bleeding may be difficult to control with clotting factors. There was no difference between alternating thrombin and fibrinogen, therefore, the two agents were given together. Histological sections demonstrate a thin fibrin layer over the ulcer base. They report that there was some hematoma formation around the

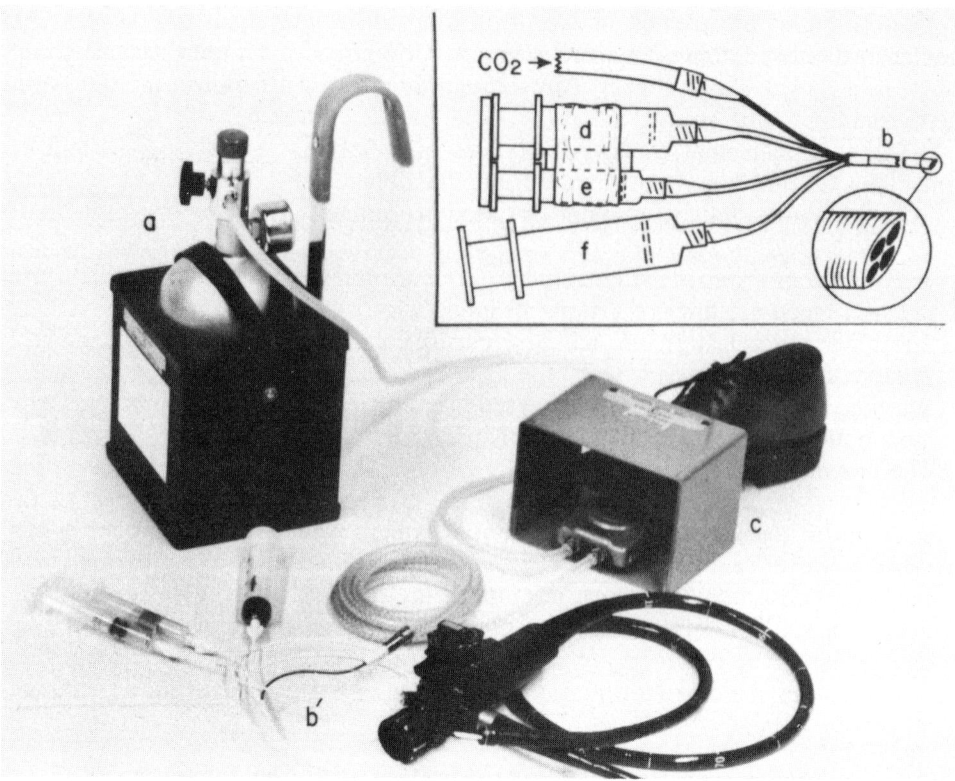

FIGURE 3. Spraying device (made by Medi-Tech, Watertown, Mass.). (a) CO_2 pressure tank with pressure reducer; (b) 2 mm diameter, 4-lumen catheter, 250 cm long; (c) foot pedal; (d) and (e) twin syringe (CP 10 m*l*, thrombin 5 m*l*); (f) saline syringe (30 m*l*).

ulcer base probably related to submucosal bleeding. An uncontrolled clinical trial appeared to have a positive effect.[108] They feel that the technique is ready for clinical testing in a controlled manner because it had demonstrated control of bleeding in both heparinized and nonheparininzed canine models.

Jensen et al.[109] studied the same clotting factors and failed to demonstrate reliable hemostasis in standard ulcers or gastric erosion whether applied at laparotomy or endoscopically. It is unclear why the results of the two groups of investigators differ. This author would be somewhat concerned about rebleeding following clot lysis. This question remains for clinical studies to determine. It is unlikely that this can be studied in animal models because it is difficult to produce chronic bleeding with or without heparinization. There is a great tendency for animal models to stop bleeding. The rebleeding rate in the dog even when heparinized is not universal. The possibility of clotting factors becoming a clinical modality in the control of GI bleeding remains to be determined. The polylumen tube, as designed by Linscheer and Fazio,[107] has merit if multiple agents are utilized in endoscopic therapy. In most of the therapeutic endeavors, a cleaning jet with a liquid, plus drying with carbon dioxide, was necessary before the application of the therapeutic agent.

IV. COLLAGEN

Recent studies by Kline et al.[110] demonstrated a significant reduction in bleeding in dogs from the standard ulcer model when treated with collagen. They showed a decrease of total blood loss of about 60% in the treated ulcers. None of the ulcers

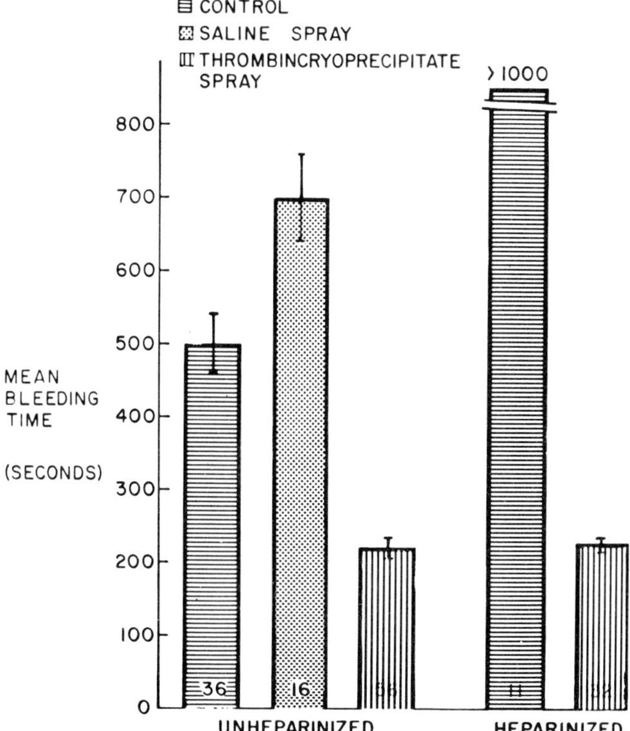

FIGURE 4. The effect of spraying treatment on bleeding is shown which illustrates the following points: (1) Washing with saline alone increases the bleeding, (2) bleeding is decreased in both heparinized and nonheparinized dogs, and (3) in neither ulcer model is the bleeding stopped immediately and completely.

treated with the dry collagen continued to bleed, compared to 29% of the control ulcers, which were bleeding actively at the end of the test period. There was no difference between the slurry mixture and the dry powder.

The agent used was Avitene.® This is a microcrystalline collagen initially described by Hait et al.[111] in 1969. It is a water-soluble hydrochloric acid salt derived from bovine skin. The cross linkage coming off the fibers preserves the structure in the microcrystals at a submicron level.[112-113] Histological examination of tissue treated with this collagen shows that it is slowly biodegradable and does not interfere with wound healing. In addition, it has been shown to be nontoxic.[114-118] Intraperitoneal administration of 5 gm/k in dogs produced no untoward effects.[116] No tetragenicity has been observed and immunological studies show it to be only weakly antigenic.[119-120] Hemostasis is thought to be achieved by activation of the intrinsic clotting mechanism. It may attract platelets and trigger their adhesiveness to the collagen fibrils, thus stimulating the platelet release mechanism. In addition, the microcrystalline collagen swells during gel formation when in contact with blood to seal small vessels like an adhesive patch.[121-124] Even after heparin and salicylate administration the hemostatic activity is retained in experimental animals.[124] Only in the severely thrombocytopenic animals with platelet counts less than 10,000 is hemostasis impaired. This agent is not effective in severe clotting disorders such as hemophilia. In studies on skin donor sites, it has been shown to decrease the amount of bleeding and does not affect wound healing. It has been reported to be effective in controlling the superficial bleeding from splenic injuries and has been used to control bleeding from the liver and anastomotic sites. Avitene® may be particularly helpful in patients undergoing surgery who have received heparin preoperatively.[124] A study by Hanisch et al.[125] showed Avitene® to be more effective in controlling prostatic hemorrhage than gelfoam. Alexander and Rabinovitz[126] studied its effect on oral wounds in animals. In dogs it was more effective than gelfoam or Surgicel® as a topical hemostatic agent. Weinstein et al.[127] studied its effect on splenic trauma. A total of 24 patients were entered into the study. Six patients required splenectomy and 18 patients had all or portions of their injured spleen salvaged. Nine of the 18 salvaged spleens required only suturing and topical application of Avitene® for hemostasis. The remaining nine had more extensive procedures including partial splenectomy. Three patients required oversewing of the spleen and bleeding surfaces with ligation of vessels without removal of the splenic tissue. There were no postoperative complications resulting from attempts at splenic salvage. Sixteen of the 18 undergoing splenorrhaphy had functional splenic tissue on postoperative scanning.

This technique is of interest because of its lack of tissue destruction, its apparent very low risk, and its ability to use standard equipment. It is unclear from the published abstracts the exact method that the authors intend for endoscopic delivery. Would this be as a powder or some type of liquid spray? The collagen is very slowly biodegradable and would not be affected by clot lysis. The equipment must be developed to quickly deliver either powder or a thick liquid to control major bleeding. The adherence of the material to a gastritis model obviously needs to be tested. Current data show reduction of bleeding in the dog ulcer model but questions remain as to whether it will stop major arterial bleeding. The collagen is very interesting but requires further laboratory work prior to clinical trials.

V. USE OF MICRO-IRON PARTICLES AND ELECTROMAGNETS

This is a unique methodology suggested by Smith et al.[128] involving the principle of ferromagnetics to tamponade. This ferro-magnet suspension consists of elemental iron powder, thrombin, carboxy-methyl-cellulose, glycerol and water. It can be injected down an endoscopic catheter to the mucosal surface of bleeding lesions. A powerful electromagnet is used to pull the material against the gastric wall. It has been shown to be effective in the control of hemorrhagic gastritis in animals. There is a problem according to Carlson et al.[129] controlling arterial bleeding in the standardized ulcer model. In their studies,[129] the technique was effective in only 48% of standard ulcers but was effective in the control of bleeding from acute gastric erosions. No tissue damage resulted from their therapy. One would anticipate difficulty in controlling ulcer bleeding by this method because of the inability of the magnetic iron to coapt large blood vessels. This technique needs a powerful electromagnet which would be relatively immobile. Its primary advantage is its ability to treat diffuse lesions. Clinical trials have shown tentative positive effects on patients. It may be a desirable therapy in diffuse lesions that are not amendable to electrocoagulation or laser discussed in previous Chapters.

VI. VASO-CONSTRICTOR AGENTS

Irrigation of the stomach with vaso-constrictors has been used in a small number of studies.[130-132] These showed a positive effect, but in an uncontrolled manner. Generally, there has been little enthusiasm for their local endoscopic use. It may be of value to transiently decrease the rate of bleeding by direct spray application prior to treating with a more definitive agent. This complicates the whole experimental design of using more than one therapy in a given patient. It seems unlikely that vaso-constricting agents will play a major role in the control of gastrointestinal bleeding by endoscopic methods.

VII. SUMMARY OF THE TOPICAL AGENTS FOR THE CONTROL OF UPPER GI BLEEDING

These methods have considerable theoretical advantage. For the most part, they have little risk and little tissue damage. They can be delivered by simple techniques. They are portable and should be inexpensive. Further exploration of a number of these techniques is warranted. They probably represent the only endoscopic method that has potential to be effective in the treatment of diffuse mucosal lesions.

In conclusion, although most of these techniques are not ready for extensive clinical testing at the present time, they appear to be fruitful areas for further investigation.

REFERENCES

1. **Grossman, M. I.,** Digestive diseases as a national problem, *Gastroenterology,* 53, 821, 1967.
2. **Crohn, B. B.,** Need for aggressive therapy in massive upper gastrointestinal hemorrhage, *JAMA,* 151, 625, 1953.
3. **Krag, E.,** Acute hemorrhage in peptic ulcer, *Acta Med. Scand.,* 80, 339, 1966.
4. **Shiller, K. F. R., Truelove, S. D., and Williams, D. C.,** Haematemesis and melena with special reference to factors influencing the outcome, *Br. Med. J.,* 2, 7, 1970.
5. **Hamalgyi, A. F.,** A critical review of 425 patients with upper gastrointestinal hemorrhage, *Surg. Gynecol. Obstet.,* 130, 419, 1970.
6. **Skillman, J. J., Gould, S. A., Chung, S. K., and Silen, W.,** The gastric mucosal barrier: Clinical and experimental studies in critically ill and normal man, and in the rabbit, *Ann. Surg.,* 172, 564, 1970.
7. **MacCraig, J. N., Strange, S. L., and Norris, T. S.,** Hemorrhage from the upper alimentary tract, *Gut,* 5, 136, 1964.
8. **Gordon, H. E.,** Diagnosis and management of gastrointestinal bleeding, *Ann. Int. Med.,* 71, 993, 1969.
9. **Stewart, J. D., Schaer, S.M., Potter, W. H., and Massover, A. J.,** Management of massively bleeding peptic ulcer, *Ann. Surg.,* 128, 791, 1948.
10. **Enquist, I. F., Karlson, K. E., and Dennis, C.,** Statistically valid 10-year comparative evaluation of 3 methods of management of massive gastroduodenal hemorrhage, *Ann. Surg.,* 162, 550, 1965.
11. **Read, R. C., Huebl, H. C., and Thal, A. P.,** Randomized study for massive bleeding from peptic ulcer., *Ann. Surg.,* 162, 561, 1965.
12. **Fogelman, J. J. and Garvey, J. M.,** Acute gastroduodenal ulceration incident to surgery and disease: Analysis and review of 88 cases, *Am. J. Surg.,* 112, 615, 1966.
13. **Sherlock, S.,** Hematemesis in portal hypertension, *Br. J. Surg.,* 51, 746, 1964.
14. **Orloff, M. J., Halasz, N. A., Lipman, C., Schwabe, A. D., Thompson, J. C., and Weidner, W. A.,** The complications of cirrhosis of the liver, *Ann. Int. Med.,* 66, 165, 1967.
15. **Editorial,** Gastrointestinal bleeding—what progress? *Lancet,* 1, 1157, 1970.
16. **Morrisey, J. F.,** Gastrointestinal endoscopy, *Gastroenterology,* 62, 1241, 1972.
17. **McGinn, F. P., Guyer, P. B., Wilken, B. J., and Steer, H. W.,** A prospective comparative trial between early endoscopy and radiology in acute upper gastrointestinal hemorrhage, *Gut,* 16, 707, 1975.
18. **Katon, R. M. and Smith, F. W.,** Panendoscopy in the early diagnosis of acute upper gastrointestinal bleeding, *Gastroenterology,* 65, 728, 1973.
19. **Northfield, T. C.,** Acute gastrointestinal hemorrhage, *Br. J. Hosp. Med.,* 8, 325, 1972.
20. **Johnson, S. J., Jones, P. F., Kyle, J. J., and Needham, C. D.,** Epidemiology and course of gastrointestinal hemorrhage, *Br. Med. J.,* 3, 655, 1973.
21. **Wilson, D. E., and Chalmers, T. C.,** Management of emergencies: acute hemorrhage from the upper gastrointestinal tract, *N. Engl. J. Med.,* 274, 1368, 1966.
22. **Lucas, C. E., Sugawa, C., Riddle, J., Rector, F., Rosenberg, B., Watt, A. J.,** Natural history and surgical dilemma of stress gastric bleeding, *Arch. Surg.,* 102, 266, 1971.
23. **Palmer, E. D.,** The vigorous diagnostic approach to upper-gastrointestinal tract hemorrhage. A 23 year prospective study of 1400 patients, *JAMA,* 207, 1477, 1969.
24. **Hedberg, S. E.,** Endoscopy in gastrointestinal bleeding. A systematic approach to diagnosis, *Surg., Clin. N. Am.,* 54, 549, 1974.

25. **Josen, A. S., Giuliani, E., Voorhees, A. B., and Ferrer, J. M., Jr.,** Immediate endoscopic diagnosis of upper gastrointestinal bleeding. Its accuracy and value in relation to associated pathology, *Arch. Surg.,* 11, 980, 1976.
26. **Katz, D., Pitchumoni, C. S., Thomas, E., and Antonelle, M.,** The endoscopic diagnosis of upper-gastrointestinal hemorrhage. Changing concepts of etiology and management, *Am. J. Dig. Dis.,* 21, 182, 1976.
27. **Cotton, P. B., Rosenberg, M. T., Waldram, R. P., and Axon, A. T. R.,** Early endoscopy of oesophagus, stomach and duodenal bulb in patients with haematemesis and melaena, *Br. Med. J.,* 2, 505, 1973.
28. **Dagradi, A. E., Rinz, A. E., and Weingarten, Z. G.,** Influence of emergency endoscopy on the management and outcome of patients with upper gastrointestinal hemorrhage, *Am. J. Gastroenterol.,* 72, 403, 1979.
29. **Cello, J. P. and Theoni, R. F.,** Gastrointestinal hemorrhage. Comparative values of double contrast upper gastrointestinal radiology and endoscopy, *JAMA,* 243, 685, 1980.
30. **Sugawa, C., Werner, M. H., Hayes, D. F., Lucas, C. E., and Watt, A. J.,** Early endoscopy. A guide to therapy for acute hemorrhage in the upper gastrointestinal tract, *Arch. Surg.,* 107, 133, 1973.
31. **Gilbert, D. A., Silverstein, F. E., Tedesco, F., Persing, J., and 677 members of the ASGE,** Endoscopy in upper gastrointestinal bleeding. Preliminary results of the National ASGE Bleeding Survey, *Gastrointest. Endosc.,* 25, 39, 1979.
32. **Gilbert, D. A.,** Clinical and endoscopic predictive features in upper gastrointestinal bleeding. ASGE Course—Endoscopy Update 1980, Salt Lake City, May 22 to 23, 1980.
33. **Silvis, S. E., Nebel, O., Rogers, G., Sugawa, C., and Mandelstam, P.,** Endoscopic complications: results of 1974 ASGE Survey, *JAMA,* 235, 928, 1976.
34. **Katz, D.,** Morbidity and mortality in standard and flexible gastrointestinal endoscopy, *Gastrointest. Endosc.,* 15, 134, 1969.
35. **Schindler, R.,** Results of the questionnaire on fatalities in gastroscopy, *Am. J. Dig. Dis.,* 7, 293, 1940.
36. **Jones, A. F., Doll, R., Fletcher, C., and Rogers, H. W.,** The risks of gastroscopy: A survey of 49,000 examinations, *Lancet,* 1, 647, 1951.
37. **Palmer, E. D. and Wirts, C. W.,** Survey of gastroscopic and esophagoscopic accidents, *JAMA,* 164, 2012, 1957.
38. **University Group Diabetes Program,** A study of the effects of oral hypoglycemia on vascular complications in patients with AODM, Diabetes, 19 (Suppl. 2), 747, 1970.
39. **Knatterud, G. L., Meinert, C. L., Klimt, C. R., Osborne, R. K., and Martin, D. B.,** Effects of oral hypoglycemic agents on vascular complications in patients with AODM, *JAMA,* 217, 777, 1971.
40. **Seltzer, H. S.,** A summary of criticisms of the findings and conclusions of the UGDP, *Diabetes,* 21, 976, 1972.
41. **Bertolasi, C. A., Tronge, J. E., Riccitelli, M. A., Villamayor, R. M., and Zuffardi, E.,** Natural history of unstable angina with medical or surgical therapy, *Chest,* 70, 596, 1976.
42. **Murphy, M. L., Hultgren, H. N., Detre, K., Thomsen, J., Takaro, T., and Participants of the Veterans Administration Cooperative Study,** Treatment of chronic stable angina: A preliminary report of survival data of the randomized Veterans Administration Cooperative Study, *N. Engl. J. Med.,* 297, 621, 1977.
43. **McIntosh, H. D. and Garcia, J. A.,** The first decade of aortocoronary bypass grafting, *Circulation,* 57, 405, 1978.
44. **Chalmers, T. C., Proudfit, W. L., Feinstein, A. R., and DiBona, G. F.,** Symposium: The scientific uses and abuses of the clinical trial: Treatment of chronic stable angina with saphenous vein bypass grafting: Randomized Veterans Administration Cooperative Study, *Clin. Res.,* 26, 229, 1978.
45. **Hoare, A. M.,** Comparative study between endoscopy and radiology in acute upper gastrointestinal hemorrhage, *Br. Med. J.,* 1, 27, 1975.
46. **The role of endoscopy in the management of upper gastrointestinal hemorrhage,** reprints may be obtained from Executive Secretary, ASGE, 13 Elm St. P.O. Box 1565, Worchester, Massachusetts 01944.
47. **Hellers, G. and Ihre, T.,** Impact of change to early diagnosis and surgery in major upper gastrointestinal bleeding, *Lancet,* 2, 1250, 1975.
48. **Sandlow, L. J., Becker, G. H., Spellberg, M. H., Allens, H. A., Berg, M., Berry, L. H., and Newman, E. A.,** A prospective randomized study of the management of upper gastrointestinal hemorrhage, *Am. J. Gastroenterol.,* 61, 282, 1973.
49. **Keller, R. T. and Logan, G. M., Jr.,** Comparison of emergent endoscopy and upper gastrointestinal series radiography in acute upper gastrointestinal hemorrhage, *Gut,* 17, 180, 1976.
50. **Graham, D. Y. and David, R. E.,** Acute upper gastrointestinal hemorrhage. New observations on an old problem, *Am. J. Dig. Dis.,* 23, 76, 1978.

51. **Allan, R. and Dykes, P.,** A comparison of routine and selective endoscopy in the management of acute gastrointestinal hemorrhage, *Gastrointest. Endosc.,* 20, 154, 1974.
52. **Morris, D. W., Levine, G. M., Soloway, R. D., Miller, W. G., Goehel, M. A., and GI Section of University of Pennsylvania,** Prospective, randomized study of diagnosis and outcome in acute upper-gastrointestinal bleeding: endoscopy versus conventional radiography, *Am. J., Dig. Dis.,* 20, 1103, 1975.
53. **Stevenson, G. W., Cox, R. R., and Roberts, C. J.,** Prospective comparison of double-contrast barium meal examination and fibreoptic endoscopy in acute upper gastrointestinal hemorrhage, *Br. Med. J.,* 2, 723, 1976.
54. **Peterson, W., Barnet, C., Smith, H., Allen, M., and Corbett, D.,** A randomized, controlled trial of endoscopy and upper gastrointestinal hemorrhage, *Gastroenterology,* 78, 1236, 1980.
55. **Katon, R. M.,** Experimental conrol of gastrointestinal hemorrhage via the endoscope: A new era dawns, *Gastroenterology,* 70, 272, 1976.
56. **Awe, W. C., Roberts, W., and Braunwald, N. S.,** Rapidly polymerizing adhesive as a hemostatic agent: Study of tissue response and bacteriological properties, *Surgery,* 54, 322, 1963.
57. **Lewers, D. T., Just-Viera, J. O., and Yeager, G. H.,** New tissue adhesives, *Md. Med. J.,* 12, 141, 1963.
58. **O'Neill, P., Healey, J. E., Clark, R.L., and Gallager, H. S.,** Nonsuture intestinal anastomosis, *Am. J. Surg.,* 104, 761, 1962.
59. **Eklund, M. K. and Kent, J. N.,** The use of isobutyl 2-cyanoacrylate as a post-extraction dressing in humans, *J. Oral Surg.,* 32, 264, 1974.
60. **Howard, D., Whitehurst, V. E., Bingham, R., and Stanback, J.,** The use of bucrylate to achieve hemostasis in tooth extraction sites, *Oral Surg.,* 35, 762, 1973.
61. **Giunta, J. L. and Sklar, G.,** Cyanoacrylate and oral wound healing in hamsters, *Arch. Oral Biol.,* 19, 845, 1974.
62. **Bhaskar, S. N.,** Tissue adhesives in dentistry: A review, *J. Can. Dent. Assoc.,* 9, 337, 1972.
63. **Bhaskar, S. N., Cutright, D. E., Beasley, J. D., and Ward, J. P.,** Oral spray of isobutyl cyanoacrylate and its systemic effect, *Oral Surg.,* 29, 313, 1970.
64. **Matsumoto, T., Hardaway, R. M., Heisterkamp, C. A., Pani, K. C., Leonard, F., and Margetis, P. M.,** Cyanoacrylate adhesive and hemostasis, *Arch. Surg.,* 94, 858, 1967.
65. **Matsumoto, T., Pani, K. C., Hardaway, R. M., and Leonard, F., N-alkyl**—α-cyanoacrylate polymers in surgery, *Arch., Surg.,* 94, 153, 1967.
66. **Matsumoto, T., Pani, D. C., Hardaway, R. M., Leonard, F., Jennings, P. B., and Heisterkamp, C. A.,** Higher homologous cyanoacrylate tissue adhesives in injured kidney, *Arch. Surg.,* 94, 392, 1967.
67. **Matsumoto, T., Hardaway, R. M., Pani, K. C., Leonard, F., Heisterkamp, C. A., and Margetis, P.,** Intestinal anastomosis with N-butyl cyanoacrylate tissue adhesive, *Surgery,* 61, 567, 1967.
68. **Matsumoto, T.,** Tissue adhesives in fatal hemorrhage from solid organs, *Mil. Med.,* 132, 951, 1967.
69. **Pani, K. C., Gladieux, G., Brandes, G., Kulkarni, R. K., and Leonard, F.,** The degradation of N-butyl acrylate tissue adhesive: II, *Surgery,* 489, 1968.
70. **Gasset, A. R., Hood, C. I., Ellison, E. D., and Kaufman, H. E.,** Ocular tolerance to cyanoacrylate monomer tissue adhesive analogues, *Invest. Ophthalmol.,* 9, 3, 1970.
71. **Aleo, J. J., and DeRenzis, F. A.,** On the possible mechanism of cyanoacrylate histotoxicity, *Pharmacol. Ther. Dent.,* 2, 21, 1975.
72. **Aaby, B. V., West, R. I., and Jahnke, F. J.,** Myocardial response to the application of tissue adhesives: Comparison of methyl-2-cyanoacrylate and butyl-cyanoacrylate, *Ann. Surg.,* 165, 425, 1967.
73. **Goetz, R. H., Weissberg, D., and Hoppenstein, R.,** Vascular necrosis caused by application of methyl-2-cyanoacrylate (Eastman 910 monomer): Seven-month follow up in dogs, *Ann. Surg.,* 163, 242, 1966.
74. **Jacobson, J. H., Jr., Moody, R. A., Kusserow, B. K., Reich, T., and Wang, M. C. H.,** The tissue response to a plastic adhesive used in combination with microsurgical technique in reconstruction of small arteries, *Surgery,* 60, 379, 1966.
75. **Lehman, R. A., Hayes, G. J., and Leonard, F.,** Toxicity of alkyl 2-cyanoacrylates: I. Peripheral nerve, *Arch. Surg.,* 93, 441, 1966.
76. **Weissberg, D. and Goetz, R. H.,** Necrosis of arterial wall following application of methyl-2-cyanoacrylate, *Surg. Gynecol. Obstet.,* 119, 1248, 1964.
77. **Woodward, S. C., Herrmann, J. B., Cameron, J. I., Brandes, G., Palaski, E. J., and Leonard, F.,** Histotoxicity of cyanoacrylate tissue adhesive in the rat, *Ann. Surg.,* 162, 113, 1965.
78. **Wilkinson, T. S., Rybka, R. F., and Paletta, F. X.,** Studies in nonsuture immobilization of skin, *South. Med. J.,* 65, 25, 1972.
79. **Hale, J. E.,** Isobutyl cyanoacrylate as a skin adhesive, *Postgrad. Med. J.,* 46, 447, 1970.
80. **Matsumoto, T., Nemhauser, G. M., Soloway, H. B., and Hamit, H. F.,** Cyanoacrylate tissue adhesives: an experimental and clinical evaluation, *Mil. Med.,* 134, 247, 1969.

81. **Levin, M. P., Cutright, D. E., and Bhaskar, S. N.,** Cyanoacrylate as a peridontal dressing, *J. Oral Med.,* 30, 40, 1975.
82. **Matsumoto, T., and Heisterkamp, C. A.,** Long-term study of aerosol cyanoacrylate tissue adhesive spray: Carcinogenicity and other untoward effects, *Am. Surg.,* 35, 825, 1969.
83. **Collins, J. A., James, P. M., Levitsky, S. A., Brandenburg, C. E., Anderson, R. W., Leonard, F., and Hardaway, R. M.,** Cyanoacrylate adhesives as topical hemostatic aids. II. Clinical use in seven combat casualties, *Surgery,* 65, 260, 1969.
84. **Regenbogen, L., Romano, A., Zuckerman, M., and Stein, R.,** Histoacryl tissue adhesive in some types of retinal detachment surgery, *Br. J. Ophthalmol.,* 60, 561, 1976.
85. **Heisterkamp, C. H., Simmons, R. L., Vernick, J., and Matsumoto, T.,** An aerosol tissue adhesive, *J. Trauma,* 9, 587, 593, 1969.
86. **Scheetz, W. L., and Matsumoto, T.,** Cyanoacrylate tissue adhesive: Thrombogenic effect, *Am. Surg.,* 36, 418, 1970.
87. **Matsumoto, T., Pani, K. C., Kovaric, J. J., and Hamit, H. F.,** Aerosol tissue adhesive spray, *Arch. Surg.,* 97, 727, 1968.
88. **Ousterhout, D. K. and Leonard, F.,** Tumor hemorrhage controlled with N-butyl alpha-cyanoacrylate, *Int. Surg.,* 51, 120, 1969.
89. **Nelson, R. A., Banitt, E. H., Kvam, D.C., Harrington, J. K., Robertson, J. E., and Buelow, J. S.,** A new fluoroalkyl cyanoacrylate surgical adhesive, *Arch. Surg.,* 100, 295, 1970.
90. **Dellevigne, W., Wolferth, C. C., Jones, N., and Matsumoto, T.,** Cyanoacrylate monomers as an adhesive, *Arch. Surg.,* 102, 493, 1971.
91. **Payne, J. T.,** A new biologic adhesive: Experimental observations, *Am. Surg.,* 36, 615, 1970.
92. **Mesrobian, A. Z. and Sklar, G.,** Gingival carcinogenesis in the hamster, using tissue adhesives for carcinogen, fixation, *J. Peridont.* 40, 603, 1969.
93. **Investigator's Brochure—MBR 4197—**a new biological adhesive, Surgical Products Division, Minnesota Mining and Manufacturing Company, St. Paul, Minnesota.
94. **Maxwell, J. A. and Goldware, S. I.,** Use of tissue adhesive in the surgical treatment of cerebrospinal fluid leaks—experience with isobutyl 2-cyanoacrylate in 12 cases, *J. Neurosurg.,* 39, 332, 1973.
95. **Zanetti, P. H. and Sherman, F. E.,** Experimental evaluation of a tissue adhesive as an agent for the treatment of aneurysms and arteriovenous anomalies, *J. Neurosurg.,* 36, 72, 1972.
96. **Orda, R., Wiznitzer, T., Goldberg, G. M., and Ezer, M.,** Repair of hepatic and splenic injuries by autoplastic peritoneal patches and butyl-2-cyanoacrylate monomer. An experimental study, *J. Surg. Res.,* 17, 365, 1974.
97. **Goldin, A. R.,** Control of duodenal haemorrhage with cyanoacrylate, *Br. J. Rad.,* 49, 583, 1976.
98. **Lahiffe, B. J., Caffesse, R. G., and Nasjleti, C. E.,** Healing of periodontal flaps following use of MBR 4197 (flucrylate) in Rhesus monkeys, *J. Periodont.,* 49, 635, 1978.
99. **Freeny, P. C. and Kidd, R.,** Transhepatic portal venography and selective obliteration of gastroesophageal varices using isobutyl 2-cyanoacrylate (bucrylate), *Dig. Dis. Sci.,* 24, 321, 1979.
100. **Keller, F. S.,** Occlusion of varices with ethyl cyanoacrylate, NIH Consensus Exercise, August 22, 1980, *Ann. Int. Med.,* in press.
101. **Keller, R. T. and Logan, G. M.,** Treatment of hemorrhagic gastritis by the endoscopic application of acrylic polymer, *Gastrointest. Endosc.,* 21, 75, 1974.
102. **Martin, T. R. and Silvis, S. E.,** The endoscopic control of GI blood loss with a tissue adhesive (MBR 4197), *Gastroenterology,* 72, 1099, 1977.
103. **Protell, R. L., Silverstein, F., Gulacsik, C., Martin, T. R., and Dennis, M. B.,** Cyanoacrylate glue (flucrylate) fails to stop bleeding from experimental gastric ulcers, *Gastroenterology,* 72, 1114, 1977.
104. **Protell, R. L., Silverstein, F. E., Piercey, J., Dennis, M., Sprake, W., Rubin, C. E.,** A reproducible animal model of acute bleeding ulcer—the "ulcer maker", *Gastroenterology,* 71, 961, 1976.
105. **Martin, T. R., Onstad, G. R., and Silvis, S. E.,** Endoscopic control of massive upper GI bleeding with a tissue adhesive (MBR 4197), *Gastrointest. Endosc.,* 24, 74, 1977.
106. **Peura, D.,** A randomized control trial of cyanoacrylate (MBR 4197), unpublished data.
107. **Linscheer, W. G., and Fazio, T. L.,** Control of upper gastrointestinal hemorrhage by endoscopic spraying of clotting factors, *Gastroenterology,* 71, 642, 1979.
108. **Linscheer, W. G.,** Uncontrolled clinical observations in bleeding patients treated with clotting factors, personal communication.
109. **Jensen, D. M., Michicado, G., and Tapia, J.,** Clotting factors fail to control bleeding from standard ulcers in gastric erosions, *Gastroenterology,* 78, 1187, 1980.
110. **Klein, F. A., Druels, R. I., Dunn, J. K., Brewer, R. I., and Schilli, R.,** Control of gastrointestinal bleeding with Avitene®, *Gastrointest, Endosc.,* 26, 70, 1980.
111. **Hait, M. R., Battista, O. A., Stark, R. B., and McCord, C. W.,** Microcrystalline collagen as a biologic dressing, vascular prosthesis, and hemostatic agent, *Surg. Forum,* 20, 51, 1969.

112. **Battista, O. A., Erdi, N. Z., Ferraro, C. F., and Karasinski, F. J.,** Novel microcrystals of polymers, Part II, *J. Appl. Polym. Sci.,* 11, 481, 1976.
113. **Hait, M. R.,** Microcrystalline collagen: A new hemostatic agent, *Am. J. Surg.,* 120, 330, 1970.
114. **Hait, M. R., Robb, C. A., Baxter, C. R., Borgmann, A. R., and Tippett, L. O.,** Comparative evaluation of Avitene® microcrystalline collagen hemostat in experimental animal wounds, *Am. J. Surg.,* 125, 284, 1973.
115. **Abbott, W. M. and Austen, W. G.,** Microcrystalline collagen as a topical hemostatic agent for vascular surgery, *Surgery,* 75, 925, 1974.
116. **Vistnes, L. M., Goodwin, D. A., Tenery, J. H., Ksander, G. A., and Gruber, R. P.,** Control of capillary bleeding by topical application of microcrystalline collagen, *Surgery,* 76, 291, 1974.
117. **Hunt, L. M. and Benoit, P. W.,** Evaluation of a microcrystalline collagen preparation in extraction wounds, *J. Oral Surg.,* 34, 407, 1976.
118. **Data on File,** Surgical Department, Alcon Laboratories, Fort Worth, Texas.
119. **Wilkinson, T., Tenery, J., and Zufi, D.,** The skin graft donor site as a model for evaluation of hemostatic agents, *Plast. Reconstr. Surg.,* 51, 541, 1973.
120. **Kortnblat, P. E., Kothbers, R. M., Menden, P., and Farr, R.,** Immune response of human adults after oral and parenteral exposure to bovine serum albumin, *J. Allergy,* 41, 226, 1968.
121. **Abbott, W. M. and Austen, W. G.,** The effectiveness and mechanism of collagen-induced topical hemostasis, *Surgery,* 78, 723, 1975.
122. **Schittek, A., Achilles, A. D., Seifter, E., Stein, J. M., and Levenson, S. M.,** Microcrystalline collagen hemostat (MCCH) and wound healing, *Ann. Surg.,* 184, 697, 1976.
123. **Mason, R. G. and Read, M. S.,** Some effects of a microcrystalline collagen preparation on blood, *Haemostasis,* 3, 31, 1974.
124. **Zucker, W. H. and Mason, R. G.,** Ultrastructural aspects of interactions of platelets with microcrystalline collagen, *Am. J. Pathol.,* 82, 129, 1976.
125. **Hanisch, M. E., Baum, N., Beach, P. D., Griffith, D. P., and Tyler, M.,** A comparative evaluation of Avitene® and Gelfoam® for hemostasis in experimental canine prostatic wounds, *Invest. Urol.,* 12, 333, 1975.
126. **Alexander, J. M. and Rabinowitz, J. L.,** Microfibrillar collagen (Avitene®) as a hemostatic agent in experimental oral wounds, *J. Oral Surg.,* 36, 202, 1978.
127. **Weinstein, M. E., Govin, G. G., Rice, C. L., and Virgilio, R.,** Splenorrhaphy for splenic trauma, *J. Trauma,* 19, 692, 1979.
128. **Smith, F. W., Heinonen, L. A., Peterson, E. C., Lobitz, J. R., and Schoemake, R.,** The use of a strong magnetic field in the control of gastrointestinal bleeding, *Gastroenterology,* 78, 1264, 1980.
129. **Carlson, D., Jensen, D. M., Machicado, G., Frasco, P., and Tapia, J.,** Treatment of experimental bleeding of gastric ulcers and erosions with ferromagnetic tamponade, *Gastroenterology,* 78, 1147, 1980.
130. **Mormino, J., Taft, F., and Powers, S. R.,** A nonsurgical approach to the treatment of upper gastrointestinal hemorrhage: A preliminary report, *Mt. Sinai J. Med.,* 44, 269, 1977.
131. **Kiselow, M. C. and Wagner, M.,** Intragastric instillation of levarternol, *Arch. Surg.,* 107, 387, 1973.
132. **LeVeen, H. H., Diaz, C., Falk, G., and Piccone, V. A.,** A proposed method to interrupt gastrointestinal bleeding: Preliminary report, *Ann. Surg.,* 175, 459, 1972.
133. **Matsumoto, T.,** Management of diffuse hemorrhage from gastric mucosa, *Am. J. Surg.,* 123, 160, 1972.
134. **Naitove, A., Mikell, F. L., and Karl, R. C.,** Topical vasopressin in the management of nonvariceal bleeding from lesions of esophagus, *Am. J. Surg.,* 127, 382, 1974.
135. **Wayne, R., Margolis, I. B., Rongone, E. L., and Beegle, R. C.,** Effect of norepinephrine on gastric wound healing, *Surg. Gynecol. Obstet.,* 143, 749, 1976.

Chapter 9

APPROACH TO THE PATIENT WITH RECTAL BLEEDING

Jerome D. Waye

TABLE OF CONTENTS

I. INTRODUCTION

Rectal bleeding is one of the commonest symptoms related to the large bowel. The presence of blood always indicates a pathologic process, and its origin must always be identified. Whether bleeding is overt and is reported by the patient or is occult and found on chemical examination of the stool, the problem for the physician is the same—the etiology must be explained. The causes for colorectal bleeding are many and vary from the most frequent site being the relatively innocuous hemorrhoid[1] to the serious problem of colon cancer.

Most patients who present with rectal bleeding do not require a total diagnostic evaluation including colonoscopy and angiography. Some patients will require all these procedures as part of an extensive series of investigations to ascertain the etiology of rectal bleeding. The physician must decide which of many investigative techniques will be the most helpful in each individual patient. This Chapter outlines the extent of investigation required for the diagnosis of rectal bleeding in each clinical setting and the proper sequencing of studies in the search for a bleeding site.

II. DEFINITION OF THE PROBLEM

A. Massive Bleeding

The approach to the patient with massive rectal bleeding is considerably different than for smaller amounts of blood loss. Massive rectal bleeding may be defined[2] as the passage of copious quantities of bloody bowel movements requiring two or more units of blood transfusion to maintain the hematocrit at 30% or bleeding which causes clinical signs of hypovolemia, such as shock, postural hypotension, tachycardia, and pallor. Immediate resuscitative efforts must be directed toward sustaining life simultaneously with the institution of plans to identify the location of the bleeding site.[3] Uncontrolled massive bleeding may be associated with a significant mortality and must be classified as a medical emergency.[1,4-6]

B. Nonmassive Bleeding

Most patients who present with frequent bloody bowel movements (occurring as often as every 15 min.) will not fulfill the above criteria for massive rectal bleeding. This group of more stable patients should be approached differently, both diagnostically and therapeutically. The actual amount of blood lost with each bowel evacuation may be moderate and, although causing great anxiety in the patient, may not be associated with an immediate life-threatening situation. In many cases, relatively small amounts of fresh blood from a rectal source such as hemorrhoids or proctitis may appear to be a large quantity. A few cubic centimeters of fresh blood may dramatically color the toilet bowel red or may arouse a panic reaction should blood soak through clothing or bed sheets before the patient is aware of its presence.

III. HISTORY

The first step in the diagnostic approach to the patient with rectal bleeding is obtaining a thorough history (Table 1). A detailed description of the color of bleeding, its relationship to bowel movements, and its frequency is the most important determinant of the diagnostic approach. The patient with massive bleeding will have frequent movements with the presence of clots and fresh blood. Massive bleeding episodes are usually not accompanied by brown stool. If after the first bowel movement brown stool is present as well as red blood, the site of bleeding is in the left colon and

Table 1
COLON BLEEDING

Significance of red bleeding associated with history
Suggests perianal site:
- Following bowel evacuation
- Dripping into bowl
- On toilet tissue
- On perineum without evacuation

Suggests further investigation:
- Streaks on stool
- Mixed with stool

usually in the recto-sigmoid region. The explanation for this statement is that bleeding which originates from the right side of the colon admixes with fecal contents; whereas passage of brown stool and red blood indicates a more distal origin for bleeding.

The physician must always consider that a common cause for rectal passage of blood is an upper intestinal site with rapid transit time. The origin is most likely to be a peptic ulcer, but certain historical clues should be sought to enable a proper decision concerning the diagnostic investigation. When an acute upper intestinal bleed causes the passage of red blood per rectum, it is always associated with signs of cardiovascular instability from the sudden loss of a massive quantity of blood. Smaller amounts of blood at a slower flow rate do not stimulate peristalsis and present as melena, rather than red bleeding. Whenever rectal bleeding is associated with evidence of hypovolemia, strong consideration must be given to a proximal source and a careful history of a potential upper gastrointestinal bleeding site must be elicited. A previous history of ulcer disease is important. Melena preceding red rectal bleeding points to a slowly bleeding upper intestinal source with a sudden increase in output. A history of alcoholism and/or cirrhosis may be obtained suggesting acute gastritis or the presence of esophageal varices. Patients must be carefully questioned about any bleeding tendency,[7] and especially whether any specific medication such as anticoagulants are being taken. Predisposing factors which increase the risk for large bowel pathology must be sought; among these are a previous history of polyps or carcinoma or a family history of large bowel polyps or cancer. Rectal manipulation or trauma should also be considered.[8]

The most common complaint regarding rectal bleeding is that of recurrent small amounts either staining the toilet tissue or seen in the bowl following defecation. Blood found only on the toilet tissue in association with a normal bowel movement always has its origin in or around the anal canal. Blood spurting (or dripping) into the toilet bowl following normal evacuation is due to a perirectal lesion; the most common of which is hemorrhoids. The symptom of rectal bleeding must not be ignored. Small amounts of bleeding attributed to hemorrhoids over years may, without change in character or frequency, be found on investigation to be originating from a rectal cancer or polyp occurring concomitantly with hemorrhoids. Blood may drip into the toilet bowl as the tumor is everted during the act of defecation.

Bright bleeding which stains the bed linen (or clothing) occurring without the patient's awareness and without a bowel movement is a frightening experience, but in the patient who maintains fecal continence, is always associated with a site in the anal canal or adjacent to it. The actual amount of blood lost is usually of small volume and selflimited, but provokes alarm because of its sudden occurrence and implies the presence of hemorrhoids or a rectal fissure.

The sight of a streak of blood on one side of a normally formed stool, or spots of blood mixed in with the stool is less dramatic than free-flowing bright bleeding, but of considerably greater diagnostic importance. Bleeding of this nature is rarely due to pathology in the rectum or anal canal and implies a specific bleeding site in the left colon which coats the formed stool as it passes by the lesion. Diverticula rarely, if ever, cause this type of bleeding. Blood streaking, spotting, or visibly mixed with stool is most often caused by a polyp or carcinoma of the descending/sigmoid colon.[9] Bleeding from a more proximal source mixes with stool and may not cause any grossly detectable evidence of blood loss and is discovered by testing for occult blood.

Occasionally, the history may be given that a reddish color is seen in the toilet water around the formed brown stool. This is usually due to leaching of red blood cells by the hypotonic water with the resultant reddish color. Blood from the proximal colon may thoroughly mix with fecal contents and be invisible until hemolysis occurs.

Pain as a symptom accompanying rectal bleeding allows a more precise diagnosis for the etiology of bleeding. When defecation causes rectal pain and bright red bleeding on the toilet tissue or dripping into the bowel, a fissure, rectal ulcer, or a thrombosed and ulcerated hemorrhoid is the predictable site.[10] The previously asymptomatic patient who gives a history of acute abdominal pain followed by loose stools and usually dark red blood is characteristically a victim of a colonic vascular insult (ischemic bowel disease).[11] If ischemia is transient, these symptoms usually subside rapidly over 12 to 24 hr. Although vascular insufficiency is most frequently associated with atherosclerotic narrowing of blood vessels,[12] young women on oral contraceptives may suffer from venous occlusion without any antecedant history.[13]

Bright-red blood diffusely coating the normal solid brown stool may occur with radiation colitis[14] even years after the radiation therapy was administered. The rectum, being fixed in its position, is the portion of the gut most commonly affected during radiotherapy for pelvic neoplasm. Radiation tissue damage may stimulate neovascularization of the mucosal surface and a propensity to bleed. Proctitis may also cause blood to coat a normal stool, but urgency is an almost invariable accompaniment. Bloody diarrhea, with or without mucus and pus, points to the presence of colonic inflammation, the most frequent cause of which is ulcerative colitis. Other specific inflammatory processes may cause diarrhea and bleeding, such as Yersinia enterocolitis, Campylobacter fetus, amebiasis, or bacterial infections.[15]

IV. PHYSICAL EXAMINATION

With the exception of a digital rectal examination, the general physical examination of patients with rectal bleeding may be of little benefit. Blood in the small bowel acts as a peristaltic stimulant. An increased bowel sound activity associated with passage of dark or bright blood per rectum is a diagnostic clue suggesting its origin in the upper intestinal tract. Physical examination of the abdomen must be meticulously performed; since further information may be gathered to assist in the location of the bleeding site. A mass in the abdomen may be associated with a carcinoma. Ascites and/or an enlarged liver may be evidence of cirrhosis. Intestinal ischemia with the left colon characteristically involved will have tenderness with or without rebound in the left upper and midabdomen.

A contracted blood volume due to acute blood loss almost invariably causes circulatory instability. Pallor, tachycardia, and diaphoresis may be seen. Postural hypotension is common in hypovolemia. Those patients who tolerate massive blood loss while lying supine may, on assuming a sitting position, develop tachycardia and hypotension.

V. LABORATORY TESTS

Blood volume determination is the most accurate parameter for measuring the amount of blood loss. Even though the hematocrit does not immediately reflect changes in blood volume, it is valuable for following the rate of bleeding. An elevated blood urea nitrogen indicates resorption of blood in the upper intestinal tract. Luekocytosis is caused by any inflammatory process, such as infection, inflammation, or ischemia. However, sudden blood loss may stimulate an immediate bone marrow response with an elevation in the peripheral white-blood cell count. Screening tests for a possible bleeding diathesis should be performed with abnormalities sought in the prothrombin time and platelet count. Tests for the detection of occult blood in the stool must be a regular part of every patient examination. A positive result cannot be ignored. These tests are readily and easily performed by either the patient or the physician.

VI. CAUSES FOR RECTAL BLEEDING

Many lesions are responsible for rectal bleeding. All of them must be considered in each patient who presents with this symptom. Most sources can be considered and discarded as untenable during the course of history-taking. Bleeding from the upper intestinal tract and right colon can be ruled out in the patient who gives a history of bright-red blood dripping into the toilet bowl following defecation, but must be given stronger consideration when the history is of the passage of dark-red or maroon stools. In spite of a history consistent with a rectal source of bleeding, a lesion of the more proximal colon must be strongly suspected when there is, in addition, a positive test for occult blood or anemia. A carefully directed history must be extracted from the patient who presents with bloody diarrhea and cramps. When the previously asymptomatic patient presents with these symptoms, an important differential diagnosis hinges on the history of cramps and abdominal pain preceding the bloody bowel movements. Severe abdominal pain followed within minutes by bloody evacuations are characteristic of an ischemic vascular insult. On the other hand, diarrhea and painful cramps which later become bloody are more indicative of an inflammatory bowel disease.[16] The causes for rectal bleeding are listed in Table 2.

VII. DIAGNOSTIC PROCEDURES

The diagnostic procedures available for the investigation of colonic bleeding are varied and include:

1. Digital-rectal examination
2. Proctosigmoidoscopy
3. Barium enema X-ray
4. Colonoscopy
5. Radionuclide technetium scanning
6. Angiography
7. Gastric aspiration with nasogastric tube
8. Upper gastrointestinal endoscopy
9. Upper gastrointestinal and small bowel X-ray examination
10. Surgery

Given the array of diagnostic procedures which can be performed, the physician must decide which should be performed on each patient, and what should be the sequence of

Table 2
CAUSES OF COLON BLEEDING

Hemorrhoids
Fissures
Diverticulosis
Polyps
Cancer
Inflammatory bowel disease
  Ulcerative colitis
  Granulomatous colitis
  Proctitis
Infectious colitis
Arteriovenous malformations
Ischemia
Radiation
Ulcers—idiopathic
Rectal Prolapse
Small bowel
  Meckel's diverticulum
  Tumor
Upper gastrointestinal source

examinations. A detailed medical history and a knowledge of the possible etiologies of bleeding will point to the proper diagnostic procedures that will be necessary in each patient and yet be cost-effective, so that not every test is ordered in every patient.

A. Digital Examination

As part of the physical examination, every patient should have a digital rectal examination. If inordinate pain is elicited upon introduction of the well—lubricated finger into the anal canal, a fissure should be considered as the etiology of bleeding. During the rectal examination, a foreign body may be palpable. In elderly infirmed patients, the digital examination may reveal a mass of impacted stool causing a stercoral ulcer. A coarsely granular feeling of the mucosa should arouse suspicion of the presence of proctitis. Rectal carcinoma can be detected as a firm, polypoid, or ridge-like mass.

The examining glove should be inspected once it has been withdrawn from the anus to derive further information to assist in the differential diagnosis of the site of bleeding. Observation of black melanotic stool usually implies that bleeding is coming from proximal to the area of the ligament of Treitz. This is not always true, since blood placed in the cecum during appendectomy has been reported to cause melena[17] if the first bowel movement occurs more than 72 hr following instillation of blood. However, it is unusual for a bleeding site in the right colon to be of sufficient quantity to produce a tarry stool and, yet, have such a slow transit time of 3 days from the cecum to the rectum. Black material on an examining glove should be tested for the presence of blood, since iron ingestion may cause an appearance similar to that of melena. Dark-red blood on the examining glove indicates a proximal colonic source, while bright-red bleeding is more indicative of a sigmoid/rectal lesion. The observation of brown stool and red blood is characteristic of bleeding from the left colon. Occasionally, the digital examination may lead to an entire change in the approach to the patient. A history of fresh red bleeding, but dark-maroon blood on the examining glove, would indicate a more proximal site.

B. Sigmoidoscopy

A sigmoidoscopic examination should be performed on every patient being investigated for rectal bleeding. In addition to being able to identify a bleeding site or see a lesion, visualization of the lowermost mucosal surface may reflect the status of the entire colon. Whenever possible, anoscopy should be performed with a separate instrument, since bleeding from hemorrhoids and fissues may be difficult to evaluate with a standard 10-in. rigid proctosigmoidoscope. The entire circumference of the anal canal can be much better observed using the anoscope with its oblique wide-caliber opening. Through the sigmoidoscope, one may evaluate mucosal pattern, the presence of proctocolitis, hemorrhoids, polyps, and carcinoma of the recto-sigmoid region. In the presence of proctitis and frequently with hemorrhoidal bleeding, the instrument may reach above the bleeding site, giving a high degree of diagnostic accuracy.

Whenever sigmoidoscopy is performed for acute bleeding, it must be recognized by the clinician that blood from the rectum may reflux proximally and, upon its return flow down from the sigmoid region, may be misinterpreted as evidence of a "bleeding site above the reach of the sigmoidoscope." This is a difficult problem and may only be resolved by passing a colonoscope through the area of bleeding and upon withdrawal identifying a distal origin of blood loss. Blood may reflux up to the area of the mid-to upper-descending colon[3] from a hemorrhoidal site in a vigorous, healthy, young person whose tight rectal sphincteric musculature prevents fecal (and blood) incontinence.

C. Barium Enema X-ray

Persistent bleeding, or the finding of positive occult blood in the stool, should be investigated with a detailed history, digital rectal examination, sigmoidoscopy, and air-contrast barium enema X-ray examination. The double-contrast barium enema will discover the majority of lesions causing rectal bleeding,[18] and proper therapy may be initiated on the basis of the diagnosis discovered on barium enema. If a polyp is found on barium enema, electrodiathermy may be set up at the time of colonoscopic examination so that polypectomy may be performed. If polypectomy is only practiced in a hospital setting, the information gained from a barium enema will permit hospitalization arrangements to be made in advance, and the diagnostic colonoscopy may then be combined with a therapeutic option. Frequently, the barium enema will reveal a carcinoma which does not require colonoscopic verification. Surgery should be the next procedure. Occasionally, no lesions are found during the standard diagnostic workup including X-ray examination. In these patients with colonic bleeding, colonoscopy should be performed.[19-21]

The barium enema plays no role in the management of patients with acute rectal bleeding.[22] Barium coats the bowel walls and precludes the subsequent use of either angiography or colonoscopy. Another reason not to use barium in investigation of massive acute bleeding is that most patients are bleeding from diverticula or arteriovenous malformations. These lesions cannot be diagnosed by routine radiography. For many years, there was a belief that barium in an enema form helped to "plug" a bleeding site and was, therefore, useful in the approach to colonic bleeding.[23] This has not been shown to have any scientific basis and, at the present time, a barium enema is not considered to be of benefit either diagnostically or therapeutically in the patient who is actively bleeding.

D. Colonoscopy

The colonoscope has been demonstrated to reach the cecum in a high percentage of cases (92 to 95%) with or without the use of fluoroscopic control.[24] Even the most tortuously shaped colon yields to the well-trained endoscopist. Only a few patients cannot be totally intubated. Failures may be encountered in patients with colons fixed by previous pelvic surgery or diverticular disease. During the course of acute bleeding, specific identification of any lesion is much more difficult than in the well-prepared, nonemergency examination. The problems of colonoscopy in acute rectal bleeding will be discussed later in this chapter. Colonoscopy is of great importance in the

Table 3
COLONOSCOPY IN UNEXPLAINED RECTAL BLEEDING

Patients (#)	Lesions Found (%)	Polyps (%)	Cancer (%)	IBD* (%)	Ref.
215	41	14	13	7	1
258	42	15	11	7	21
306	30	14	8	4	25
561	42	14	11	10	26
239	40	16	10	10	27

*IBD = inflammatory bowel disease.

investigation of patients with chronic, unexplained rectal bleeding.[1,6] When colonoscopy is performed under these circumstances and "routine" diagnostic maneuvers including barium enema have failed to find a lesion, approximately 30 to 40% of patients will have a specific lesion discovered by endoscopy.[1,21,25-27] Several studies have revealed that approximately 15% of patients with unexplained bleeding will have a colon polyp, approximately 10% will be bleeding from a carcinoma, 5% will have an arteriovenous malformation, and 7% will have undiagnosed inflammatory bowel discasc (Table 3).

E. Radionuclide Scanning

Technetium-99m scanning is a relatively new noninvasive diagnostic modality that provides rapid information on whether a lesion is actively bleeding at the time of the procedure.[28,29] The technique involves intravenous injection of technetium radioisotope which rapidly clears from the circulatory system. In the actively bleeding patient, a collection of intraluminal radioactive material occurs at the bleeding site. This is a sensitive, highly reliable test but is relatively nonspecific. For example, a bleeding site in the area of the hepatic flexure may either be in the colon or in the duodenal bulb. Sequential examinations may increase specificity by demonstrating appropriate peristaltic flow of radioactive material in the pattern of the colon or the small bowel. The ease of this examination and its rapidity (information may be obtained in 15 min.) have prompted some centers to refuse angiography unless active bleeding has been demonstrated on an immediately preceding radionuclide scan.

F. Angiography

Abdominal angiography is helpful in brisk bleeding when the rate of blood loss is more than 0.5m*l*/min.[30] In the presence of such active bleeding, extravasation of dye from the vascular compartment to the intraluminal space occurs, leaving a persistent stain after the vascular flush disappears. When bleeding is at a slower rate, insufficient dye collects to be of diagnostic value. The procedure requires an expert angiographer. A precise localization of the site of bleeding may be accomplished, although a specific diagnosis may not be possible.[31] In nonbleeding patients, an arteriovenous malformation may be identified as a vascular blush or by the presence of a large draining vein.

G. Gastric Aspiration by Nasogastric Tube

It has been reported that the passage of a nasogastric tube in all patients with gastrointestinal bleeding provides fairly accurate information concerning the presence of an upper gastrointestinal bleeding site.[32] In a series of 1190 patients, only 1% were found to have an inaccurate diagnosis of an upper intestinal bleeding site as determined by the passage of a nasogastric tube with aspiration of gastric contents. However, in that same journal, an editorial[33] pointed out that, when specific patients were selected as being at high risk from upper gastrointestinal hemorrhage, as many as 20% of bleeding duodenal ulcers had no evidence of bloody reflux into the stomach and, therefore, will have a spuriously negative nasogastric aspirate.

H. Upper Gastrointestinal Endoscopy

With the advent of smaller-caliber, more easily tolerated upper intestinal panendoscopes capable of examining the entire esophagus, stomach and duodenum, passage of a flexible fiberoptic endoscope into the stomach is less traumatic than the passage of a nasogastric tube. Whenever upper gastrointestinal bleeding is seriously considered as a cause for colonic hemorrhage, an upper gastrointestinal endoscopic examination should be the first line of investigation, since information obtained from passage of the nasogastric tube may be misleading.[33] Whenever upper gastrointestinal bleeding occurs, the endoscopic examination has been shown to be the best diagnostic procedure for the location of the site of bleeding.[34] An endoscopic examination may be performed quickly at the bedside of the bleeding patient and yields considerably more diagnostic information than either passage of a nasogastric tube or an upper gastrointestinal barium X-ray series.

I. Upper Gastrointestinal X-ray Series

Apart from angiographic visualization of small bowel blood vessels, current technology has not permitted a simple and efficient method of visualizing the small intestine. For patients with recurrent bleeding whose bleeding rate is slow, or whose angiogram is negative, a small bowel X-ray series should be carefully performed. Tumors of the small bowel are unusual, but do occur and may be detected by barium studies. In the acutely bleeding patient, barium should not be given for it interferes with subsequent diagnostic evaluations such as angiography and intestinal endoscopy.

J. Surgery

Exploratory surgery for massive intestinal bleeding is rarely performed because of the spectrum of diagnostic studies currently available.[18,22] Angiography has demonstrated that bleeding from diverticulosis frequently occurs from the right side of the colon, although there are many more diverticula in the sigmoid region. When massive bleeding occurs, either radionuclide scanning or angiography should be performed as the fourth step following history, digital rectal examination, and proctosigmoidoscopy. When these studies are unavailable or unrevealing, "blind" subtotal colectomy may be necessary and may be a life-saving procedure.

VIII. THE SEQUENCE OF DIAGNOSTIC TESTS IN COLONIC BLEEDING

The basic diagnostic evaluation in every patient consists of the **history**, **digital rectal examination**, and **sigmoidoscopy**. After the basic evaluation has been performed, the type of further investigation will depend on assessment of whether major bleeding has occurred or whether it is a nonmassive episode. The history is the best tool for making this distinction. When left colon bleeding occurs, defecatory responses are frequently stimulated by the presence of blood in the rectum, although the total volume of bleeding may be relatively small. Because of this, bleeding originating from the colon tends to give signs of hypotension late in the course, as opposed to the early development of hypotension when rectal blood loss is a symptom of upper intestinal bleeding.

A. Nonmassive Acute Rectal Bleeding

An important differential in patients with a history of frequent red bowel movements without signs of hypotension is whether abdominal pain is present. Painless bleeding is caused by hemorrhoids, cancer, polyps, diverticular disease, or arteriovenous malformation. The patient should be asked whether bleeding is accompanied by the passage of brown stool. If there is brown stool and red bleeding, the site is in the left colon or rectum. Bleeding from the left colon will not be mixed with stool formed in the more proximal portion of the bowel. The source in these patients is usually hemorrhoids or left-sided diverticular bleeding. Patients may not be able to answer the question of whether brown stool is present, and the physician again must decide whether the frequent passage of bloody bowel movements indicates bleeding from the right or left colon. Fortunately, most bleeding ceases spontaneously no matter what the origin.

1. Blood Dripping Into Toilet Bowel Following Defecation

Additional procedures—barium enema optional. This symptom indicates a site of bleeding in or near the anal canal. If pain occurs, there may be a fissure which was torn open by the passage of stool which can be seen with an anoscope/proctoscope. In the absence of pain, this type of bleeding is most likely due to hemorrhoids which have become everted with the passage of stool. The history which usually accompanies this symptom is one of recurrent bleeding episodes which stop spontaneously. Bleeding seen on the toilet tissue following defecation is of similar perirectal origin and should have the "basic diagnostic evaluation." Not all such bleeding should be attributed to hemorrhoids, since proctitis, rectal polyps, or rectal carcinoma may occasionally present in this fashion. Every patient must have a rectal examination and sigmoidoscopy to explain this symptom. Preferably, an exploratory barium enema should also be performed to examine the whole colon, although the history of many patients may not prompt this study. Colon cancer is one of the most common cancers in the U.S. and, although the etiology of rectal bleeding may be explained, the symptom which has stimulated that patient to enter the health care system provides sufficient reason to have the patient's colon examined. The barium enema X-ray examination is an excellent general screening test for colon pathology and can, in most instances, detect significant polyps, carcinoma, and abnormalities of the large bowel. If a positive test for occult blood is obtained from a patient with this history in the absence of visible bleeding, a barium enema then becomes a mandatory examination.

2. Bright Red Blood Staining Bed Linen/Undergarments Without Defecation

Additional procedures—barium enema optional. Bleeding of this nature, without an active attempt to open the rectal sphincter, is always associated with a bleeding site external to the rectal sphincter muscles. This means that the site is in or external to the anal canal. The usual etiology is a ruptured hemorrhoid, and the site may be seen on direct inspection with an anoscope. Even though the etiology of such bleeding is obvious on proctosigmoidscopic examination, all patients should have a barium enema X-ray examination so that lesions elsewhere in the colon will not be overlooked.

3. Rectal Bleeding with Abdominal Pain

Additional procedures—angiography—subsequent barium enema. When bloody bowel movements are associated with the sudden onset of abdominal pain in a previously asymptomatic patient, the most likely etiology is ischemic bowel disease. Sigmoidoscopic examination, if negative, should be followed by angiographic evaluation. A subsequent barium enema may reveal the typical "thumb-printing" along the edges of the colon. The most frequent location for ischemia is in the area of the

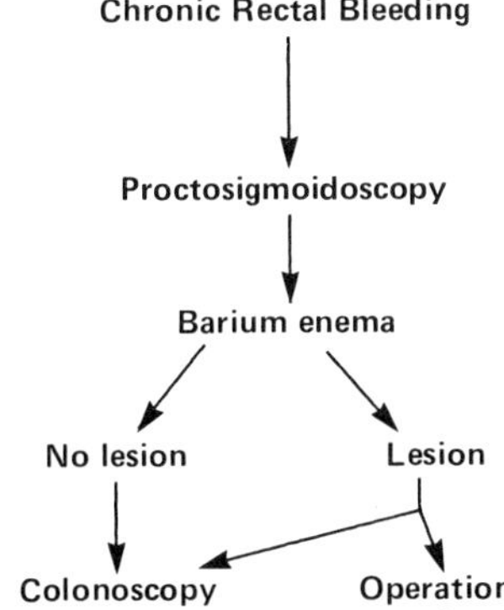

FIGURE 1. Chronic rectal bleeding.

splenic flexure; however, the sigmoidoscopic examination itself may reveal evidence of a dusky mucosa when ischemia occurs low in the left colon.

4. Rectal Bleeding and Diarrhea

Additional procedures—stool cultures—barium enema. Most diarrheal diseases begin without bleeding but may subsequently bleed. Ulcerative colitis usually has a nonbleeding phase before the characteristic symptoms develop. The sigmoidoscope may enable the correct diagnosis to be made. If the patient is quite ill, therapy may be instituted without any additional diagnostic procedures except stool evaluation for ova and in culture. In the absence of a toxicitic patient, a barium enema should be the next diagnostic procedure to allow definition of the entire colon and for evaluation of the extent of disease.

B. Chronic Colonic Bleeding (Figure 1)

1. Streaks of Blood on the Surface of the Stool

Additional procedures—barium enema—if negative, colonoscopy. This is a significant symptom that requires exploration. Every effort must be made to explain the symptom satisfactorily. Whenever this complaint is obtained, careful attention must be given to the strong possibility that a lesion exists in the area of the rectosigmoid colon. Although a hemorrhoid or fissure may cause this symptom, a cancer or polyp in the left colon may deposit a linear streak of blood on the surface of a formed stool as it passes the lesion. This type of bleeding does not occur as a result of diverticulosis. If a lesion is seen on double-contrast barium enema, a decision must be made concerning proper therapy. If no lesion is identified, colonoscopic examination must be performed. The sigmoid colon is a difficult area for the radiologist to adequately visualize. It is in this area that hidden lesions may be expected. The X-ray-negative patient with a significant history will have a 15% incidence of polyps and a 10% incidence of carcinoma. A significant history means:

1. Blood streaking or spotting the stool
2. A positive test for occult blood
3. Unexplained iron deficiency anemia

2. Spots of Blood Mixed with the Stool

This symptom has the same significance as streaks of blood on the surface of the stool and should be investigated in a similar fashion.

3. Red Blood on the Toilet Tissue, Associated with the Presence of a Light-Red Color of Blood Emanating from the Surface of a Brown-colored Stool and Staining the Water Immediately Around It

Additional procedure—barium enema—if negative, colonoscopy. This symptom is almost always associated with an organic lesion in the left colon or distal transverse colon. Blood mixes with a superficial portion of the stool and, being present in small amounts and mixed with surface mucus, is not visibly red when spread over the surface of the stool, but hemolyzes and causes a reddish color. As the stool passes the anal canal, it leaves a film of blood which may be seen on the toilet tissue.

C. Occult Blood in the Stool, in the Absence of Any Evidence of Visible Bleeding

Additional procedures—barium enema—if negative, colonoscopy. This finding usually indicates a lesion in the right colon which loses small amounts of blood that mix with the stool and is then not visible to the naked eye. In these instances, cancer of the colon is a common cause, but polyps and arteriovenous malformations may also cause occult bleeding. Even if hemorrhoids are seen on sigmoidoscopy, the bleeding should not be attributed to them. A barium enema must be performed. If negative, colonoscopy should follow. Angiography or radionuclide scanning is not usually helpful in these circumstances since the rate of bleeding is low.

D. Massive Bleeding With Signs of Hypovolemia (Figure 2)

Additional procedures—radionuclide scanning and/or angiography—upper gastrointestinal endoscopy if an upper intestinal bleeding site is suspected.

To meet the criteria for massive bleeding, the patient must pass copious quantities of bloody bowel movements with either clinical evidence of hypotension or require two units of blood transfusion to maintain the hematocrit at 30%. Bleeding of this severity may be caused by a variety of conditions but usually involves the three major causes listed below, although carcinoma may occasionally bleed massively.[36]

1. Diverticular bleeding
2. Arteriovenous malformation
3. Upper gastrointestinal bleeding

Diverticular disease accounts for the majority of all massive colon bleeds,[37,38] and 3% of all patients with symptomatic diverticular disease will sustain a massive rectal hemorrhage.[5,39,40] Although there are many more diverticuli in the sigmoid colon than in the right colon, diverticulosis of the right colon has been demonstrated to be the origin of rectal bleeding in a substantial number of cases.[41,42] The diagnosis of massive bleeding from diverticular disease is best made on radionuclide scanning or angiography, since the presence of blood in the bowel tends to obscure visualization during the use of the colonoscope. Most patients with acute rectal bleeding tend to stop spontaneously.[35] Only 5% of patients with massive bleeding from diverticular disease will require surgery on an emergency basis to stop bleeding.[43]

Arteriovenous malformations usually occur in the right colon and may be associated with the degenerative process of aging. These A-V communications tend to bleed suddenly without warning and produce no symptoms for the patient other than frequent bowel movements of dark-red blood. The bleeding is usually voluminous. It may stop as suddenly as it starts, but may require resection of the right colon to control hemorrhage. Localization of the bleeding site requires radionuclide scanning or angiography.[41,44] The angiographic demonstration of a prominent draining vein from an area of arteriovenous malformation makes the diagnosis more definite. Rarely are large bowel arteriovenous

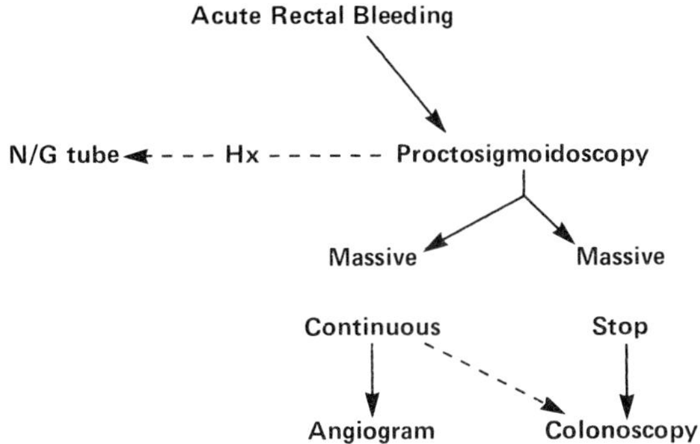

FIGURE 2. Acute rectal bleeding.

malformations associated with other vascular anomalies in that patient. Once bleeding has stopped, the patient may be safely colonoscoped during an interim nonbleeding period with full preparation, including cathartics and enemas, 48 hr following the bleeding episode.

Small arteriovenous malformations appear to the endoscopist as a collection of fine, reddish blood vessels localized to a specific area on the wall of the ascending colon.[45,47] These malformations may be either small or extensively interlaced, covering a wide area of the right colon.

Although angiography may be quite helpful in localizing the site of massive rectal bleeding, colonoscopy has been reported to be of variable benefit in the massively bleeding patient.[48] Rossini[49] states that blood in the bowel acts as a cathartic, and that the multiple evacuations associated with acute, voluminous rectal bleeding cleanse the colon so that enemas are not necessary. It is frequently helpful to pass a sigmoidoscope with a wide-caliber suction apparatus to evacuate clots in the rectal ampulla where they tend to accumulate. The colonoscope may be passed under direct vision up to the bleeding lesion or beyond the area of bleeding into a nonbloody segment of the colon.[50] As soon as the instrument has passed beyond the segment of active bleeding, the procedure need not be continued, since identification of the bleeding area is the desired endpoint of the examination, not full and total colonoscopy. Other investigators have found that blood clinging to the walls of the colon during episodes of active bleeding obscure mucosal markings and make it difficult to ascertain which of multiple bloody areas may be bleeding.[6,51] Cleaning the bowel sufficiently for adequate visualization is almost impossible. It has been advocated that a dental Water Pik® be adapted to use through the biopsy port of the instrument with the ability to squirt a powerful jet of water at the mucosa to cleanse it of blood and residue.

Bleeding from the upper intestinal tract is usually accompanied by the passage of dark-red stool or port-wine-colored bowel movements, but bright-red bleeding may be present.[2] Whenever dark blood is passed per rectum, the site is almost always proximal colon or upper intestinal tract. If the bleeding site is a Meckel's diverticulum,[52] or originates elsewhere in the small bowel, there may be no clues to that etiology.[39] A technetium Meckel's scan may be helpful. On the other hand, upper intestinal bleeding may be accompanied by an episode of melena for 1 to 2 days prior to the episode of brisk bleeding from a source such as a peptic ulcer. Patients should be questioned about previous bowel movements, as well as ingestion of drugs known to be associated with upper GI bleeding, such as salicylates, antirheumatic therapy, reserpine, or corticosteroids. A history of previous peptic ulcer disease must be carefully elicited, and special attention should be directed toward the presence of alcoholism, previous liver disease, previous intestinal bleeding episodes, and any other factors which may have predisposed to upper intestinal bleeding. In these patients with massive rectal bleeding from an upper intestinal source, a considerable amount of blood is present in the intestinal tract with a rapid transit time. This leads to hyperactivity of the small bowel with easily audible borborygmus and signs of hypovolemia, such as postural hypotension, tachycardia, and pallor. Blood in the intestinal tract may cause an elevated blood urea nitrogen (BUN). In spite of a strong suspicion of an upper intestinal bleeding site, a sigmoidoscopic examination should be performed in every patient to permit observation of the rectal mucosa.[35] It is possible that the frequent passage of bloody stools, although dark in color, may be the initial manifestation of ulcerative colitis which can be diagnosed through the sigmoidoscope. Following a negative sigmoidoscopic examination in a patient with a high suspicion for an upper intestinal bleeding site, an upper intestinal panendoscope should be passed into the stomach and duodenal bulb to acertain the presence and site of bleeding.

IX. SUMMARY

A step-by-step schema has been presented for the investigation of patients who present with the symptom of rectal bleeding. The cornerstone of an accurate diagnosis rests on a thorough and complete history obtained from the patient. Although each of the many possibilities must be considered in every patient with rectal bleeding, the differential diagnosis may be markedly narrowed by an accurate history and pinpointed by the appropriate diagnostic procedure. A stepwise approach to every patient who presents with rectal bleeding will enable a prompt and precise diagnosis.

REFERENCES

1. **Teague, R. H., Manning, A. P., Thornton, J. R., Salmon, P. R. and Read, A. E.,** Colonoscopy for investigation of unexplained rectal bleeding, *Lancet,* 1, 1350, 1978.
2. **Kirkpatrick, J. R.,** Massive rectal bleeding in the adult, *Dis. Colon Rectum,* 12, 248, 1969.
3. **Moody, F. G.,** Rectal bleeding, *N. Engl. J. Med.,* 290, 839, 1974.
4. **Hoar, C. S. and Bernhard, W. F.,** Colonic bleeding and diverticular disease of the colon, *Surg. Gynecol. Obstet.,* 99: 101, 1954.
5. **Young, J. M. and Howorth, M. B., Jr.,** Massive hemorrhage in diverticulosis, *Ann. Surg.,* 146, 128, 1954.
6. **Hedberg, S. E.,** Endoscopy in gastrointestinal bleeding, *Surg. Clin. N.A.,* 54, 549, 1974.
7. **Balint, J. A., Sarfeh, I. J., and Fried, M. B.,** in *Gastrointestinal Bleeding. Diagnosis and Management,* John Wiley & Sons, New York, 1977, 23.
8. **Turell, R.,** Laceration to anorectum incident to enema, *Arch. Surg.,* 81, 953, 1960.
9. **Waye, J. D.,** Colitis, cancer, and colonoscopy, *Med. Clin. N.A.,* 62, 211, 1978.
10. **Shackelford, R. T.,** Hemorrhoids and their surgical treatment, in *Diseases of the Colon and Anorectum,* **Turell, R., Ed.,** W. B. Saunders, Philadelphia, 1959, 851.
11. **Marston, A., Pheils, M. T., Thomas, M. L. and Morson, B.** Ischaemic colitis, *Gut,* 7, 1, 1966.
12. **Bergan, J. J.,** Recognition and treatment of intestinal ischemia, *Surg. Clin. N.A.,* 47, 109, 1967.
13. **Kilpatrick, Z., Silverman, J., Betancourt, E., Farman, J., and Lawson, J.,** Vascular occlusion of colon and oral contraceptives, *N. Engl. J. Med.,* 269, 622, 1968.
14. **Collock, B. and Hume, A.,** Radiation injury to the sigmoid and rectum, *Surg. Gynecol. Obstet.,* 108, 306, 1959.
15. **Williams, C. B. and Waye, J. D.,** Colonoscopy in inflammatory bowel disease, *Clin. Gastroenterol.,* 7, 701, 1978.

16. **Korelitz, B. I. and Janowitz, H. D.,** Ulcerative colitis—general considerations, in *Diseases of the Colon and Anorectum,* **Turell, R., Ed.,** W. B. Saunders, Philadelphia, 1959, 662.
17. **Luke, R. G., Lees, W., and Rudick, J.,** Appearances of the stools after the introduction of blood into the caecum, *Gut,* 5, 77, 1964.
18. **Veidenheimer, M. C., Corman, M. L. and Coller, J. A.,** Colonic hemorrhage, *Surg. Clin. N.A.,* 58, 581, 1978.
19. **Knoepp, R. H. and McCulloch, J. H.,** Colonoscopy and the diagnosis of unexplained rectal bleeding, *Dis. Colon Rectum,* 21, 590, 1978.
20. **Knutson, C. O. and Max, M. H.,** Value of colonoscopy in patients with rectal blood loss unexplained by rigid proctosigmoidoscopy and barium contrast enema examinations, *Am. J. Surg.,* 130, 84, 1980.
21. **Tedesco, F. J., Waye, J. D., Raskin, J. B., Morris, S. J., and Greenwald, R. A.** Colonoscopic evaluation of rectal bleeding, *Ann. Int. Med.,* 89, 908, 1078.
22. **Reuter, S. R. and Bookstein, J. J.,** Angiographic localization of gastrointestinal bleeding, *Gastroenterology,* 54, 876, 1968.
23. **Adams, J. T.,** The barium enema as treatment for massive diverticular disease, *Dis. Colon Rectum,* 17, 439, 1974.
24. **Williams, C. B. and Teague, R. H.,** Progress report: colonoscopy, *Gut,* 14, 990, 1973.
25. **Brand, E. J., Sullivan, B. H., Jr., Sivak, M. V., Jr., and Rankin, G. B.,** Colonoscopy in the diagnosis of unexplained rectal bleeding, in press.
26. **Hunt, R. H.,** Rectal bleeding, *Clin. Gastroenterol.,* 7, 719, 1978.
27. **Swarbrick, E. T., Fevre, D. I., Hunt, R. H., Thomas, B. M., and Williams, C. B.,** Colonoscopy for unexplained rectal bleeding, *Br. J. Med.,* 2, 1685, 1978.
28. **Alavi, A., Dann, R. W., and Baum, S.,** Scintigraphic detection of acute gastrointestinal bleeding, *Radiology,* 124, 753, 1977.
29. **Winzelberg, G. G., McKusick, K. A., and Strauss, H. W.,** Evaluation of gastrointestinal bleeding by red blood cells labelled in vivo with technetium-99m, *J. Nucl. Med.,* 20, 1080, 1979.
30. **Nusbaum, M., Baum, S., and Blakemore, W. S.,** Clinical experience with the diagnosis and management of gastrointestinal hemorrhage by selective mesenteric catheterization, *Ann. Surg.,* 170, 506, 1969.
31. **Hall, T. J.,** Meckel's bleeding diverticulum diagnosed by mesenteric arteriography, *Br. J. Surg.,* 62, 882, 1975.
32. **Luk, G. D., Bynum, T. E., and Hendrix, T. R.,** Gastric aspiration in localization of gastrointestinal hemorrhage, *JAMA,* 241, 576, 1979.
33. **Blackstone, M. O. and Kirsner, J. B.,** Establishing the site of gastrointestinal bleeding, Editorial, *JAMA,* 241, 599, 1979.
34. **NIH Consensus Exercise,** The role of endoscopy in upper gastrointestinal hemorrhage, *National Institutes of Health,* Washington, D.C., in press.
35. Profuse bleeding from the colon, Editorial, *Lancet,* 2, 85, 1974.
36. **Abrams, B. and Lynn, H. B.,** Rectal bleeding in children, *Am. J. Surg.,* 104, 831, 1962.
37. **Behringer, G. E. and Albright, N. L.,** Diverticular disease of the colon: a frequent cause of rectal bleeding, *Am. J. Surg.,* 125, 419, 1973.
38. **Cathcart, P. M., Cathcart, R. S., and Rambo, W. M.,** Management of massive lower gastrointestinal bleeding, *Am. Surg.,* 43, 217, 1977.
39. **Peters, H. E., Jr.,** Massive hemorrhage from the lower intestinal tract, *West J. Surg.,* 41, 646, 1956.
40. **Turnbull, G. C.,** Massive hemorrhage from diverticula of the colon, *Q. Bull. Northwestern Univ. Med. School,* 22, 292, 1948.
41. **Baum, S., Athanasoulis, C. A., and Waltman, A. C.,** Angiographic diagnosis and control of large bowel bleeding, *Dis. Colon Rectum,* 17, 447, 1974.
42. **Casarella, W. J., Kanter, I. E., and Seaman, W. B.,** Right-sided colonic diverticula as a cause of acute rectal hemorrhage, *N. Engl. Med. J.,* 286, 450, 1972.
43. **Welch, C. W. and Hedberg, S.,** Gastrointestinal hemorrhage. I. General considerations of diagnosis and therapy, *Adv. Surg.,* 7, 95, 1973.
44. **Baum, S., Nusbaum, M., and Blakemore, W. S.,** The preoperative radiographic demonstration of intra-abdominal bleeding from undetermined sites by percutaneous selective celiac and superior mesenteric artiography, *Surgery,* 58: 797, 1965.
45. **Bartelheimer, W., Remmele, W., and Ottenjahn, R.,** Coloscopic recognition of hemangiomas in the colon ascendens, *Endoscopy,* 4, 109, 1972.
46. **Rogers, B. H. G. and Adler, F.,** Hemangiomas of the cecum. Colonoscopic diagnosis and therapy, *Gastroenterology,* 71, 1079, 1976.
47. **Skibba, R. M., Hartong, W. A. and Mantz, F. A.,** Angiodysplasia of the cecum: colonoscopic diagnosis, *Gastrointest. Endosc.,* 22, 177, 1976.

48. **Montori, A., Messinetti, S., Viceconte, G., Miscusi, G. Viceconte, G. W., and Pastorino, C.,** Diagnostic and operative colonoscopy in emergency diseases of the colon, *Surg. Ital.,* 6, 1, 1976.
49. **Rossini, F. P. and Ferrari, A.,** Emergency coloscopy, *Acta Endocrinol. Radiocin.,* 2, 165, 1976.
50. **Deyhle, P., Blum, A. L., Neusche, H. J., and Jenny, S.,** Emergency colonoscopy in the management of the acute peranal hemorrhage, *Endoscopy,* 6, 229, 1974.
51. **Schmitt, M. G., Jr., Wu, W. C. Geenen, J. E. and Hogan, W. J,** Diagnostic colonoscopy, *Gastroenterology,* 69, 765, 1975.
52. **Sheehy, T. W. and Floch, M. H.,** *The Small Intestine: Its Function and Diseases,* Harper & Row, New York, 1964, 419.

Chapter 10

ELECTROCOAGULATION OF VASCULAR ABNORMALITIES OF THE LARGE BOWEL

B. H. Gerald Rogers

TABLE OF CONTENTS

I. VASCULAR ABNORMALITIES

A. Introduction

For the purposes of this Chapter, vascular abnormalities of the cecal area will be defined as the small, bright red, flat, mucosal lesions usually seen in the cecum. Although they can be seen elsewhere in the large bowel, they do have a strong predilection for the cecal area, and tend to occur on the antimesenteric side opposite the ileocecal valve. Although the size can vary from pinpoint to over 2 cm in diameter, clinically significant lesions are usually between 3 and 10 mm in diameter. The blood vessels which make up the vascular abnormality are packed so closely together that the center of the lesion appears to be one solid, red mass. Although it is quite variable, the lesion usually has a rounded shape. Radiating vessels from the solid center sometimes give it a stellate appearance. It can occur singly, but usually two or three smaller, less-developed lesions are seen close to the largest. Biopsy of the lesion will usually show abnormal, dilated vessels with thin walls located in the mucosa between colonic glands. Less frequently, thick-walled vessels will be seen. Associated atheroemboli in the lamina propria are uncommon. Almost always, the patient will be elderly, with associated valvular heart disease, atherosclerotic cardiovascular disease, pulmonary disease, hypertension, or diabetes mellitus. Presentation is typically painless bleeding manifested by maroon-colored stools. Well-developed lesions will be elevated 1 to 2 mm above the surrounding mucosa and have a flat top. It is important to differentiate these small vascular abnormalities from larger vascular lesions which can affect the large bowel, such as varices, lymphangiomas, and capillary hemangiomas. The small lesions can be treated safely with endoscopic electrocoagulation. The role of endoscopic therapy for the larger lesions remains to be defined.

B. Historical Review

Not until the advent of angiography was it shown that small vascular abnormalities of the large bowel could result in significant hemorrhage. The first patient in whom the bleeding site was searched for and identified by angiography was a 69-year old woman with repeated massive hemorrhages from the rectum for 20 years, reported by Margulis et al.[1] During laparotomy, a mesenteric angiographic examination was performed by injecting the ileocecal artery. A bleeding vascular abnormality in the ascending colon was identified by the intraluminal extravasation of contrast material and a plexus of abnormal vessels. There was immediate opacification of the inferior mesenteric vein suggesting shunting. Baum et al.[2] were first to demonstrate a small vascular abnormality on the lateral aspect of the cecum in the intact patient. The lesion was not visible with conventional, superior mesenteric arteriography, but was seen by using magnification. A large arterial feeder could be seen extending to the abnormality. On the same exposure, a large, early-appearing, draining vein could be seen extending from a vascular lake. Edie and Brennan reported the first case of successful surgery for a vascular abnormality of the ascending colon which was diagnosed preoperatively by angiography.[3] The patient was a 72-year-old woman with unexplained, recurrent, bright-red rectal bleeding. Angiography showed a single vascular abnormality in the ascending colon. At surgery, the lesion was impossible to demonstrate by palpation or inspection of the serosal surface. Right colectomy cured her bleeding. Klein et al.[4] published the first convincing photomicrographs of a small vascular abnormality involving the mucosa of the large bowel in a surgical specimen. It showed the typical thin-walled, dilated vessels coursing between colonic glands.

Evidently, the first small vascular abnormality of the large bowel demonstrated in the living patient was reported by Bockus et al. in 1953[5]. The case was that of a 75-year old man who was investigated because of recurrent bloody stools of 18-months duration. After all diagnostic techniques had failed to reveal the cause, he was explored when actively bleeding. At surgery, the cecum was turned inside-out. It showed a "dark red, rosebud-like lesion, measuring 3 mm in diameter, resembling a hemangioma with a white fleck in the center." A right colectomy was performed and there was no bleeding in the succeeding 19 months of follow-up. Multiple sections of the surgical specimen failed to reveal conclusive evidence of the vascular abnormality. Bartelheimer et al.[6] were first to recognize the lesion colonoscopically. They reported a 70-year old woman with profuse gastrointestinal bleeding which occurred over a period of 7 years. In spite of intense diagnostic procedures including exploratory laparotomies, the source of bleeding could not be elucidated. Only total colonoscopy combined with biopsy verified multiple vascular abnormalities in the cecum. Rogers and Adler were first to report electrocoagulation for therapy of these lesions.[7] They reported five cases of vascular abnormalities in the cecum demonstrated by colonoscopy after more conventional diagnostic methods had failed. The lesions were bright-red and flat, and clearly seen through the colonoscope. They were all successfully treated with electrocoagulation. All five patients had some type of associated cardiac or vascular disease. Also published with this article were the first photographs of endoscopic biopsies which demonstrate the histology of the vascular abnormality.

Small vascular abnormalities of the large bowel were difficult to detect prior to angiography or colonoscopy. They are rarely seen at surgery because of their location in the mucosa. The lesions have been extremely difficult to demonstrate in the surgical pathology specimen because they are small, flat, and inconspicuous in the fixed state. Alfidi et al.[8] were first to demonstrate the lesion with a corrosive cast. This method confirmed the angiographic diagnosis, but had the disadvantage of destroying the tissue in the process. Baum was first to use a silicone-rubber solution to study the lesion.[9] He injected the surgical specimen with the solution and allowed it to harden. The specimen was then subjected to a clearing procedure in which the tissue water was replaced by a material with a low index of refraction, such as glycerin or methylsalicylate. With this technique, the tissue parenchyma remained intact, although it was poorly visible. In the final product, therefore, only the rubber-filled vascular channels were evident and could be viewed under a dissecting microscope. Later, the tissue could be processed through routine histologic procedures for microscopic confirmation. The first photograph of such an injected specimen came from a 75-year old man who had passed black stools 7 days prior to admission. He was known to have chronic, mild azotemia. A biopsy of the kidney had disclosed acute and chronic pyelonephritis, with atheromatous emboli. Hypertension had been known to be present for 5 years. Four years previously, he had a lacunar stroke. Selective superior mesenteric angiography showed a cluster of abnormally dilated vessels in the area of the cecum. The patient underwent a right colectomy. The surgical specimen was treated as outlined above. When examined with the dissecting microscope, it showed an abnormal cluster of vessels resembling a coral reef extending up from the depths and replacing the normal mucosa. The entire abnormal area did not occupy more than 3 mm of tissue. The specimen was then processed in the usual manner for microscopic examination. It showed dilated, thin-walled blood vessels in the mucosa and submucosa. Without the localization by injection technique, this small lesion would almost certainly have been missed.

It is no wonder that small vascular abnormalities of the large bowel went virtually unrecognized in the past. In 1949, Gentry et al.[10] reported 106 cases of vascular tumors and malformations of the bowel among the 1,400,000 case records of the Mayo Clinic. In their series, only Case 4 can be recognized as a typical small vascular abnormality affecting the large bowel. It was found in the cecum of a 67-year old man who died from hypertension, arteriosclerosis, and hemiplegia. The lesion was 1 × 1.3 × 1 cm and was found incidentally at autopsy. Boley et al.[11] showed that the lesions were more likely to be multiple and also occurred in elderly patients without a history of bleeding. Twelve colons taken from patients who had a clinical and angiographic diagnosis of bleeding from a vascular abnormality of the large bowel were studied by the injection technique. Only three of the specimens showed a single vascular abnormality. The other 9 showed 2 or more lesions, including one with more than 25. The colon with the greatest number of mucosal lesions came from the oldest patient, who was 84 years of age. Boley's group also studied 15 right colons resected from patients with carcinoma. None of these patients had a history of gastrointestinal bleeding or of large bowel obstruction, and all were over 60 years of age. Single mucosal vascular abnormalities were identified in 4 of the 15 colons. The lesions were small when compared to those seen in patients with clinically diagnosed bleeding. Large, dilated, tortuous submucosal veins were noted in 8 of the 15 colons, including the 4 with mucosal lesions. It was concluded that an enlarged submucosal vein was one of the earliest steps in the formation of these vascular abnormalities. These findings indicate that these lesions are present in a significant portion of the population over 60 years of age, with or without bleeding. Boley's group concluded that these small vascular abnormalities may be the most common source of bleeding from the large bowel. Thus, over a period of 30 years, the small vascular abnormality of the large bowel came to be recognized as a common lesion, whereas before it was thought to be quite rare.

Clinicians were aware of the increased incidence of gastrointestinal bleeding in patients with aortic stenosis before small vascular abnormalities of the large bowel were demonstrated. Only after angiography had demonstrated that the vascular lesions in patients with aortic stenosis was the association clarified. In 1958, Heyde wrote to the editor of the *New England Journal of Medicine* stating that he had seen 10 patients with aortic stenosis over the previous 10 years with gastrointestinal bleeding for which he could discover no cause. All patients were elderly and ranged in age from 60 to 80.[12] Schwartz responded by noting also a relationship between aortic stenosis and unexplained gastrointestinal bleeding in an elderly patient.[13] Williams was also impressed with the massive, unexplained, recurrent gastrointestinal hemorrhage that occurred in patients with aortic stenosis.[14] He did a review of 1443 consecutive gastrointestinal bleeders and found 95 (6.5%) were judged to have no demonstrable source for their blood loss. Of this group, 25% had aortic valvular lesions, mainly calcific stenosis, a significant difference from matched controls. In addition, the majority of patients with unexplained bleeding were in the seventh and eighth decades of life. In 1965, Jacobsen recommended a blind right colectomy for a suspected bleeding vascular abnormality in the ascending colon of a 70-plus-year old woman with marked aortic stenosis and unexplained gastrointestinal bleeding.[15] He had gotten this idea from Dr. Richard B. Cattell of the Lahey Clinic, who had cured a similar patient by surgical excision of the right colon.

Early angiographic studies paid little attention to diseases associated with the vascular abnormality.[4,16-18] Boss and Rosenbaum,[19] in 1971, reported the case of a 77-year-old man who had continuous gastrointestinal bleeding of obscure cause which was present for the 6 years prior to his death. He had severe aortic stenosis, and at autopsy it was clear that the bleeding was coming from the right colon. In 1974, Galloway et al.[20] showed the cause of bleeding in patients with aortic stenosis was a vascular abnormality in the right colon. Angiographic studies demonstrated the lesions in three consecutive patients with lower gastrointestinal tract bleeding of unknown cause. Right colectomy resulted in cessation of bleeding. It is interesting that one of three patients had idiopathic hypertrophic subaortic stenosis. The observation was important because prior to that time, it was thought by some that only patients with calcific aortic stenosis were subject to increased gastrointestinal bleeding. An association between the colonoscopically visualized vascular abnormality and aortic stenosis was made by Rogers and Adler in 1976.[7] In addition, an association was made between other types of cardiac and vascular disease, including mitral insufficiency, atherosclerotic vascular disease, and coronary artery disease. In 1977, Baum et al.[21] reported 34 patients who had a vascular abnormality of the right large bowel, 17 of whom had a history of cardiac disease. Nine had a clinical diagnosis of aortic stenosis. Three had combined valvular disease, and five had atherosclerotic coronary disease. In 1979, Gelfand et al.[22] reported five patients with aortic stenosis who had multiple, massive hemorrhages from the lower gastrointestinal tract which defied diagnosis by conventional methods. Mesenteric angiography, however, disclosed the origin of bleeding. In four patients, vascular abnormalities were found in the right colon and one in the jejunum. Right hemicolectomy and partial jejunectomy resulted in a cure in all. Boley et al.[23] reported nine patients with aortic stenosis among 32 in whom vascular abnormalities of the right colon were identified by angiography. In 1980, Rogers reported a colonoscopic series of 24 patients with small vascular abnormalities in the colon.[24] Twenty of the 24 had associated cardiac, vascular, or pulmonary disease. Three of them had aortic stenosis.

Thus, it is clear from the literature that there is a definite relationship between aortic stenosis and hemorrhage from vascular abnormalities of the right large bowel. In addition to aging, there seems to be a definite correlation between this vascular abnormality and other disease states, including atherosclerotic coronary disease, valvular heart disease other than aortic stenosis, atherosclerotic vascular disease, long-standing hypertension, diabetes mellitus, and chronic obstructive pulmonary disease. It is interesting to note that the earliest small vascular abnormality of the cecum recognizable in the literature was described in a 67-year-old man who had hypertension, arteriosclerosis, and hemiplegia.[10] A grade II systolic murmur was noted in the 75-year-old man first reported to have a vascular abnormality in the cecum at surgery.[5] In the first case report of small vascular abnormality seen colonoscopically, the patient was a 70-year-old woman who had symptoms of beginning circulatory failure.[6] Genant and Ranniger reported two cases in 1972,[25] one of whom was a 65-year-old patient with a heart murmur. In one of the four cases reported by Crichlow et al.[26] in 1975, chronic obstructive pulmonary disease and congestive heart failure were noted. In 1976, Skibba et al.[27] reported a vascular abnormality seen colonoscopically in the cecum of a 69-year-old man with a grade II/VI systolic ejection murmur. The cardiograph showed left axis deviation. In 1977, Thanik et al.[28] reported a 56-year-old man with angina who was found to be bleeding from a vascular abnormality of the cecum at colonscopy. In 1978, Richardson et al.[29] reported 39 patients with bleeding vascular abnormalities. Twenty-nine of this group were 50 years of age or older. Of these 29, 12 had aortic stenosis and 11 other patients had other forms of cardiac disease, usually manifested as congestive heart failure requiring digitalis therapy. In 1980, Tedesco et al.[30] reported 15 patients with vascular abnormalities of the colon. Three of the patients had chronic obstructive pulmonary disease. One had angina, one had mitral valvular disease, and another had had a mild myocardial infarction 5 years previously. All were 56 years of age or older. In 1980, Thompson[31] noted the majority of his patients had diabetes mellitus. Heart disease and generalized atherosclerosis were also common.

From the historical perspective, a high incidence of unexplained lower intestinal bleeding was first recognized in patients with aortic stenosis. Angiographic studies showed most of those patients to be bleeding from a small vascular abnormality in the area of the cecum. As more patients were studied, it became clear that the lesion was not only present in patients with aortic stenosis, but also in patients with other forms of cardiovascular disease, pulmonary disease, hypertension, and diabetes mellitus. It is also clear from both colonoscopic and angiographic studies that the lesions can occur in otherwise clinically healthy patients. At this time, it is impossible to know whether all of these small vascular abnormalities are similar or have a common etiology. However, any theory of formation must take all of this data into consideration.

C. Terminology

1. Hemangioma

In 1949, Gentry et al.[10] classified their single vascular abnormality of the cecal area as a capillary hemangioma. Since it was found in a patient who had hypertension, arteriosclerosis, and hemiplegia, it can be considered a lesion of the type dealt with in this Chapter. When Bockus et al.,[5] in 1953, reported a vascular abnormality of the cecum, they described it as a "dark-red, rosebud-like lesion, measuring 3 mm in diameter, resembling a hemangioma with a white fleck in the center". Unfortunately, they were not able to conclusively demonstrate the lesion microscopically. In 1971, Upson et al.[32] classified a small vascular abnormality of the cecum which was diagnosed by angiography as a hemangioma, because of the widely dilated vascular channels within the submucosa and serosal regions, composed of both venous and arterial components. In 1972, Bartelheimer et al[6] described the first colonoscopically visualized lesion as a hemangioma. The basis for this decision was a combination of its endoscopic and mircroscopic appearances. Endoscopically, many sharply demarcated, reddish, ovoid patches of about 1 cm in diameter were evident on the medial wall of the cecum. Microscopically, the mucosa contained many vessels characterized by a thin wall and a wide lumen. The walls of these vessels consisted only of a flat endothelial layer and a basal membrane. In 1976, Rogers and Adler[7] used the term *hemangioma* to be in step with Bartelheimer et al.[6] In addition, the lesion most closely fell into the category of simple, capillary hemangioma as outlined by Gentry et al.[10] By definition, *hemangioma* is a benign tumor made up of newly formed blood vessels. The small vascular abnormalities which occur in the cecal area of elderly patients do appear to be made up of newly formed blood vessels, but whether or not they are actually neoplastic, as implied in the term *hemangioma,* has not been settled. Presently, it is believed that these lesions are not neoplastic and, therefore, the use of the term can be misleading.

2. Arteriovenous Malformation

Arteriovenous malformation is a term commonly used by radiologists in describing the small vascular abnormality seen in the right colon on angiography. *Arteriovenous anastomosis,*[3] *arteriovenous shunt,*[16] and *arteriovenous fistula*[2] are all synonyms for *arteriovenous malformation.* Hagihara et al.[33] gave the angiographic definition of an arteriovenous malformation in 1977. It consists of a slightly enlarged feeding artery, a vascular lake, and an early draining vein. The first small vascular abnormality located in the cecum reported by Baum et al.[2] was called an *arteriovenous malformation* and an *arteriovenous fistula.* Magnification radiography was necessary to demonstrate the large feeding artery, small vascular lake, and early draining vein. Moore et al.[34] studied 17 patients with arteriovenous malformations and categorized them into three types: Type 1 arteriovenous malformations were solitary, localized lesions within the right colon which occurred in seven patients 55 years of age or older. None were palpable or visible at operation. Type 2 occurred in seven patients. They were larger and occasionally visible at surgery. They were most commonly found in the small intestine and thought to be probably of congenital origin. All of their symptoms began before 50 years of age. Type 3 were those associated with hereditary hemorrhagic telangiectasia. All of the arteriovenous malformations were diagnosed on the basis of typical angiographic findings, as outlined above, or microscopic examination of excised tissue. Arteriovenous malformation is a very general term and can include many vascular abnormalities besides those small ones found in the cecal area.

Many other authors have used the same term to describe their angiographic findings.[26,35,36] Mitsudo et al.[37] have studied these lesions thoroughly, utilizing injection techniques, plus light microscopy and scanning electron microscopy. They have shown that what appeared to be a vascular lake angiographically, is actually a conglomeration of dilated, thin-walled venules and capillaries. They did find evidence for arteriovenous shunting, but it appeared to be a minor part of the lesion. Thus, the angiographic and microscopic findings do not seem to correlate. The most significant sign angiographically is shunting which is demonstrated by the early draining vein,[38] whereas microscopically, the evidence for shunting is minimal. By definition, *arteriovenous malformation* is an acceptable term to describe the abnormality seen angiographically, if shunting is present. When doing so, one must realize the arteriovenous malformation may represent only a small part of the vascular abnormality. The term should not be used to describe the lesion as seen endoscopically because the colonoscopist sees the blood-filled, dilated venules and capillaries. It should not be used to describe the microscopic findings unless thick-walled vessels and arterialized veins are seen.

3. Angiodysplasia

Galdabini used this term to describe a small "coral reef" vascular abnormality of the ascending colon,[39] which Baum had previously referred to as an *arteriovenous malformation.*[9] Baum et al.[21,40] accepted *angiodysplasia* and have used it to describe such lesions in the right colon. This is a confusing term because by definition, *dysplasia* is an abnormality of development such as is seen in congenital defects.[41] In pathology, the term *dysplasia* usually refers to an alteration in size, shape, and organization of adult cells. It is best known from its use in describing cellular deviations from the normal in the epithelium in the uterine cervix.[41]

Evidently, a variety of conditions can give rise to the angiographic diagnosis of angiodysplasia and, therefore, the term suffers because it is nonspecific. Tarin et al.,[42] in 1978, reported 12 consecutive patients studied with angiography in whom a diagnosis of angiodysplasia was made. Microscopic examination of the resected specimens, however, revealed a variety of lesions other than the classical angiodysplasia as described by Baum and Galdabini. Their conclusion was that although the term angiodysplasia was useful clinically and radiologically, it should not be taken to denote a single pathological entity.

Unfortunately, the term *angiodysplasia* has been used in association with Osler-Weber-Rendu disease. Prior to the adoption of the term by Baum and Galdabini, Halpern et al.,[43] in 1968, used angiography to study a series of four patients with hereditary hemorrhagic telangiectasia. All four patients had vascular abnormalities of the abdominal viscera, which were thought to be an integral part of hereditary hemorrhagic telangiectasia, and were described as angiodysplasia. No histology was available.

The term *angiodysplasia* has gained acceptance in the medical community and has been used widely. However, small vascular abnormalities of the cecal area are not presently believed to be dysplastic in any sense of the word. In addition, the term is nonspecific, as observed by Tarin et al.[42] For these reasons, it appears wise to abandon this term.

4. Vascular ectasia (Angiectasis)

Boley et al.[11] studied colons from patients with the clinical and angiographic diagnoses of cecal vascular lesions. Surgical specimens were studied by injection and clearing, and also by histological sections. Minimal lesions showed ectasia and distortion of only a few capillary rings of the superficial mucosal circulation. The most extensive lesions replaced the normal vascular architecture with dilated, thin-walled, tortuous, distorted vessels resembling the coral reef, as described by Baum.[9] Surprisingly, the most prominent and consistent finding was not the mucosal lesion, but the presence of markedly ectatic and tortuous submucosal veins. They found no evidence for neoplasm, nor any morphological changes associated with congenital arteriovenous malformation. On the basis of these findings, the term *vascular ectasia* was introduced to describe the typical small vascular abnormality of the right colon. They were thought to be degenerative lesions of aging.[11] Athanasoulis et al.[40] think *vascular ectasia* is a rather unfortunate combination of Latin and incorrect Greek. *Vascular* is Latin and *ectasia* is Greek. Evidently, the Greek meaning for *ectasia* is stretching, and to satisfy purists, the term *vascular ectasia* should be abandoned or substituted with the etymologically correct term, *angiectasis.* He also noted that in the majority of cases studied by his group, some of the component vessels are narrowed, rather than dilated. In a more recent report of the pathologic character of the vascular abnormalities described by Boley's group, Mitsudo reported the findings of 26 right colons resected from patients with a clinical and angiographic diagnosis of bleeding from a colonic area of vascular ectasia.[37] Most cases demonstrated the typical dilated vessels previously described in their original paper.[11] One patient, however, had a vascular abormality which occurred at the mouth of a diverticulum. It had large, thick-walled arteries and several thick-walled, nondilated veins resembling a congenital arteriovenous malformation. Thus, what appeared clinically and angiographically to be a vascular ectasia, turned out to be an arteriovenous malformation on microscopic examination.

Vascular ectasia is a proper term when microscopic exam shows dilated vessels, but it is fallacious to believe that all vascular abnormalities seen on angiography or colonoscopy will turn out to be of this single type. *Angiectasis,* a refined synonym for *vascular ectasia,* can also be used properly to describe dilated vessels. In addition, the term *angiectasis* has the advantage of being etymologically homogeneous and briefer than the term *vascular ectasia.*

5. Vascular Malformation

Vascular malformation was the term used by Margulis et al.[1] to describe the first vascular abnormality diagnosed during interoperative angiography. Galloway et al.[20] used the term when describing their three cases of vascular abnormalities of the right colon associated with aortic stenosis. Recently, Richardson et al.[29] used the term to describe the lesions found in a combined angiographic and colonoscopic series. The term is noncontroversial because it is simply descriptive. By definition, *vascular malformation* means deformed vessels. Malformation can refer to both deformity of congenital origin and of mature tissues.[41] Therefore, the use of this term does not indicate etiology or pathogenesis.

6. Vascular Dysplasia

Genant and Ranniger used this term to describe their two cases of angiographically demonstrated vascular abnormalities of the right colon.[25] They chose this term because they found it extremely difficult to differentiate clinically and histologically between neoplasms (hemangioma), arteriovenous malformations (hamartomas), and simple telangiectasias. They noted that the terms were used indiscriminately and interchangeably in the literature. Therefore, they chose the term *vascular dysplasia* to encompass all vascular abnormalities. Unfortunately, *dysplasia* suffers from the connotations of congenital defect and cellular deviation as given in detail under angiodysplasia. In light of the present understanding of the small vascular abnormality of the cecal area, the term *vascular dysplasia* is inappropriate.

7. Angioma

Bentley used this term when describing the diagnostic problem of the bleeding cecal vascular abnormality.[44] One difficulty with this term is that it does not differentiate between types of blood vessels involved in the lesion, since an angioma could be made up of either blood or lymph vessels. *Angioma* suggests neoplasia, like *hemangioma,* and for the same reasons is incorrect.

8. Telangiectasia

Waye has used the term *telangiectasia* to describe vascular abnormalities of the right colon seen colonoscopically.[45] By definition, *telangiectasia* is a thin, web-like vessel which is stretched.[41] Most of the vascular abnormalities seen colonoscopically will show these findings on biopsy. The term, however, has been strongly associated with hereditary hemorrhagic telangiectasia, and when used, suggests Osler-Weber-Rendu disease. Therefore, it would be confusing to apply it to the vascular abnormality of the cecal area, since the clinical syndromes are so different.

9. Resolution

In a recent article, Gelfand et al.[46] used the terms *vascular malformation, angiodysplasia, vascular dysplasia, mucosal ectasia, submucosal ectasia,* and *vascular ectasia* interchangeably, without defining any of them. All of these terms have been used to describe the small vascular abnormality seen in the cecal area. All have some relevance, but none are completely satisfactory. Continued indiscriminate use of these terms will not further the understanding of this disease. It is clear from the work of the angiographer that most of the small vascular abnormalities which affect the large bowel have an early draining vein, strongly suggestive of an arteriovenous malformation. Many of these lesions have been proven to be the "coral reef" abnormality described by Baum and Galdabini, and labeled as *angiodysplasia.*[9,39] From the work of Boley's group, it is clear the characteristic feature of most of these lesions is dilation or *vascular ectasia*[11]. When the colonoscopist is confronted with a small vascular lesion in the large bowel, it is impossible to be certain whether it is the "coral reef" lesion of Baum, an arteriovenous malformation, a hemangioma, or some other vascular abnormality. Therefore, it is proposed that the colonoscopist withhold judgment as to the nature of the vascular abnormality until there is biopsy proof of its nature. If the biopsy shows thin-walled, abnormally dilated vessels in the mucosa, then the diagnosis would be vascular ectasia, or angiectasis. If the biopsy shows thick-walled vascular spaces, then the diagnosis of arteriovenous malformation should be entertained. If both components are present, then both should be taken into consideration when reaching a diagnosis. Other diagnoses would depend upon appropriate histological findings. This resolution of the problem is similar to the present approach to polyps of the large bowel. The term polyp can be used to describe all protrusions into the lumen of the bowel. The histology of a colonic polyp can only be suspected until microscopic evidence is at hand. A similar approach to mucosal vascular abnormalities of the large bowel seems in order.

D. Colonoscopic Diagnosis

1. Clinical Setting

The clinical setting should alert the colonoscopist to the possibility of a small vascular abnormality in the cecal area. The diagnosis should be suspected in any elderly patient whose gastrointestinal blood loss has been undiagnosed by other means. The patient will usually be 55 years of age or older. Most patients will present with gross rectal bleeding which is usually bright-red when rapid, and dark-red or maroon when slower. These patients can present with black stools because slow bleeding from the right colon can result in melena. Some will present with other symptoms and be found to be anemic. If the anemia is caused by a vascular abnormality, the stools will probably be intermittently positive for occult blood. Almost all patients will have some obvious associated disease. Associated conditions include atherosclerotic heart disease, valvular heart disease, atherosclerotic vascular disease, chronic obstructive pulmonary disease, hypertension, or diabetes mellitus. Many patients will have more than one condition. Even if there is no obvious associated condition, the patient will almost always be in the elderly age group. The lesions will be found about equally in males and females.

Physical examination is likely to show pallor, spooning of the nails, hypertension, evidence for an old CVA, increased anterior-posterior diameter of the thorax, cardiac murmur, decreased peripheral pulses, or other findings consistent with the associated diseases previously discussed. Usually, by the time a patient with gastrointestinal blood loss is being considered for colonoscopy, most of the routine diagnostic procedures will have been completed. Contrast X-ray studies of the entire gastrointestinal tract will be normal or show abnormalities not related to the patient's blood loss. If angiography has shown a vascular abnormality in the right large bowel prior to colonoscopy, then the colonoscopist should expect to find a mucosal lesion which corresponds with the angiographic findings. However, even if precolonoscopy angiography is negative, the diagnosis should still be considered and colonoscopy performed. Regardless of what investigations have been done previously, the only way to exclude a small mucosal vascular abnormality of the cecal area is to do total colonoscopy in the well-prepared patient. Also, colonoscopy may disclose other significant lesions, such as carcinoma, polyps, or inflammatory bowel diseases which may explain the patient's blood loss.

2. Endoscopic Findings

The small mucosal vascular abnormality of the large bowel will be found primarily in the cecum and proximal ascending colon. The largest and most highly developed lesion is usually found in the cecum on its antimesenteric aspect opposite the ileocecal valve and a little below it. This area should be carefully inspected endoscopically in all patients who are suspected of harboring the lesion. It may be single, but more often there are several, additional, smaller lesions found close to the largest. The abnormalities may be scattered throughout the entire large bowel, but are less frequent and less well-developed as one proceeds distally from the cecum. If the clinical setting strongly suggests a small vascular abnormality of the large bowel and it is endoscopically negative, inspection of the distal terminal ileum should be carried out because the lesions have been reported there.[47]

The lesion is easy to recognize endoscopically in the living patient because it is perfused by oxygenated blood which gives it a bright-red color. Any lesion seen endoscopically which is bluish should be considered to be some other kind of vascular abnormality such as a varix. Biopsy or electrocoagulation of such lesions is not recommended. The center of a well-developed lesion is composed of a mass of vascular tissues so dense that individual blood vessels cannot be discerned. At the margin of the lesion, individual vessels may be seen trailing off and disappearing into the mucosa. These vessels radiate from the center and, therefore, frequently give it a stellate appearance. If there are no radiating vessels, the shape is usually ovoid or circular. The shape can be very irregular, especially when two large lesions are located close together and vessels are seen coursing between them. Lesions 2 or 3 mm in diameter frequently have a triangular shape. The size varies from pinpoint to over 2 cm in diameter. The lesion responsible for bleeding is usually well-developed and 3 mm or more in size. Most will not be bleeding when viewed endoscopically. The surface of the lesion is glistening when intact. A white fleck located near the center is occasionally seen and indicates erosion. The presence of erosion increases the likelihood that the lesion has bled recently. Most lesions will be flat and flush with the surrounding mucosa. Extremely well-developed ones will be slightly raised 1 or 2 mm and are more likely to be eroded. Elevation above the surrounding mucosa is difficult to see unless the lesion is viewed tangentially.

Small mucosal vascular abnormalities of the large bowel are quite friable. Just touching them frequently results in brisk, bright-red bleeding. This is easily differentiated from a varix which gives the cushion sign when touched. The colonoscopist will have no difficulty recognizing large vascular abnormalities of the colon. They usually occur in a much younger age group, show phleboliths on X-ray, and grossly deform the lumen resulting in a characteristic appearance on X-ray. Endoscopically, the appearance is of a large, irregular mass composed of small vessels perfused by oxygenated blood and large vessels carrying venous blood.[48] Endoscopic therapy is not recommended for these large lesions.

3. Histologic Confirmation

Endoscopic biopsy is necessary for histologic confirmation of small vascular abnormalities visualized colonoscopically. Although vascular lesions have been biopsied with ordinary pinch forceps,[6] it is recommended that the insulated electrocoagulating forceps, as described by Williams, be used.[49] This allows simultaneous electrocoagulation and biopsy. Details of the technique will be given in the following section. Because of its long-term implications, the necessity of histologic confirmation cannot be emphasized too strongly. Spontaneous ecchymoses or endoscope-induced submucosal hemorrhages are indistinguishable endoscopically from small vascular abnormalities. Therefore, without histologic proof, the diagnosis is tenuous. Since small vascular abnormalities can occur also in the small bowel and stomach, histologic confirmation of the diagnosis in the colon has important implications, especially if the patient continues to lose blood after all the lesions in the large bowel have been destroyed or removed. If properly obtained, the specimen will show large, abnormal, dilated vascular channels in the mucosa coursing between colonic glands. The vascular channels will be lined by a thin wall composed primarily of endothelial cells. Occasionally, an erosion demonstrating the bleeding site will be seen. This histology is compatible with the "coral reef" lesion of Baum,[9] or the vascular ectasia of Boley.[11] An arteriovenous malformation seen endoscopically may be more prominently elevated and less vascular in appearance. Biopsy will show vessels with thick walls and relatively narrow lumens. It is not unusual to find vessels with both thin and thick walls in the same lesion. Atheromatous emboli will be found infrequently, and are diagnosed by the cholesterol clefts seen in the mucosa and submucosa. The implication here is that the patient may have atheromatous emboli in other parts of the body, which could explain other symptoms.

Most pathologists will miss a small vascular abnormality of the bowel without coaching from the colonoscopist. Pathologists are in the habit of looking for malignancy or inflammation in such biopsies. Therefore, they focus their attention in the epithelial cells of the colonic glands. In a vascular abnormality, these cells will be absolutely normal. The pathologist is also attuned to looking for inflammation, primarily in the lamina propria. Small vascular abnormalities of the large bowel are almost never associated with any type of inflammation. Review of the microscopic slides with the pathologist will be necessary in most cases to make the proper diagnosis.

E. Electrocoagulation

1. Technique

Good visualization of the lesion is a prerequisite for proper therapy. Needless to say, adequate preparation is a necessity. The best position to view the lesion is perpendicularly. Slight deviations from the perpendicular are tolerable, but attempting to treat the lesion from a tangential view is fraught with difficulties. Good preparation tends to eliminate explosive gases such as hydrogen and methane. Sparking during colonoscopic electrosurgery can ignite these gases and result in a disastrous explosion.[50] This author uses carbon dioxide throughout the entire procedure so that even if preparation is not perfect, electrocoagulation can be safely completed. This is important because sometimes it is a long, hard struggle to pass the colonoscope all the way to the cecum. The adequacy of preparation of the right colon cannot be determined until it is reached. It would be very frustrating to find a lesion and not be able to treat it because of residual feces.

Safe, familiar electrosurgical equipment in good-working order should be used. This author uses the Williams® electrocoagulating biopsy forceps (A.C.M.I.®, Cat. #9115). These insulated biopsy forceps can be used to obtain tissue for microscopic examination and simultaneously electrocoagulate the remaining surrounding mucosa. All patients in this author's series were examined by A.C.M.I.® colonoscopes. The colonoscope with the joy-stick control is ideally suited for scanning the cecum. Light source, electrosurgical unit, and carbon dioxide insufflation are all provided by the Wappler Pnuemotome 200.

The largest lesion is dealt with first. It is the most likely source of the patient's bleeding, and any reduction in its mass of vascular tissue should decrease the chance for further bleeding. Also, if the electrocoagulation session is terminated prematurely, the greatest good would have been accomplished with the allotted time. The electrocoagulating biopsy forceps are passed through the channel and protruded beyond the tip of the colonoscope far enough so the operator can see the insulation. This prevents short circuiting of current through the instrument. Size of the lesion is estimated by the open forceps, which have a diameter of 8 mm. A small bite of the lesion is taken with the forceps and elevated from the surrounding mucosa to produce a tent-like pyramid with the lesion at its apex. Too small a bite will simply pull vascular tissue away from the lesion and initiate profuse bleeding—too large a bite will result in ineffective electrocoagulation and increases the possibility of hemorrhage. After the lesion has been grasped and elevated, 10 W of current are applied. This is the lowest power setting on the Pneumotome. As soon as the tissue at the apex of the "tent" turns white, the biopsy is obtained by quickly pulling the forceps into the scope. If there is no effect after 2 sec. of applied current, the power is increased to 15 W. In some patients, 25 W is necessary, particularly if they are obese. Ideally, not more than 2 sec. is required for application of current, although sometimes 4 sec. is used. The longer the application and higher the power setting, the more likely there will be a transmural burn and possible perforation. Electrosurgical therapy works best when the site is not flooded with blood, feces, or residual enema fluid. The first specimen obtained is the one most likely to confirm the diagnosis histologically. After the first specimen is taken, residual vascular tissue is grasped, elevated, and treated in the same fashion. This eventually results in some bleeding and distortion of the tissues so that the task becomes more and more difficult. It is, therefore, advantageous to make the entire procedure as quick and bloodless as possible.

It should be emphasized that when taking a biopsy with the electrocoagulating forceps, careful attention to details is necessary in order to obtain satisfactory material. When the forceps have mucosa in its grasp, the high—frequency current causes heat to build up in the tissue beyond the forceps because of the increased resistance at that point. The forceps themselves do not become hot unless heat generated in the tissue diffuses back into them. For this reason, it is important to withdraw the specimen as quickly as possible after the mucosa has been electrocoagulated in order to prevent this back-diffusion of heat, which may cause coagulation of the biopsy specimen.

Mounting the biopsy specimen properly is important in obtaining good orientation for microscopic study. After the specimen has been obtained, the forceps are opened perpendicularly over a small piece of Millipore® filter paper. A needle is used to disengage the specimen from the forceps and transfer it to the filter paper. This should be done in such a way that the mucosal surface is oriented away from the paper. The specimen tends to stick to the filter paper and can be dropped directly into formalin. The pathology technician is then instructed to mount the specimen so that cutting will result in a cross section of the mucosa. Millipore® paper is used because it can be processed right along with the mucosal specimen without damage to the microtome knife. Although the electrocoagulating biopsy forceps is preferred, the dome-tip electrode can also be used (A.C.M.I.® Cat. #253-165). The disadvantages of using the electrode include the tendency for the electrode to break away coagulated tissue during withdrawal after treatment. This can be prevented somewhat by cleaning the electrode and applying Pam®* between every second electrocoagulation. Another disadvantage of the electrode is that when it is pressed against the bowel wall, the resulting pressure tends to thin it out, which results in conditions more favorable for a transmural burn. On the contrary, the electrocoagulating biopsy forceps elevate the mucosal lesion away from the underlying muscularis propria, which tends to prevent a transmural burn. Therefore, when using the dome-tip electrode, applications of current are given with light pressure. Consequently, there is less tissue destruction and more than one course of therapy may be necessary in order to eradicate the lesions. Another disadvantage is the lack of tissue for microscopic examination.

2. *Personal Cases with Commentary*

The 35 cases included in this series are virtually all those in whom this author has found small mucosal vascular abnormalities of the large bowel. This series dates from August of 1971 to August of 1980 and includes approximately 4000 colonoscopies. Excluded from this series are congenital vascular abnormalities found in children or young adults which only incidentally involved the large bowel.[48] Also excluded are varices and telangiectases which occur after radiation. All cases of hereditary hemorrhagic telangiectisia have been excluded except for one case (15) in which the patient appears to have both conditions.

As this author gained more experience with this lesion, identification has been more frequent. Two years of colonoscopy passed before the first case of a vascular abnormality of the cecum was found. Only after learning to identify the lesion endoscopically could the diagnosis be made with any frequency. Recognition of the syndrome in which the lesion is found was also helpful. Consequently, the proportion of cases recently identified is greater.

Case 1: This 62-year-old woman was referred because of recurrent rectal bleeding of 8-years duration. The sigmoid colon had been resected because of multiple diverticula, which were thought to be a source of bleeding. Her hemorrhages continued unabated. Colonoscopy by another gastroenterologist was said to be

*Pam® is a cooking oil made by Boyle-Midway Inc., New York and is available in most grocery stores.

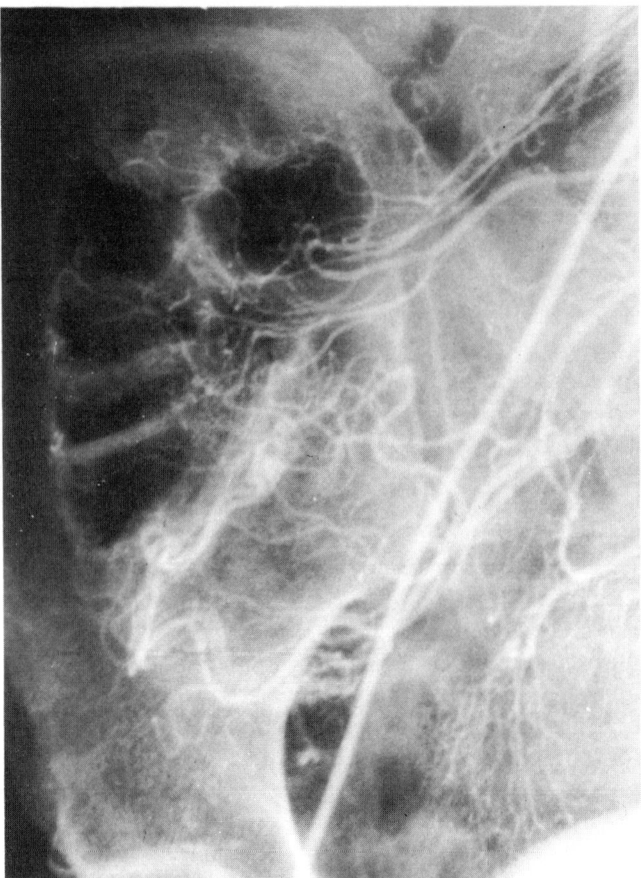

FIGURE 1. Vascular abnormality in the cecum demonstrated by angiography (Case 1). (From Rogers, B. H. G. and Adler, F., *Gastroenterology,* 71, 1079, 1976.

negative. Characteristically, the patient's bleeding was painless and followed a definite pattern. She first experienced borborygmi, then gaseousness, followed by passage of burgundy-colored blood per rectum. She noted that certain activities, such as bending over while working in her garden, seemed to exacerbate the bleeding. She had a known heart murmur since her college days. Her cardiac condition did not limit her activity, although she noted she was sometimes short of breath. On examination, she had cardiomegaly. There was a grade III/VI systolic murmur present at the apex which radiated to the left axilla. The electrocardiograph showed left ventricular hypertrophy. At colonoscopy, an 8-mm vascular abnormality was found on a large semilunar fold in the cecum. Two other smaller lesions were found close by. Biopsy was not attempted for fear of precipitating another hemorrhage. The lesions were electrocoagulated using the dome-tip electrode. Three more electrocoagulations were necessary before her bleeding was brought under control. Repeat colonoscopy 1 year after her initial endoscopy showed no residual lesion. In retrospect, the superior mesenteric angiogram, which was performed prior to her referral, did demonstrate the vascular abnormality in the cecum (Figure 1).

The patient's hemoglobin levels were restored to normal by treatment with oral iron. Anemia has not recurred.

Comment:

Prior to this patient's initial colonoscopic electrocoagulation, she had been hospitalized several times and received numerous transfusions. Since her original treatment 7 years ago, she has never required another transfusion. A total of four colonoscopic electrocoagulations were necessary to bring her hemorrhages under control. Part of this difficulty was inexperience. Part was due to use of the dome-tip electrode which is not as effective as the electrocoagulating biopsy forceps now used.

Case 2: This 62-year-old woman presented with intermittent passage of black and burgundy-red stools for 9 months. She also had paresthesias of the lower extremities and intermittent claudication. Translumbar aortography showed arteriosclerosis obliterans with severe, nearly total occlusion of the distal abdominal aorta approximately 2 cm above the bifurcation. She was also found to be anemic, with a hemoglobin of 8.4 g/d*l*. Stools were 4+ positive for occult blood. X-ray studies of the gastrointestinal tract and proctosigmoidoscopy failed to reveal the source of bleeding. It was decided that further investigation of her gastrointestinal bleeding was necessary before a surgical bypass could be performed for her vascular disease. Upper intestinal endoscopy showed a hiatal hernia only. At colonoscopy four, bright-red, mucosal vascular abnormalities were seen in the base of the cecum. The largest was 1 cm in diameter. All were electrocoagulated with the dome-tip electrode. It was noted that just touching the vascular abnormalities with the electrode caused fairly profuse bleeding. The patient was discharged from the hospital on the following day, and 3 months later had her aorto-ilio Dacron bypass. Shortly after the patient's surgery, she had one more episode of bright-red rectal bleeding, but none since (6 years).

Comment:

Friability is a characteristic of small mucosal vascular abnormalities of the large bowel. It is used to help distinguish them from ecchymoses.

Case 3: This 70-year-old woman was referred because of intermittent tarry stools of 2-year's duration, which caused anemia and progressive worsening of her angina. During the 2 years prior to referral, the patient had had 6 gastrointestinal work-ups using conventional techniques without elucidation of the source of bleeding. The patient had a known heart murmur for many years. On examination, it was a soft, blowing, systolic murmur at the apex which radiated to the axilla. Ischemic changes in the anterior wall of the electrocardiogram became less prominent after transfusions. Echocardiography was consistent with idiopathic hypertrophic subaortic stenosis. Cardiac catheterization confirmed the diagnosis and also showed minimal mitral insufficiency. Coronary arteriography revealed severe disease. At colonoscopy, three mucosal vascular abnormalities were noted in the cecum. The largest was 1 cm in diameter. Each was electrocoagulated with the dome-tip electrode. She was discharged home on the following day. She did well with minimal angina while taking Inderal® until 3 years later, when massive rectal bleeding occurred. After transfusions, colonoscopy revealed a 5 × 8-mm lesion close to the opening of the appendix. Close by was a smaller lesion. The larger lesion was biopsied and in the process it was noted that the center appeared to contain some fibrous tissue which caused it to assume a plate-like configuration when elevated. The lesions were then destroyed with electrocoagulation. The biopsy showed angiectasis. The patient has done well for 3½ years.

Comment:

The center of this patient's lesion appeared to have some fibrous tissue which gave it a plate-like configuration when manipulated. Scarring is one of the characteristics of a vascular abnormality as it ages. Scarring could also be a result of the initial electrocoagulation.

The author's second and third cases of mucosal vascular abnormalities of the cecum came within 3 days of each other. Both had dramatic cardiovascular pathology although of a different type than the first case. The clinical constellation was striking and strongly suggested a syndrome. A careful search of the cecum has since been made for vascular abnormalities in patients with unexplained lower intestinal bleeding.

Case 4: A 73-year-old man was referred because of abdominal pain and diarrhea. Past history included hypertension, a cerebral vascular accident, and chronic peptic ulcer disease of many years duration. Stools were 4+ positive for occult blood. The hemoglobin was 11.7 g/d*l*. Colonoscopy was performed because of a large, 2-cm polyp in he sigmoid which was found and removed. An unexpected finding was a bright-red, flat, mucosal vascular abnormality at the base of the cecum approximately 6 × 8 mm in diameter and slightly raised from the surrounding mucosa (Figure 2). The lesion was biopsied and treated with the electrocoagulating biopsy forceps. Microscopic examination of the biopsies showed vascular spaces lined by thick walls and normal endothelium (Figure 3). In addition, vascular spaces lined by thin walls were seen.

Approximately 2 years later, in August 1977, the patient was investigated because of hematemesis and

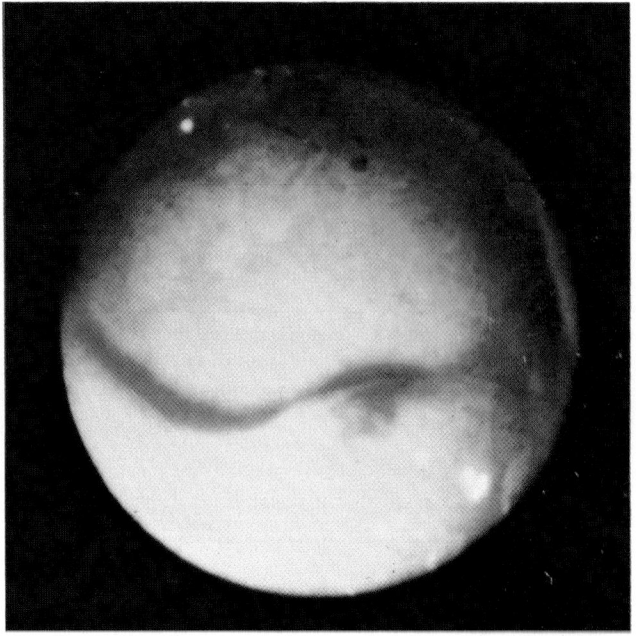

FIGURE 2. Endoscopic view of small vascular abnormality of the cecum, which is slightly raised above the surrounding mucosa (Case 4). (From Rogers, B. H. G. and Adler, F., *Gastroenterology,* 71, 1079, 1976 With permission.)

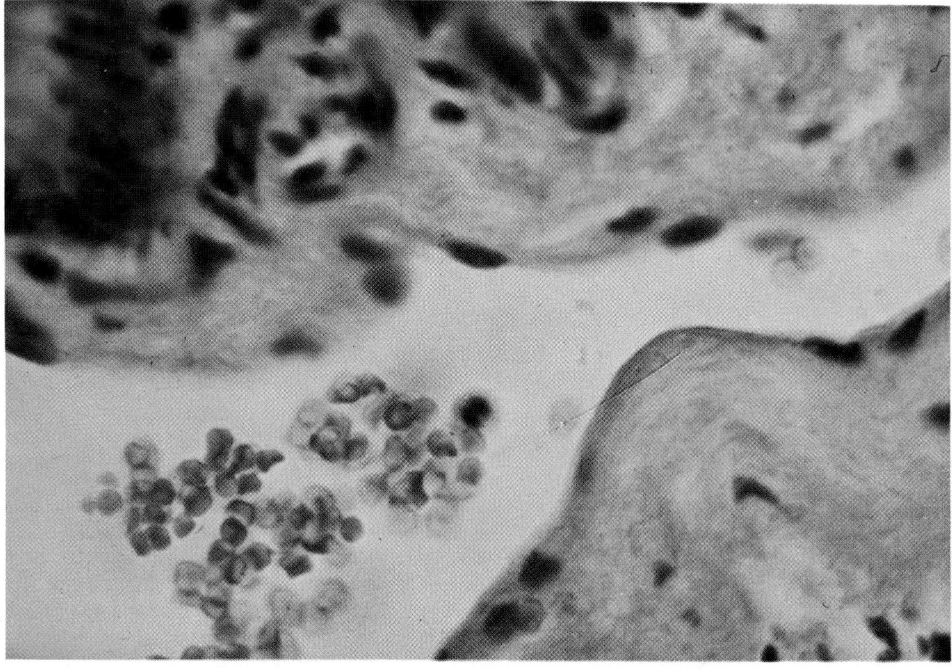

FIGURE 3. Microscopic view of biopsy which shows a large, thick-walled, vascular space lined by normal epithelial cells in the lamina propria (Case 4). (Original magnification × 400.) (From Rogers, B. H. G. and Adler, F., *Gastroenterology,* 71, 1079, 1976. With permission.)

melena and found to have an active duodenal ulcer on endoscopy. The patient was treated medically and did well until January 1978 when he was admitted again because of epigastric pain and anemia. Endoscopy showed a pinpoint narrowing of the second portion of the duodenum which created a partial outlet obstruction of the stomach. Prior to surgical correction, colonoscopy was performed. In the base of the cecum and opposite the ileocecal valve was a stellate, pale but definite vascular abnormality. It was approximately 8 × 6 mm in diameter. Close by was another vascular abnormality 3 × 6 mm. Both lesions were biopsied and electrocoagulated. The patient recovered from his peptic ulcer surgery and has done well since.

Comment:

Total colonoscopy was performed initially at the time of polypectomy to rule out other polyps or carcinoma. The vascular abnormality was an unexpected finding. It is impossible to know whether the patient's anemia was due to bleeding from the large polyp or from the vascular lesion in the cecum. The vascular lesions seen at the second colonoscopy had developed during the 3 years since the first exam. The second colonoscopy was done simply to make sure the patient did not have bleeding from a vascular abnormality of the cecum in his postoperative period.

Case 5: This 82-year-old man was referred because of unexplained anemia. He had a 9-year history of hypertension. He had developed angina about 18 months prior to admission.

There was a grade III/VI systolic murmur heard best at the apex, which radiated into the left axilla. His nails were spoon-shaped. The stools were strongly positive for occult blood. The chest X-ray showed the transverse diameter of the heart to be at the upper limits of normal. Upper intestinal endoscopy was negative. Colonoscopy showed a 6 × 8-mm irregularly shaped, bright-red, superficial vascular abnormality on the lateral wall of the cecum, midway between its base and the level of the ileocecal valve (Figure 4). The lesion was biopsied and electrocoagulated with the Williams biopsy forceps.[49] Preparation was less than ideal and complete visualization of the cecum was impossible. Therefore, the patient was reexamined on the following day. Preparation was better and complete visualization of the cecum was possible. No additional lesion was seen. Only a shallow ulcer at the site of the electrocoagulation was found. Since then, his hemoglobin has been maintained without therapy for 5 years.

Comment:

Shortly before encountering this case, the Williams® electrocoagulating biopsy forceps became commercially available (A.C.M.I.®, Stamford, Connecticut). They are ideally suited to deal with small vascular abnormalities because they make it possible to obtain a specimen suitable for microscopic examination and to destroy all or part of the lesion simultaneously. The Williams® forceps have been used in all the following cases.

Case 6: This 55-year-old woman was referred because of recurrent episodes of gastrointestinal bleeding. She had been known to be hypertensive for at least 33 years. Mild chronic renal failure had been diagnosed 6 months earlier. When she presented at the emergency room, her hemoglobin was 3.9 g/d*l*. A harsh systolic murmur was present in the aortic area which radiated into the carotids. The BUN was 61 and the creatinine was 10.2. UGI endoscopy was normal. Her stools were positive for occult blood. A chest X-ray showed cardiomegaly. Mesenteric angiography suggested numerous arteriovenous malformations within the vasculature of the rectosigmoid colon. Colonoscopy showed five vascular abnormalities 4 to 6 mm in size, scattered from the cecum to the distal transverse (Figure 5). In addition, there were multiple 1 to 2-mm lesions seen in the sigmoid colon at 35 cm, which corresponded to the angiographic findings. All were electrocoagulated except some of the tiny ones in the sigmoid. Microscopic examination showed angiectasis. She has had no significant bleeding for 4½ years.

Comment:

This is one of the most florid cases in this series. The vascular abnormalities seemed larger and more prominent in the cecum and ascending colon, and became paler and less prominent towards the splenic flexure. In the sigmoid all were quite small. This pattern has been seen in almost every patient who has multiple vascular abnormalities of the large bowel.

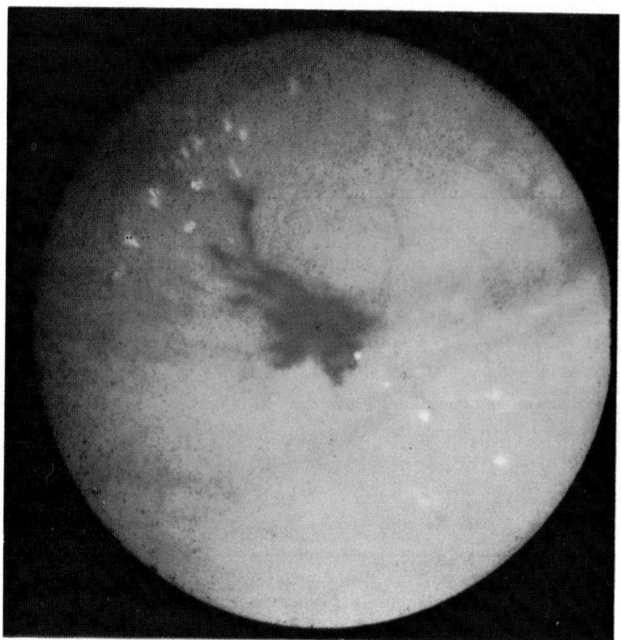

FIGURE 4. Bright-red, flat, irregular vascular abnormality of the cecum (Case 5). (From Rogers, B. H. G. and Adler, F., *Gastroenterology,* 71, 1079, 1976. With permission.)

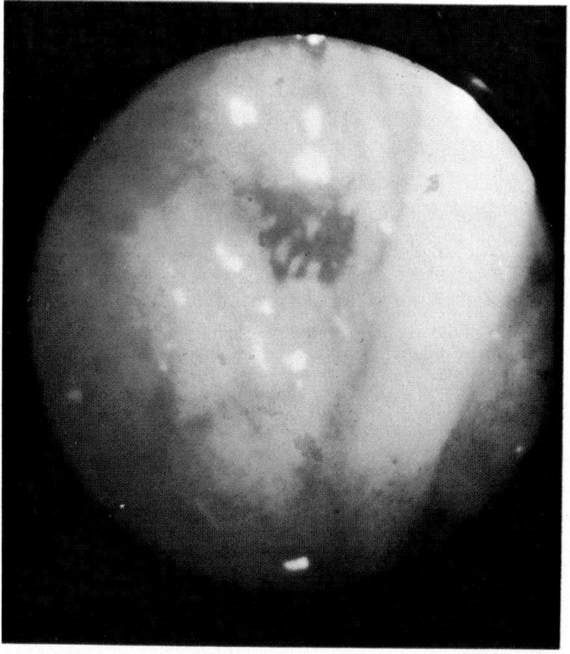

FIGURE 5. Endoscopic view of stellate vascular abnormality of the transverse colon (Case 6).

Case 7: This 70-year-old man was referred because of intermittent, bright-red, rectal bleeding of 2-years duration. The bleeding was relatively painless, although the patient had noted an associated uncomfortable sensation in the lower-right quadrant. He was found to have a bicuspid aortic valve and calcific aortic stenosis, which was proven on cardiac catheterization. Physical examination showed findings typical of aortic stenosis, but was otherwise normal. At the time of admission, his rectal bleeding had ceased and all stools for occult blood had been negative except one, which was found to be 4+. The electrocardiograph was compatible with left ventricular hypertrophy. Colonoscopy showed a 1-cm vascular abnormality on the lateral wall of the cecum opposite the ileocecal valve. It was treated with electrocoagulation. Simultaneously obtained biopsy confirmed the vascular abnormality. Rectal bleeding ceased. Two and one half years later, he returned because of the sudden loss of vision in the lower-left quadrant of his left eye. Fundoscopic examination showed an atheromatous plaque lodged in the superior temporal retinal artery. His vision never returned in spite of treatment with aspirin and Persantine®. A year later, the patient noted the onset of pain in his lower-right quadrant after walking two blocks. Examination of the abdomen was unremarkable. The patient was then hospitalized for reevaluation for possible replacement of his aortic valve. Although the patient had had no rectal bleeding since his original electrocoagulation 3½ years previously, it was felt wise to eliminate any residual or newly formed vascular abnormalities which may have occurred. Accordingly, total colonoscopy was performed. No vascular abnormality in the cecum or anywhere else in the large bowel was found. Shortly thereafter, he had his aortic valve replaced with an Edwards porcine heterograft. The patient did well postoperatively with no gastrointestinal bleeding in spite of anticoagulation with Coumadin®. Postoperatively, he could walk as far as he wanted without developing pain in the lower-right quadrant.

Comment:

This is a classic case of calcific aortic stenosis and gastrointestinal bleeding from a vascular abnormality of the cecum. The lesion was completely destroyed, except for the biopsy, with 10 W. of current applied for 2 sec. Because of his severe aortic stenosis, it was felt that certainly he would have formed more lesions in the cecum in the three and one half subsequent years. However, at follow-up colonoscopy, no lesion could be found. The atheroembolus to the retinal artery was a significant observation because such emboli may play an etiologic role in the development of some mucosal vascular abnormalities.[39] It is interesting that the patient's abdominal angina which appeared on walking was localized in the right-lower quadrant over the cecum, precisely where his vascular abnormality had been located.

Case 8: This 64-year-old woman was referred because of a mucosal vascular abnormality of the cecum which had been found at colonoscopy. The patient had a history of bright-red rectal bleeding which had started approximately 3 years previously. At the time of diagnostic colonoscopy, probing the lesion induced bleeding. The only abnormality on physical examination was a blood pressure of 150/90. At the time of therapeutic colonoscopy, a 5 × 8-mm lesion was found directly opposite the ileocecal valve. It was treated in the usual fashion. Biopsy showed typical changes. The patient has had no bleeding for 3½ years.

Case 9: A 72-year-old woman was referred because of two episodes of hematochezia. Her cardiovascular-pulmonary system was clinically normal. At colonoscopy, in the area of the splenic flexure, an 8-mm polyp with an erythematous and hemorrhagic head was noted. It was removed and found to be a tubular adenoma. In the cecum, a large pale, 1.2-cm poorly developed vascular abnormality was noted. It was biopsied and destroyed by electrocoagulation. Biopsy showed angiectasis. The patient has had no bleeding for 3 years.

Comment:

The poorly developed lesion found in the cecum of this patient was an incidental finding. The hemorrhagic polyp was thought to be the source of bleeding.

Case 10: This 79-year-old man was referred because of anemia and shortness of breath for 1 year. A complete GI series had failed to reveal the source of bleeding. In spite of treatment with iron, his hemoglobin had fallen to 7.4. Physical examination showed a harsh grade III/VI systolic murmur which was heard over the entire precordium. Chest X-ray showed cardiomegaly. Stools for occult blood were 3+ positive on one occasion and negative on another. An electrocardiograph showed a right-bundle branch block and supraventricular premature contractions. Colonoscopy showed a large, irregular 2 × 1.5-cm vascular abnormality on the lateral wall of the cecum opposite the ileocecal valve. Another small lesion was seen at the base of the cecum.

In addition, a 4 × 6-mm lesion was seen in the ascending colon. All lesions were treated in the usual way and biopsied. One year later, he returned because of anemia. Repeat colonoscopy showed five small lesions in the cecum and ascending colon. All were treated in the usual fashion. Since then, his hemoglobin has been maintained with oral iron (17 months).

Comment:

This patient is thought to be bleeding from vascular abnormalities outside the large bowel. Because of his age and general medical condition, an attempt at eradicating them will not be made unless his anemia cannot be controlled with iron therapy.

Case 11: This 65-year-old woman was referred because of passing dark-red blood per rectum. The patient had suffered two myocardial infarctions, 6 and 4 years previously. Physical examination of the heart showed it to be enlarged with diminished heart sounds and no murmur. A colon X-ray was nondiagnostic. The electrocardiograph was abnormal because of right bundle-branch block. Colonoscopy showed a 5 mm bright-red lesion just below the ileocecal valve and somewhat lateral. A white fleck at the center suggested that it was eroded (Figure 6). The lesion was biopsied and destroyed in the usual fashion. Microscopic examination showed angiectasis. In addition, the ulcerated surface was confirmed. She has had no bleeding for 2½ years.

Comment:

In this case, the eroded vascular abnormality strongly suggested the lesion was the source of the patient's bleeding.

Case 12: A 75-year-old man was referred because of multiple vascular abnormalities found in the right large bowel at colonoscopy. Biopsy had shown vessels with thick walls in the mucosa. The patient suffered from atherosclerotic heart disease with mitral insufficiency and congestive heart failure. He had angina pectoris and adult-onset diabetes mellitus. He was being treated for subacute bacterial endocarditis when he developed frank gastrointestinal bleeding. Angiography showed one area of vascular abnormality in the large bowel. At therapeutic colonoscopy, six lesions were found in the cecum and ascending colon. They ranged in size from pinpoint to 6 mm in diameter. The largest lesions were in the cecum and their size diminished in direct proportion to the distance from it. A very early, poorly developed lesion was found in the distal transverse portion. Five of the larger lesions were destroyed by electrocoagulation. He has had no rectal bleeding in 2½ years.

Comment:

This case illustrates how colonoscopy can be much more sensitive in detecting vascular abnormalities than angiography. One lesion was detected by angiography, whereas seven were detected by colonoscopy. This patient also demonstrated that whatever is causing the vascular abnormalities to form is strongest in the cecum. The further the lesions are from the cecum, the smaller they become. Although all of the lesions in this patient were flat, the large, well-developed lesions were slightly elevated above the surrounding mucosa. The thick-walled vessels seen on biopsy are suggestive of arteriovenous malformation.

Case 13: This 70-year-old man was referred because of two episodes of bright-red rectal bleeding 6 weeks apart. A colon X-ray had shown diverticula which were assumed to be the source of bleeding. The patient's past history included a left carotid endarterectomy done 10 years previously. He was being treated for hypertension. Physical examination showed a grade II/VI systolic murmur over the precordium. The chest X-ray showed a tortuous aorta. His cardiograph showed changes compatible with coronary insufficiency. At colonoscopy, five vascular abnormalities were found in the cecum. The most prominent was just below the ileocecal valve and about 8 mm in diameter. It had a circular shape and the center was ulcerated. It was flat, but slightly raised from the surrounding mucosa. Close by were other lesions which ranged in size from 2 to 10 mm. They were not ulcerated and not raised above the surrounding mucosa. As many of the lesions as possible were biopsied and electrocoagulated. Bleeding and tissue changes prevented evaluation as to whether or not complete treatment had been rendered. Seven months later, repeat electrocoagulation of the cecal lesion was carried out. The patient had a third therapeutic colonoscopy 15 months after his initial one because of recurrent painless bleeding. Two more small vascular abnormalities were found in the cecum and treated. He has had no bleeding for 1 year.

Comment:

This patient illustrates the challenge of the patient who has multiple vascular abnormalities in the cecal mucosa. Invariably, there is some bleeding and tissue distortion as the result of biopsy and electrocoagulation. This tends to obscure the field so that sometimes it is difficult to be certain about adequate treatment. Overtreatment can result in perforation. Therefore, it is always wise to err on the side of undertreatment. Completeness of therapy can be determined at follow-up colonoscopy, which can be done either electively or when bleeding resumes.

Case 14: This 81-year-old man was referred because of massive lower gastrointestinal bleeding. He had had similar episodes in the past which always resolved spontaneously. Vague lower abdominal discomfort and gaseousness were associated with the bleeding. He had known colonic diverticula, which were thought to be the cause of hemorrhage. He had atherosclerotic heart disease with a documented myocardial infarction and a 20-year history of angina. At colonoscopy, numerous wide-mouthed diverticula were noted in the sigmoid. In the cecum, an 8-mm vascular abnormality of the mucosa with central ulceration was found on the lateral aspect of the base of the cecum. A group of smaller lesions were located close by. All were treated by electrocoagulation. Biopsy showed angiectasis. He has had no bleeding for 2 years.

Case 15: A 65-year-old man was referred because of unexplained iron—deficiency anemia. The patient had a history of episodic epistaxis every 1 to 2 weeks over the last year, but they never lasted for more than 5 to 10 min. A bone marrow examination showed complete depletion of iron stores. It was felt by the consulting hematologist that the patient's nose bleeds were not severe enough to explain the iron-deficiency anemia. He had no hematemesis, melena, or hematochezia. He had chronic obstructive pulmonary disease with an increased anterior-posterior diameter of the chest and P-pulmonale on his electrocardiograph. An excoriation of the right side of the nasal septum was noted. There were two small vascular abnormalities on the tip of the tongue. Colonoscopy showed a 1.2-cm, flat vascular abnormality on the lateral wall of the ascending colon at 80 cm. Across from this lesion on the medial wall was a smaller, 4-mm vascular abnormality. Scattered elsewhere in the colon were small lesions ranging from pinpoint up to 2 mm in diameter. The two large lesions in the ascending colon and some of the smaller ones were biopsied and electrocoagulated. Biopsy from the larger lesion showed angiectasis (Figure 7). Biopsies from the smaller lesions were all negative, except one which showed a cluster of small vascular channels lined with normal-appearing endothelial cells. After electrocoagulation of the lesion in the ascending colon, his hemoglobin rose from 8.3 to 10 g%. even though his epistaxis continued.

Comment:

This case is an example of the relatively large vascular abnormality which can occur in the right colon in patients with hereditary hemorrhagic telangiectasia (Osler-Weber-Rendu syndrome). The abnormal vascular channels in the mucosa seen on biopsy were similar to the findings of other cases of angiectasis in this series.

Case 16: This 60-year-old man was referred for follow-up colonoscopy 1 year after resection for carcinoma of the rectum. The patient had been a known hypertensive for 5 years. He had organic brain disease of undetermined etiology and diabetes mellitus. He had atherosclerotic heart disease treated with digoxin. Colonoscopy was performed through the descending colostomy. The only finding was a 4-mm, flat, circular vascular abnormality unexpectedly found in the cecum on the anterio-medial wall. It was electrocoagulated in the usual way. Biopsy showed angiectasis (Figure 8).

Comment:

This is an example of an early vascular abnormality which apparently had caused no bleeding. It is important to remove such lesions, because doing so may prevent future bleeding. If bleeding does develop, an established diagnosis would be very helpful in guiding future investigations and therapy.

Case 17: This 65-year-old woman was referred because of a possible polyp seen on barium enema. No associated clinical disease was evident. She was found to have a biopsy-proven, 5-mm vascular abnormality in the cecum at colonoscopy.

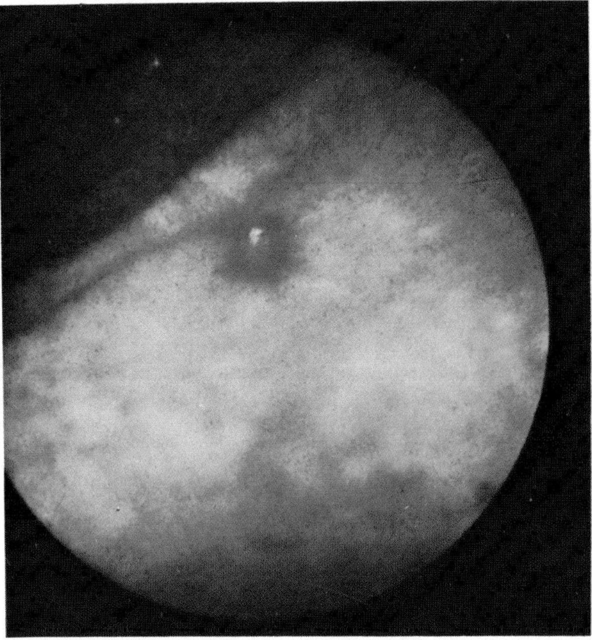

FIGURE 6. Endoscopic view of ulcerated, small vascular abnormality of the cecum (Case 11).

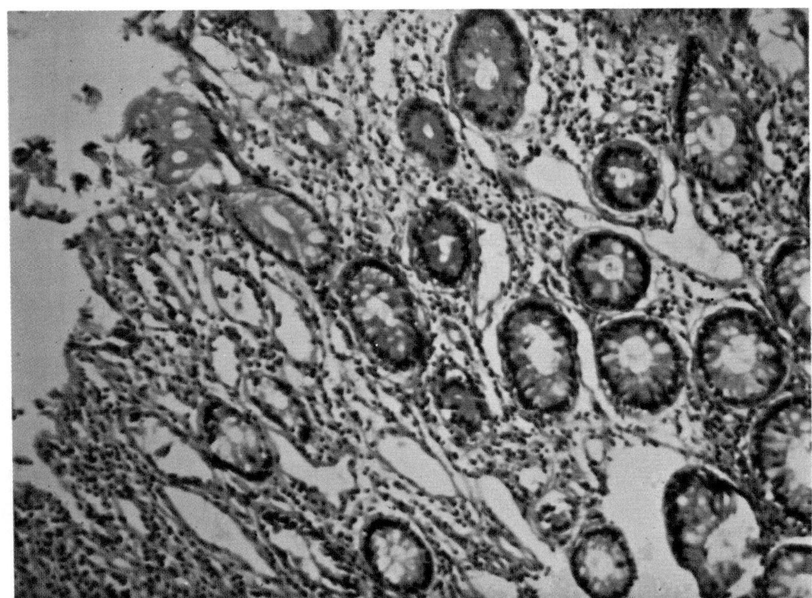

FIGURE 7. Microscopic view of vascular abnormality of ascending colon (Case 15). The lamina propria is laced with thin-walled, dilated vessels. The surface is ulcerated. (Original magnification ×40.)

Case 18: This 66-year-old man was referred because of one episode of voluminous rectal bleeding. The bleeding was painless and bright red. The patient was clinically normal with no evidence for heart, vascular, or pulmonary disease. Colonoscopy showed a 6-mm vascular abnormality close to the mouth of the appendix. It was somewhat elevated from the surrounding mucosa and was electrocoagulated. Biopsy showed angiectasis. The patient has had no bleeding since (1½ years).

Case 19: A 76-year-old man was referred because of recurrent LGI bleeding of 13-years duration. A diagnosis of arteriovenous malformation of the right colon was made 10 years previously by mesenteric angiography. A right colectomy was recommended, but the patient declined. In the following year, a diagnosis of well-differentiated, transitional cell carcinoma of the urinary bladder was made. Subsequently, the patient had repeated cystoscopies, resections, and fulgurations of the bladder tumor. At his last cystoscopy, on March 29, 1979 no evidence for recurrent tumor was present. During the intervening 10 years, the patient was treated for moderately severe hypertension. He had episodes of gross rectal bleeding in 1967, 1969, 1974, 1975, 1978, and 1979. In between episodes of gross rectal bleeding, his stools were usually found to be strongly positive for occult blood. On one occasion in 1976, the stool was negative. He was treated with several courses of oral iron. In 1976, he began to suffer transient ischemic attacks and endoscopic electrocoagulation was recommended, but the patient declined because he felt that his bladder cancer would result in his death. The patient was finally persuaded to have a colonoscopy in April, 1979. In the cecum on the lateral aspect was a large, double-stellate vascular abnormality which covered an area of approximately 1.5 × 2 cm. Another, less well-developed lesion was found on the ileocecal valve. The larger lesion was electrocoagulated and biopsied. Microscopic examination of the biopsy showed angiectasis. Postcolonoscopy, the patient was placed on iron, and his hemoglobin gradually rose to a level of 13.4 g. He has had no further evidence of bleeding.

Comment:

This patient demonstrates the natural history of a symptomatic vascular abnormality of the cecal area. He was reported as case II by Genant and Ranniger.[25] The diagnosis of a right colonic vascular abnormality was made 10 years before it was treated endoscopically. During that time, the patient suffered repeated episodes of gross rectal bleeding, weakness and lethargy due to anemia, and eventually transient ischemic attacks. Since his endoscopic electrocoagulation, his hemoglobin has risen to normal levels and he has become asymptomatic. This case is important because it demonstrates what can happen to patients with untreated vascular abnormalities of the right colon.

Case 20: This 73-year-old woman was referred for evaluation of her anemia. Her past history included long-standing atherosclerotic heart disease with angina and congestive heart failure. A chest X-ray showed cardiomegaly and the electrocardiograph showed atrial fibrillation with left ventricular hypertrophy. At colonoscopy, there was a 5-mm bright-red, flat mucosal vascular abnormality. Other, smaller, less well-developed lesions were seen in the ascending, descending, and sigmoid portions of the colon. The lesion was electrocoagulated. Biopsy showed angiectasis. The patient is now maintaining her hemoglobin by taking oral iron for 1½ years.

Case 21: This 91-year-old man was referred because of recurrent episodes of melena of 3-years duration. The patient developed angina pectoris when his hemoglobin fell. At colonoscopy, several small mucosal vascular abnormalities were noted in the cecum and ascending colon. The largest was 4 mm in diameter. Several smaller lesions were seen in the sigmoid. All of the larger lesions were treated with electrocoagulation. Biopsy confirmed the vascular nature of the lesions. However, preparation was poor and completeness of therapy could not be confirmed. Colonoscopy was repeated 5 months later because of recurrent bleeding. Four small vascular abnormalities 1 to 2 mm in diameter were found in the cecum. They were electrocoagulated even though they probably were not contributing to the patient's bleeding. The terminal ileum was intubated for about 12 cm and no vascular abnormality could be seen.

Comment:

This patient appeared to be bleeding from a site other than vascular abnormalities of the large bowel. Other possible sites include his known diverticula or a vascular abnormality in the small bowel.

Case 22: This 81-year-old woman was referred because of a profound iron—deficiency anemia. She had a history of atherosclerotic heart disease with myocardial infarction and congestive heart failure. She had a

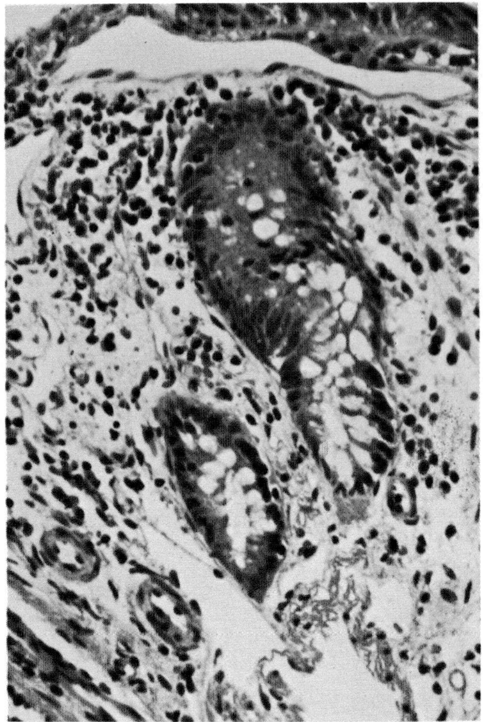

FIGURE 8. Microscopic view of biopsy showing thin-walled vascular space in lamina propria (Case 16). One of the spaces is directly beneath the thinned-out surface epithelium which could be easily traumatized and lead to bleeding. (Original magnification × 200.)

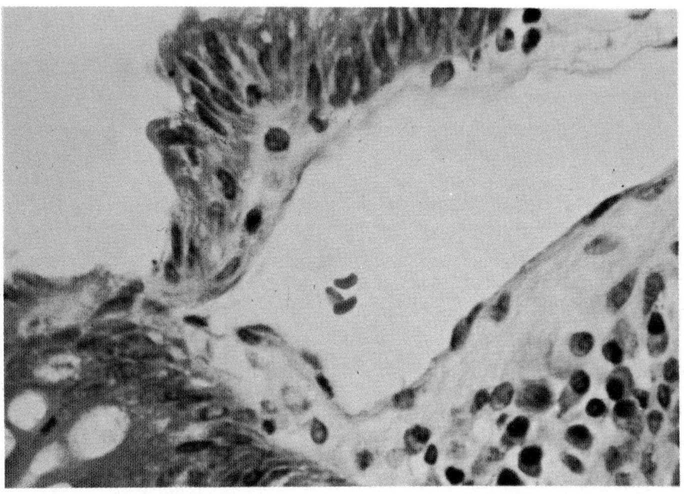

FIGURE 9. Microscopic view of large, thin-walled vascular space located just under the colonic epithelium (Case 27). (Original magnification × 400.)

grade II/VI late, blowing, systolic murmur which was heard best at the apex. At colonoscopy, on the lateral wall of the base of the cecum, a 1.5 × 0.8 cm-mucosal vascular abnormality was found. The lesion was electrocoagulated. Biopsy showed angiectasis. Her anemia responded to oral iron and was no longer a problem. She expired 1 year later due to a coronary occlusion.

Comment:

It would have been a mistake to perform a right colectomy on this elderly patient. The operation carries a significant risk and would have diminished the quality of her last year of life.

Case 23: This 58-year-old man was referred because of passage of bright-red blood when forcing a constipated stool. He had been a diabetic for 3 years for which he took 25 units of insulin each morning. In addition, he was thought to have cirrhosis of the liver. He was being treated for hypertension and angina. X-rays showed extensive arteriosclerotic changes in the abdominal and pelvic vessels. The electrocardiograph was consistent with coronary artery disease. At colonoscopy, there were two small, 1.5 × 2-mm, irregular vascular abnormalities at the base of the cecum. Both were biopsied and electrocoagulated. Intubation of the terminal ileum to 10 cm failed to reveal additional vascular abnormalities. Microscopic examination of the biopsies showed angiectasis. Small internal hemorrhoids were noted on pulling the colonoscope through the anus.

Comment:

The vascular abnormalities of this patient were thought to be an incidental finding at colonoscopy. Rectal bleeding was apparently from hemorrhoids.

Case 24: This 64-year-old man was referred for follow-up colonoscopy after endoscopic polypectomy 5 years previously. The patient had generalized atherosclerotic vascular disease and a history of a CVA. At colonoscopy, a 5-mm mucosal vascular abnormality was seen on the lateral wall of the cecum opposite the ileocecal valve and just a little below it. A smaller one was located close by. Both were biopsied and electrocoagulated. Microscopic examination showed angiectasis.

Comment:

As in Case 23, this lesion was an incidental finding in a patient with generalized vascular disease.

Case 25: This 50-year-old woman with an irritable digestive tract was referred for colonoscopy to rule out organic disease. She had no clinically evident associated disease. Endoscopy showed a 6-mm, flat, erythematous area on the medial aspect of the ascending colon. Biopsy showed angiectasis.

Comment:

This lesion was an incidental finding in a younger patient without associated, clinically evident, organic disease.

Case 26: This 81-year-old woman was referred because of painless, maroon—colored, rectal bleeding which came on just prior to admission. Ten years previously, the patient had a partial gastrectomy and a gastroenterostomy for peptic ulcer disease. Esophagogastroduodenoscopy showed three small gastric ulcers and marked gastritis in the remnant. The patient had atherosclerotic heart disease, hypertension, and diabetes mellitus. At colonoscopy, a 6-mm, flat vascular abnormality was found on a fold in the cecum across from the ileocecal valve. 25W of current were applied for 3 sec. Four other smaller lesions were found close by and treated in the same fashion. Biopsy confirmed the vascular nature of the abnormality. She did well for 3 months and then returned to the hospital with septicemia. She went into hepatorenal failure and expired.

Comment:

The maroon-colored stools strongly suggested a bleeding point in the right colon. In addition the associated diseases increased the possibility of a vascular abnormality in the right colon which was found at colonoscopy. Even though the patient had potential bleeding points in the gastric remnant, it was believed that they were not contributing to the rectal bleeding. The source of her terminal septicemia was never determined, but it was too remote from her endoscopy to consider it a complication.

Case 27: A 75-year-old woman was referred because of occult gastrointestinal bleeding. She had profound anemia with a reticulocyte count of 5.4%. Upper GI X-rays were reported to show antral gastritis and a channel ulcer. Upper intestinal endoscopy failed to confirm the X-ray findings. The patient was known to have coronary artery disease and hypertension. Vascular abnormality of the cecal area was considered and colonoscopy recommended. Careful examination of the cecum at first failed to reveal any abnormality, but on withdrawing the colonoscope over the ileocecal valve, a bright-red lesion was noted on its cecal aspect. This was confirmed on several passes, but electrocoagulation was impossible because the lesion could not be visualized in a stable position. A biopsy was taken as the lesion was sliding-by, which showed angiectasis (Figure 9). Five days later she passed bright-red blood with clots. She was taken to surgery, where a right hemicolectomy was performed. The surgical pathology specimen showed a small defect on the cecal aspect of the ileocecal valve where the endoscopic biopsy was taken. Sections through the same area showed an ulcer and intramucosal angiectasis. She has had a normal hemoglobin level for 10 months.

Comment:

The value of colonoscopy in this case was the endoscopic visualization of the lesion and biopsy with histologic confirmation. It is the only case in which this author has visualized a vascular abnormality in the cecal area and was not able to treat it. Whereas it is usually very difficult to localize the vascular abnormality in the surgical pathology specimen, in this case, the small ulceration from the endoscopic biopsy guided the pathologist to the precise site.

Case 28: This 72-year-old woman was referred because of three episodes of lower gastrointestinal bleeding over the previous year. She had hypertension, diabetes mellitus, and cirrhosis of the liver. Angiography at another hospital had shown an area of possible cecal vascular abnormality with extravasation of contrast material into the right colon. At colonoscopy, a 6 × 8-mm, flat, nonulcerated vascular abnormality was located along the medial wall of the ascending colon just above the ileocecal valve. Another 2 × 2-mm lesion was located in the ascending colon. Both were electrocoagulated. Biopsy confirmed their vascular nature. It was thought that the lesions were an unlikely source of the patient's bleeding. She was, therefore, explored shortly thereafter, and had a systemic—portal shunt plus removal of mesenteric and ileal varices. She had another episode of rectal bleeding and colonoscopy was repeated. No mucosal vascular abnormalities remained. In the transverse colon and rectum, bluish, bulging, mucosal abnormalities thought to be varices were found.

Comment:

This case is an example of a patient thought to be bleeding from varices of the gastrointestinal tract. She was found to have incidental mucosal vascular abnormalities of the ascending colon.

Case 29: This 82-year-old man was referred because of iron-deficiency anemia due to occult gastrointestinal blood loss. Colonoscopy had been attempted four years previously because of gross rectal bleeding, but the endoscope could not be passed through the sigmoid because of apparent adhesions. Angiography was then performed and showed a vascular abnormality in the right large bowel. The patient then underwent a right colectomy. After surgery, gross rectal bleeding ceased completely, but then anemia developed insidiously. On examination, he had a harsh systolic murmur heard over the precordium which radiated into the neck. Upper intestinal endoscopy showed five bright-red, vascular abnormalities in the second portion of the duodenum. The largest one was about 4 mm in diameter and was located on a circular fold. The lesions were electrocoagulated. Biopsy confirmed their vascular nature. The patient now maintains a normal hemoglobin on oral iron.

Comment:

This patient is an example of a case where only surgical therapy can be effective. In spite of the best available skill, total colonoscopy is not possible in all patients. Pathologic alteration or anatomic variation can prevent reaching the cecum. Right colectomy had cured the patient's gross rectal bleeding. When blood loss resumed, it was occult. The appearance of vascular abnormalities in the small bowel is of concern.

Case 30: This 88-year-old woman was referred because of two unsuccessful attempts at endoscopic electrocoagulation of cecal vascular abnormalities. The patient had hypertension for many years which was never well-controlled. She had a grade IV/VI harsh holosystolic murmur heard over the apex, without radiation. Her chest X-ray showed cardiomegaly. The electrocardiograph showed borderline, left-ventricular hypertrophy with strain. At colonoscopy, a 2 × 3-mm lesion was found on the lateral wall of the cecum. Close by was a larger but paler, 6 × 7-mm lesion. Two smaller lesions were found close to the splenic flexure. All were electrocoagulated. Biospy confirmed their vascular nature. She has had no bleeding for 6 months.

Comment:

When a patient has multiple small vascular abnormalities of the cecal area, it is difficult to treat all of them at one setting. Almost invariably there is some bleeding and tissue distortion which interferes with evaluation of completeness of therapy. The patient should be told that further therapy may be needed should bleeding resume. Small amounts of residual tissue may be left behind. As long as they do not result in either occult or gross bleeding, they can be ignored.

Case 31: This 78-year-old woman was referred because of a history of lower GI bleeding and an increasing transfusion requirement of 4 years duration. She had received 20 units of blood in the previous 8 months. She had the murmur of aortic stenosis. At colonoscopy, two stellate, vascular abnormalities were found in the cecum. They had diameters of 8 and 6 mm, respectively. Both were treated in the usual fashion and biopsy confirmed their vascular nature. She received no subsequent transfusion and she is no longer anemic.

Comment:

This is a classic case of aortic stenosis and small vascular abnormality of the right colon.

Case 32: A 71-year-old man was referred because of anemia due to gastrointestinal blood loss. He had generalized atherosclerosis and surgery on both carotid arteries. In addition, he had an aneursym of the abdominal aorta. On a fold opposite the ileocecal valve a 6 × 4-mm, flat, cherry-red, mucosal vascular abnormality was seen. Three biopsies and electrocoagulations were carried out. All were given 25 W for 4, 3, and 2 sec. respectively. Biopsy showed the vascular abnormality and, in addition, atheromatous emboli in the lamina propria.

Comment:

This is the first case in which atheromatous emboli were found in a mucosal biopsy of a vascular abnormality of the cecal area. They were first reported in association with this lesion by Galdabini.[39] They also have been reported by Mitsudo et al.[37]

Case 33: This 72-year-old man was referred because of a CEA of 210. He had a left colectomy 2 years previously for carcinoma. At colonoscopy, no malignancy was seen. An incidental finding was a 4 × 4-mm, poorly developed, vascular abnormality in the cecum. It was treated in the usual fashion. Biopsy confirmed the vascular nature of the abnormality.

Case 34: This 71-year-old man was referred because of a suspected polyp in the transverse colon. He was hypertensive. At colonoscopy, two small polyps were found. An incidental finding was three small vascular abnormalities in the ascending colon just above the ileocecal valve. The largest had a diameter of 4 mm. They were treated in the usual fashion. Biopsy confirmed the vascular nature of the abnormality.

Case 35: An 87-year-old woman was referred because of a vascular abnormality found in the cecum on colonoscopy. The patient had complained of dizziness and was found to be anemic with a hemoglobin of 9.8 g/d*l*. Stools were intermittently positive for occult blood. Mesenteric angiogram demonstrated the lesion. A right colectomy had been considered, but because of the patient's general medical condition, endoscopic electrocoagulation was considered. She had severe hypertension, Parkinson's disease, mild chronic renal failure, and atherosclerotic heart disease. Therapeutic colonoscopy showed the lesion to be located in the cecum opposite the ileocecal valve. It was composed of a group of smaller 2 to 3-mm lesions, which had a conglomerate diameter of about 1.5 cm. The overall shape was circular. Multiple electrocoagulations were necessary. Biopsy confirmed its vascular nature. Two weeks later, two stool specimens were negative for occult blood.

Comment:

This patient was treated endoscopically only because she was not a good surgical candidate. It is this author's belief that surgery should be reserved for those lesions which cannot be treated endoscopically.

3. Analysis of Cases

Of the 35 patients which made up this series, 18 were men and 17 were women. The average age at presentation was 72 with a range of 50 to 91. Ten of the vascular abnormalities were incidental findings. Of the remaining 25, 16 presented with gross bleeding and 9 with anemia. Thirty of the 35 patients had some clinically obvious cardiac, vascular, or pulmonary disease. Many patients had more than one condition. Breakdown of the primary diagnoses is as follows: atherosclerotic heart disease 11, hypertension 6, atherosclerotic vascular disease 5, aortic stenosis 4, mitral insufficiency 2, idiopathic hypertrophic subaortic stenosis 1, chronic obstructive pulmonary disease 1. In addition, three of these patients had diabetes mellitus. Five patients did not have any of these associated diseases.

All 35 patients had their vascular abnormalities located primarily in the right large bowel. Thirty-four had colonoscopic visualization of their lesions. Thirty were located primarily in the cecum and four in the ascending colon. In six cases, smaller, poorly developed lesions were also found in the left colon; in one the lesion was in the distal transverse, in one the splenic flexure, and in three, the sigmoid. In three cases, the largest lesion was ulcerated near the center. Only one case was found to be bleeding at the time of colonoscopy. Six cases had angiography and all were positive. Angiography usually underestimated the number of lesions. Although Case 15 appears to have hereditary hemorrhagic telangiectasia, this elderly patient was included because upper and lower gastrointestinal endoscopy showed typical vascular abnormalities in the cecum and ascending colon only. All patients had biopsy confirmation of the vascular abnormality except Cases 1 and 2.

4. Results

Attention will be focused on those patients in this series who had electrocoagulation for vascular abnormalities thought to be a source of blood loss. Excluded from the 35 cases are ten who had incidental findings and two who went to surgery without endoscopic therapy. Of the remaining 23, two have died. Case 22 had a successful electrocoagulation but died of a coronary occlusion 1 year later. Three months after treatment, Case 26 died of complications of septicemia. Both deaths were unrelated to bleeding from vascular abnormalities or from complications of endoscopic therapy. Of the remaining 21 patients who are alive after colonoscopic therapy for vascular abnormalities of the large bowel, all are doing well and none have required surgery for their bleeding. Follow-up ranges from 7 years to 2 weeks and averages 32 months. Cases 10, 20, and 21 continue to lose blood from their GI tracts; although all abnormal vascular tissue has been eradicated from the large bowel mucosa. It is believed that these three patients are bleeding from vascular abnormalities in the small bowel. Only one treatment was necessary to control the bleeding of 16 of the patients in this group of 21. Three patients required two treatments and one required three. Only the first patient has required five treatments. There have been no complications from colonoscopy or electrocoagulation in this entire group of 35 patients.

5. Experience of Others

Only a few reports have appeared in the literature on the electrocoagulation of small vascular abnormalities of the large bowel. Nüesch et al.,[51] in 1979, reported a series of six patients in whom vascular abnormalities were diagnosed either by angiography or by colonoscopy. All lesions were found in the cecum or ascending colon. They were all treated by endoscopic electrocoagulation. In the follow-up period, which varied between 3 months and 4 years, only one patient had intermittent occult fecal blood loss. No patient had a severe recurrence of bleeding and no colon resection was necessary. It was these authors' conclusion that endoscopic electrosurgical therapy was a valuable alternative to surgery and that it had low-risk and high-efficiency. Stewart et al.,[52] in 1979, reported one case out of 34 treated by endoscopic electrocoagulation. The patient had no bleeding in the subsequent 3 years. Endoscopic electrocoagulation was carried out because the patient was considered a high surgical risk due to cardiac disease. At colonoscopy, a 1-cm lesion was seen. Tedesco et al.,[30] in 1980, reported three patients who had endoscopic electrocoagulation for their vascular abnormalities. One patient had recurrent bleeding within 3 months and had a right colectomy. The two other patients had no recurrent bleeding in 6 to 12-months follow-up.

6. Complications

This author has treated 33 patients with small vascular abnormalities of the large bowel by using electrosurgical techniques. There has been no associated morbidity nor mortality. Biopsy was avoided completely in the first few patients for fear of producing a hemorrhage.[7] After institution of therapy with the electrocoagulating forceps, these lesions have been biopsied and electrocoagulated without difficulty. It should be realized that the mucosal lesion as demonstrated by Baum is made up of tiny vessels, even though they are abnormally dilated on microscopic exam.[9] The large submucosal vein described by Boley et al.[11] is apparently beyond the reach of the endoscopic biopsy forceps. No patient in this series had an immediate postelectrocoagulation hemorrhage nor the necessity for a blood transfusion. Even so, it may be wise to have the patient typed and cross-matched for one or two units of packed cells prior to endoscopic electrocoagulation.

Since the cecum has the thinnest wall of the entire large bowel, there is always the concern for a transmural burn and eventual perforation. Several patients in this series complained of discomfort in the right-lower quadrant when the electrosurgical current was applied. This was disturbing, but resulted in no subsequent problems. When this did occur, less power was used for a shorter period of time in subsequent electrocoagulations.

F. Other Forms of Therapy

1. Surgical

Rational surgical therapy is dependent upon the preoperative demonstration of the vascular abnormality by angiographic or colonoscopic means. Blind right colectomy is no longer recommended for lower gastrointestinal bleeding of undetermined cause. Unfortunately, what appears to be a vascular abnormality on angiography may turn out to be something quite different or even unrelated to the patient's bleeding.[21,42] Colonoscopy should be attempted prior to exploration in any patient in whom bleeding from a vascular lesion is suspected. Colonoscopy may show unexpected lesions such as carcinoma or inflammatory bowel disease, thereby altering the therapeutic approach. Even if angiography is positive, the surgeon should make a careful search at laparotomy for alternative lesions to explain the bleeding.[40] The biggest disadvantage of surgery is the associated operative morbidity and mortality in a group of elderly patients with associated cardiac, vascular, and pulmonary disease. At exploration, the surgeon will rarely be able to identify the lesion. Although in some cases it is visible,[53,54] identification of the lesion becomes extremely difficult unless injection techniques are used.

Unfortunately, the injection technique is laborious and long. Few departments of pathology are willing to undertake such an effort. As a result, much time can be wasted in searching for the lesion in the fixed specimen. In this author's Case 29, the lesion could not be found in the surgical specimen, even though three separate 1-hr sessions were devoted to searching for it. The most straightforward way to obtain histologic confirmation is by colonoscopic biopsy. Baum et al.,[21] in 1977, reported a group of 34 patients who were found to have vascular abnormalities of the cecum and right colon. Ten of these patients had surgery. Seven of the patients were found to be bleeding from lesions other than the vascular abnormality. In the remaining 17 patients, laparotomy failed to demonstrate any gross abnormality and a right hemicolectomy was performed on the basis of angiographic findings. Thirteen of these patients have not bled postoperatively during follow-up periods ranging from 8 months to 7 years. The remaining four patients continued to bleed following surgery. Two of the four had postoperative arteriograms which suggested similar lesions in the remaining segments of the colon which were not appreciated on the earlier examination.

Richardson et al., [29] in 1978, reported 39 patients who were treated surgically. One patient died in the postoperative period. Three other patients died from other causes leaving 35 patients for follow-up. Four of their patients have developed recurrent bleeding. The bleeding developed after 9 months in one patient, but it was at least 18 months after resection before it occurred in the other three. All recurrences developed in elderly patients. Repeat angiography was performed in all cases and showed small bowel lesions in three patients. Two of the patients were considered inoperable and were treated with Premarin® in low doses. In one patient, relatively good control was achieved with only one subsequent episode of melena. The other patient has had intermittent attacks of bleeding requiring transfusions. Two of the patients had repeat operations because of persistent bleeding. The recurrence rate for this group of patients was 4 of 35 (11.4%).

Follow-up ranged from 6 months to 8 years. One postoperative death occurred in an elderly patient following development of a subhepatic abscess. Three other patients subsequently died of problems unrelated to their vascular abnormalities; one following a pulmonary resection for carcinoma, one secondary to liver failure, and one with congestive heart failure and pneumonia.

Boley et al.,[23] in 1979, reported a series of 32 patients in whom vascular abnormalities were seen in the right large bowel on angiography. Colon resection was performed in 29. 27 patients had a right colectomy and two patients had a subtotal or total abdominal colectomy. One patient died of a myocardial infarction after right colectomy. One patient died of uremia and cardiac disease after subtotal colectomy. The operative mortality for this group was 2 out of 29, or 7%. The one patient who survived after subtotal colectomy has not rebled after 64 months. 23 of the 27 patients who survived a right colectomy have not had rebleeding after an average of 34 months. Four patients have had rebleeding.

Tedesco et al.,[30] in 1980, reported on eight patients who underwent surgical resection for vascular abnormality of the large bowel. Follow-up ranged from 6 to 15 months. Six of the patients had no further bleeding during that time. One patient bled 8 weeks after resection of the cecum, proximal right colon, and terminal ileum. Colonoscopy revealed a vascular abnormality in the remaining portion of the ascending colon.

In this author's series of 35 cases, only two have gone to surgery. Case 27 was treated surgically because the vascular abnormality was located on the cecal aspect of the ileocecal valve and could not be visualized long enough to treat with endoscopic electrocoagulation. She was treated with a right colectomy and has had no bleeding in the subsequent 10 months. Case 29 had a right colectomy because the colonoscope could not be passed all the way to the cecum. Surgery stopped his rectal bleeding, but 4 years later he was found to have iron-deficiency anemia due to gastrointestinal blood loss. Upper intestinal endoscopy showed multiple vascular abnormalities of the second portion of the duodenum which were treated with electrosurgery.

There are some conclusions which can be drawn from the combined surgical experience in dealing with this disease to date. The surgeon should not be surprised to find another cause of the patient's gastrointestinal blood loss at laparotomy, even though there was a preoperative diagnosis of vascular abnormality of the right colon. Careful inspection of the entire gastrointestinal tract should be carried out prior to a right colectomy. If a right colectomy is performed, the surgeon should not expect microscopic confirmation of the diagnosis unless injection techniques are used by the pathologist to demonstrate the lesion. The published surgical mortality for this group of patients is up to 7%. The recurrence of bleeding after surgery is at least 10%. If bleeding does recur after right colectomy, new or missed lesions should be suspected in another part of the gastrointestinal tract. Repeat study of the patient with both upper and lower endoscopy and angiography should be helpful in localizing the bleeding site.

2. Photocoagulation

Mucosal vascular abnormalities of the large bowel appear to be ideal candidates for photocoagulation with the argon laser. The argon laser produces a very shallow coagulation in the mucosa because it is rapidly absorbed by hemoglobin. This should result in destruction of the superficial, mucosal portion of the vascular abnormality. Theoretically, it would be easy to treat all lesions visualized because no bleeding should be produced during photocoagulation. The disadvantages of this method are the cost of the laser and the dangers inherent in using it. In addition, unless a separate biopsy were taken, microscopic confirmation of the diagnosis would be lacking.

3. Vasopressin

Athanasoulis,[40] in 1978, recommended vasopressin infusion as a temporizing maneuver if the patient was actively bleeding at the time of angiography. Vasopressin may be infused either directly into the superior mesenteric artery or systemically at dose rates of 0.2 units per min. Such infusions may control bleeding.

4. Treatment of Associated Disease

If aortic stenosis is somehow causing vascular abnormalities of the large bowel, it is reasonable to assume that treatment of the aortic stenosis might be beneficial. This was noted by Love et al.[55] in 1980. Two cases of gastrointestinal bleeding associated with calcific aortic stenosis relieved by aortic valve replacement were reported. Angiography was done in both patients and in neither was a lesion seen in the right large bowel. In the first case, early venous filling in the rectosigmoid was seen. In the second case, angiography was normal. Neither patient had endoscopic confirmation of the lesion. Follow-up was 2 years and 10 months, respectively.

Weaver et al.,[56] in 1980, cautioned against expecting gastrointestinal bleeding to cease in patients with aortic stenosis who have their valves replaced. In their first patients, gastric lesions recurred or remained 9 months after replacement of the aortic valve by a porcine xenograft. Their second case had recurrent gastrointestinal bleeding after the calcified aortic valve was replaced. Upper intestinal endoscopy showed areas of vascular abnormality. These were treated by endoscopic coagulation and were followed by an interval of hemoccult-negative stools. Bleeding eventually recurred to a lesser degree and was controlled by a reduction in anticoagulation. It was recommended that when valve replacement is necessary, a porcine xenograft should be considered so that anticoagulation may be minimal or may be withheld.

In 1979, Bourdette and Greenberg,[57] reported a patient with gastric vascular abnormalities and recurrent gastrointestinal bleeding who had aortic stenosis. The patient's aortic valve was replaced with a porcine xenograft. Occult blood was noted in the stools postoperatively. Endoscopy, sometime after valve replacement, continued to show gastric vascular abnormalities although gastrointestinal bleeding eventually stopped.

Thus, it is not clear from the literature whether or not improvement of the cardiovascular status of a patient by replacement of the stenotic aortic valve will have a beneficial effect on the associated vascular abnormality of the gastrointestinal tract. At the present time, it would seem wise to recommend replacement of the aortic valve on the basis of reasons other than bleeding from the gastrointestinal tract. As in this author's one patient who has subsequently had his aortic valve replaced, electrocoagulation can control the bleeding (Case 7). He had no bleeding during the 4 years which passed between electrocoagulation of his cecal vascular abnormality and the replacement of his valve. Postoperatively, he has been anticoagulated with Coumadin® without gastrointestinal blood loss.

5. Observation

Small, poorly developed, vascular abnormalities of the large bowel make up a significant portion of this author's series. If there were no associated anemia and no history of significant or recurrent bleeding, it could be argued that the lesions should have been left alone. Boley et al.[11] recommended no therapy for vascular abnormalities of the cecum and colon in patients who had not bled or were not anemic from chronic blood loss. Tedesco et al.[30] made these recommendations on the basis of the colonoscopic findings in 14 patients. This entire issue should be resolved rationally on the basis of risk vs. benefit. Obviously, surgical intervention is not indicated unless the patient is anemic or has bled. At the time of colonoscopy, an incidental, small, poorly developed, mucosal vascular abnormality can safely be ignored. This is especially true if the colonoscopist is confronted with other more important tasks such as removing polyps. However, if properly performed, the risk of biopsy and electrocoagulation of a lesion is minimal. The benefits are two-fold. The diagnosis will be confirmed by the microscopic examination of the tissue removed and future bleeding may be prevented.

G. Theory of Formation

The pathogenesis of mucosal vascular abnormalities of the gastrointestinal tract of elderly patients is unknown and all theories of formation are speculative. Heald and Ray considered them to be hamartomas.[58] Baum et. al.[59] postulated that they may be the end result of chronic submucosal arteriovenous shunting secondary to a transient increase in intraluminal pressure, and may represent a chronic form of ischemic bowel disease. Galdabini postulated the lesion was secondary to ischemia caused by atheromatous emboli.[39] Galloway et al.[20] noted the underlying similarity in their cases of aortic stenosis was decreased perfusion pressure secondary to outlet obstruction of the left ventricle. On the basis of injection studies, Boley et al.[11] postulated that the vascular lesions develop as a degenerative process of aging. In addition, Laplace's principal was invoked to explain the predilection for the cecum, where increased pressure in the wall was believed to cause a mechanical obstruction of the draining veins and result in dilation. This appears to be an erroneous application of the principle. Laplace's law says that the greater the diameter of a cylinder, the greater will be the force pulling its wall apart if the pressure within the cylinder remains constant. When this principle is applied to the vessels which perforate the walls of the cecum, it indicates that the opening through which vessels pass will be pulled apart, thereby making them wider. This is exactly opposite to the squeezing effect implied by Boley et al.

This author's theory is that the lesions are acquired because of local chronic hypo-oxygenation of the microcirculation. Hypo-oxygenation is postulated to result from the associated cardiac, vascular, or pulmonary disease. Heart and peripheral vascular disease would decrease available oxygen to peripheral tissues by decreasing blood flow. Long-standing hypertension with arteriosclerosis and diabetes mellitus, with its involvement of the microcirculation, may produce the same effect. Chronic obstructive pulmonary disease would decrease available oxygen to peripheral tissues by desaturation of hemoglobin. Localized hypoxemia of the microcirculation would lead to capillary proliferation and dilation, eventually leading to a clinically recognizable vascular abnormality. This is seen in Takayasu's arteritis, where it can cause a proliferative response around the optic disc downstream from a vascular occlusion.[60] Perhaps an angiogenesis factor is being produced by the local ischemia.[61] Ischemic necrosis or mechanical abrasion of the surface of the lesion would result in gastrointestinal bleeding. The lesions tend to form in the mucosa of the gastrointestinal tract because its contents have a very low partial pressure of oxygen, which exacerbates the local hypoxemia already produced by the associated disease. Anatomy, physiology, and vascular supply of the cecum all probably contribute to it being the most frequent site of involvement. The cecum is the widest point of the lower intestinal tract. It is physiologically normal for the cecum to contain a large, anaerobic mass of feces. The combined oxygen requirements of the metabolically active mucosa and adjacent oxygen sink should produce an area of high-oxygen need. The vascular supply of the cecum may also be a factor in producing localized ischemia, since cecal arteries are end arteries and the most distal branches of the superior mesenteric. Therefore, the cecum can be viewed as a large oxygen sink at the end of a long and precarious vascular supply. This is inconsequential in healthy, young people, but in elderly patients with cardiac, vascular, or pulmonary disease, it could lead to a localized area of chronic mucosal hypo-oxygenation and subsequent vascular proliferation. This theory explains why acquired vascular abnormalities affect the mucosa of the gastrointestinal tract, especially the cecum, and why they are associated with cardiac, vascular, and pulmonary disease. There are important implications if this theory can be proven to be true. Presently, there is no recognized demonstrable lesion of ischemic bowel disease short of infarction. Acquired mucosal vascular abnormalities of the cecal area may represent such a lesion.

H. Conclusions and Recommendations

In the clinical setting of lower gastrointestinal blood loss of obscure source in elderly patients, mucosal vascular abnormality of the cecal area should be included in the differential diagnosis, especially if hypertension, diabetes mellitus or cardiac, vascular, or pulmonary disease is also present. Colonoscopy is usually the easiest method for demonstrating the lesion in the living patient. When properly performed, electrocoagulation with biopsy during endoscopy is safe and effective. In addition, histologic confirmation of the vascular nature of the lesion is obtained. If endoscopic therapy has eradicated all abnormal vascular tissue from the large bowel, and if blood loss persists, then a bleeding point higher in the gastrointestinal tract should be suspected. An attempt at examining the distal terminal ileum with the colonoscope should be made. Esophagogastroduodenoscopy should be performed in anticipation of demonstrating a mucosal vascular abnormality in the upper GI tract, where electrocoagulation can also be performed. If both upper and lower endoscopy are negative, selective angiography of the superior mesenteric artery should be recommended. Angiography is also recommended if the colonoscopist fails to reach the cecum. Surgical therapy is recommended for all lesions demonstrated angiographically which are beyond the reach of the endoscopist. However, at exploration, the surgeon would be wise to seek other causes which may explain the patient's blood loss.

II. HEREDITARY HEMORRHAGIC TELANGIECTASIA AND OTHER VASCULAR ABNORMALITIES

The vascular lesion of hereditary hemorrhagic telangiectasia (Osler-Weber—Rendu disease) is very small and rarely more than 3mm in diameter. Patients with this disease are easily recognized because of repeated nosebleeds beginning early in life, a positive family history, and small telangiectasias seen on the mucous membrane of the mouth. Clinically, it is easy to differentiate from the elderly patient with the recent onset of lower gastrointestinal bleeding who has a vascular abnormality of the cecal area and an associated cardiac, vascular, or pulmonary disease. The patient with hereditary hemorrhagic telangiectasia may have numerous small lesions in the upper intestinal tract. The patient with the small vascular abnormality of the cecal area will have one large, 5 to 10-mm lesion in the cecum with smaller lesions close by. Although it may be easy to differentiate the two syndromes clinically, endoscopic and pathologic differentiation of a single lesion may be impossible. Wolff et al.[53] noted that the microscopic pathology of the characteristic small vascular abnormality which occurs in the right colon of elderly patients is indistinguishable from the telangiectasia of Osler-Weber—Rendu disease. Halpern et al.[43] reported four cases of hereditary hemorrhagic telangiectasia studied with angiography. Of their patients, Case 3 had a typical angiographic abnormality of the cecal area. Case 15 of this author's series appeared to have both syndromes. Further study will be necessary to determine whether this is related or fortuitous. If a patient with hereditary hemorrhagic telangiectasia is bleeding from the gastrointestinal tract, then endoscopic electrocoagulation is indicated. The same technique which was outlined for the cecal lesion should be used and applied to both the lower and upper intestinal tract. Electrocoagulation of large vascular abnormalities such as varices and congenital abnormalities is not recommended.

ACKNOWLEDGEMENTS

I am indebted to the following physicians from the Chicago area for referring their patients: Case 1, Dr. Melvin Goldberg; Cases 2 and 3, Dr. Fred Adler; Case 4, Dr. John Anagnos; Case 5, Dr. Martin Shobris; Cases 6 and 26, Dr. Stanley Yachnin; Case 7, Dr. Louis Johnston; Case 8, Dr. Stephen Winter; Case 9, Dr. George Poulos; Cases 10 and 15, Dr. John Philipp; Case 11, Dr. Svetislav Paunovic; Case 12, Dr. Richard Breuer; Case 13, Dr. Michael Ballin; Case 14, Dr. Sally Glickman; Case 16, Dr. Sumner Kraft; Cases 17 and 21, Dr. Joseph Kirsner; Case 18, Dr. Nicholas Frankovelgia; Case 19, Dr. Roger Lundquist; Case 20, Dr. John Givens; Cases 22 and 23, Dr. George Byfield; Case 24, Dr. Raymond Galt; Case 25, Dr. Mark Siegler; Case 27, Dr. Richard Nierenberg; Case 28, Dr. Charles Winans; Case 29, Dr. Anderson Hedberg; Case 30, Dr. Richard Horswell; Case 31, Dr. Bernard Levin; Case 32, Dr. Richard Saavedra; Case 33, Dr. Harry Kalsch; Case 34, Dr. David Skinner, and Case 35, Dr. Sheldon Cogan.

I am indebted to the following physicians from the Chicago area for their assistance in obtaining photomicrographs of the biopsy specimens: Drs. John Passman and Jesus Vega, Grant Hospital; Drs. Jose Bolanos and Prospero Pilar, Christ Hospital; Dr. Iris Cosnow, Ravenswood Hospital; and Dr. Robert Riddell, University of Chicago. Dr. Reza Parsavand, Highland Park Hospital, provided the photograph of the angiogram of Case 1.

I am indebted to my endoscopic assistants, Mrs. Elizabeth Tolva, R.N., Mrs. Ellen Ramos, R.N., Miss Trinidad Bayona, R.N., Mrs. Leoncia Burkart, R.N., Mrs. Jerry All, R.N., Miss Aleli Andrada, R.N., and Miss May B. Celiz, R.N. for their help with colonoscopy, and to my secretary, Miss Catherine Smith for the typing.

REFERENCES

1. **Margulis, A. R., Heinbecker, P., and Bernard, H. R.,** Operative mesenteric arteriography in the search for the site of bleeding in unexplained gastrointestinal hemorrhage, *Surgery,* 48, 534, 1960.
2. **Baum, S., Nusbaum, M., Kuroda, K., and Blakemore, W. S.,** Direct serial magnification arteriography as an adjuvant in the diagnosis of surgical lesions in the alimentary tract, *Am. J. Surg.,* 177, 170, 1969.
3. **Edie, R. N. and Brennan, J. T.,** Colonic hemorrhage from arteriovenous anastomosis; report of a case, *Arch. Surg.,* 99, 674, 1969.
4. **Klein, H. J., Alfidi, R. J., Meany, T. F., and Poirier, V. C.,** Angiography in the diagnosis of chronic gastrointestinal bleeding, *Radiology,* 98, 83, 1971.
5. **Bockus, H. L., Ferguson, L. K., Thompson, C., and Roth, J. L. A.,** Management of gastrointestinal hemorrhage of undetermined origin, *JAMA,* 152, 1228, 1953.
6. **Bartelheimer, W., Remmele, W., and Ottenjann, R.,** Coloscopic recognition of hemangiomas in the colon ascendens, *Endoscopy,* 4, 109, 1972.
7. **Rogers, B. H. G. and Adler, F.,** Hemangiomas of the cecum: colonoscopic diagnosis and therapy, *Gastroenterology,* 71, 1079, 1976.
8. **Alfidi, R. J., Hunter, T., Hawk, W. A., Winkelman, E. I., and Esselstyn, C. B, Jr.,** Corrosion casts of arteriovenous malformations, *Arch. Path.,* 96, 196, 1973.
9. **Baum, S.,** Case records of the Massachusetts General Hospital; case 36-1974, Scully, R. E. and McNeely, B. U., Eds., *N. Engl. J. Med.,* 291, 569, 1974.
10. **Gentry. R. W., Dockerty, M. B., and Clagett, O. T.,** Vacuslar malformations and vascular tumors of the gastrointestinal tract, *Int. Abstr. Surg.,* 88, 281, 1949.
11. **Boley, S. J., Sammartano, R., Adams, A., DiBiase, A., Kleinhaus, S., and Sprayregen, S.,** On the nature and etiology of vascular ectasias of the colon; degenerative lesions of aging, *Gastroenterology,* 72, 650, 1977.
12. **Heyde, E. C.,** Gastrointestinal bleeding in aortic stenosis, (correspondence), *N. Engl. J. Med.,* 259, 196, 1958.
13. **Schwartz, B. M.,** Additional note on bleeding in aortic stenosis, (correspondence), *N. Engl. J. Med.,* 259, 456, 1958.
14. **Williams, R. C., Jr.,** Aortic stenosis and unexplained gastrointestinal bleeding, *Arch. Intern. Med.,* 108, 859, 1961.
15. **Jacobson, B. M.,** Case records of the Massachusetts General Hospital; case 49-1965, Castleman, B. and McNeeley, B. U., Eds., *N. Engl. J. Med.,* 273, 1096, 1965.
16. **Reuter, S. R. and Bookstein, J. J.,** Angiographic localization of gastrointestinal bleeding, *Gastroenterology,* 54, 876, 1968.
17. **Baum, S., Nusbaum, M., Kuroda, K., and Blakemore, W. S.,** Direct serial magnification arteriography as an adjuvant in the diagnosis of surgical lesions in the alimentary tract, *Am. J. Surg.,* 117, 170, 1969.
18. **Clark, R. A. and Rosch, J.,** Arteriography in the diagnosis of large bowel bleeding, *Radiology,* 94, 83, 1970.
19. **Boss. E. G. and Rosenbaum, J. M.,** Bleeding from the right colon associated with aortic stenosis, *Dig. Dis.,* 16, 269, 1971.
20. **Galloway, S. J., Casarella, W. J., and Shimkin, P. M.,** Vascular malformations of the right colon as a cause of bleeding in patients with aortic stenosis, *Radiology,* 113, 11, 1974.
21. **Baum, S., Athanasoulis, C. A., Waltman, A. C., Galdabini, J., Schapiro, R. H., Warshaw, A. L., and Ottinger, L. W.,** Angiodysplasia of the right colon: a cause of gastrointestinal bleeding, *Am. J. Roentgenol.,* 129, 789, 1977.
22. **Gelfand, M. L., Cohen, T., Ackert, J. J., Ambos, M., and Maydag, M.,** Gastrointestinal bleeding in aortic stenosis, *A. J. Gastroenterol.,* 71, 30, 1979.

23. **Boley, S. J., Sammartano, R., Brandt, L. J., and Sprayregen, S.,** Vascular ectasias of the colon, *Surg. Gynecol. Obstet.,* 149, 353, 1979.
24. **Rogers, B. H. G.,** Mucosal vascular abnormalities of the gastrointestinal tract occurring in elderly patients and associated with cardiac, vascular and pulmonary disease: endoscopic diagnosis and therapy, *Gastrointest. Endosc.,* 26, 134, 1980.
25. **Genant, H. K. and Ranniger, K.,** Vascular dysplasias of the ascending colon, *Am. J. Roentgenol.,* 115, 349, 1972.
26. **Crichlow, R. W., Mosenthal, W. T., Spiegel, P. K., and House, R. K.,** Arteriovenous malformations of the bowel, *Am. J. Surg.,* 129, 440, 1975.
27. **Skibba, R. M., Hartong, W. A., Mantz, F. A., Hinthorn, D. R., and Rhodes, J. B.,** Angiodysplasia of the cecum: colonoscopic diagnosis, *Gastrointest. Endosc.,* 22, 177, 1976.
28. **Thanik, K. D., Chey, W. Y., and Abbott, J.,** Vascular dysplasia of the cecum as a repeated source of hemorrhage: role of colonoscopy in diagnosis, *Gastrointest. Endosc.* 23, 167, 1977.
29. **Richardson, J. D., Max, M. H., Flint, L. M. Jr., Schweisinger, W., Howard, M., and Aust, J. B.,** Bleeding vascular malformations of the intestine, *Surgery,* 84, 430, 1978.
30. **Tedesco. F. J., Griffin, J. W., Jr., and Khan, A. Q.,** Vascular ectasia of the colon: clinical, colonoscopic and radiographic features, *J. Clin. Gastroenterol.,* 2, 233, 1980.
31. **Thompson, N. W.,** Vascular ectasias and colonic diverticula: common causes of lower gastrointestinal hemorrhage in the aged, in *Gastrointestinal Hemorrhage,* Fiddian-Green, R. G. and Turcotte, J. G., Eds., Grune & Stratton, New York, 1980, 375.
32. **Upson, J. F., Brunnell, I., and Kokkinopoulis, E.,** Hemangioma of the cecum, diagnosis by angiography, *JAMA,* 217, 1104, 1971.
33. **Hagihara, P. F., Chuang, V. P., and Griffen, W. O.,** Arteriovenous malformations of the colon, *Am. J. Surg.,* 133, 681, 1977.
34. **Moore, J. D., Thompson, N. W., Appelman, H. D., and Foley, D.,** Arteriovenous malformations of the gastrointestinal tract, *Arch. Surg.,* 111, 381, 1976.
35. **Cooperman, A. M., Kelly, K. A., Bernatz, P. E., and Huizenga, K. A.,** Arteriovenous malformation of the intestine: an uncommon cause of gastrointestinal bleeding, *Arch. Surg.,* 104, 284, 1972.
36. **Singh, A., Shenoy S., Kaur, A., Sachdanand, S., and Alford, J. E.,** Arteriovenous malformation of the cecum: report of 6 cases, *Dis. Colon Rectum,* 20, 334, 1977.
37. **Mitsudo, S. M., Boley, S. J., Brandt, L. J., Montefusco, C. M., and Sammartano, R. J.,** Vascular ectasias of the right colon in the elderly: a distinct pathologic entity, *Hum. Pathol.,* 10, 585, 1979.
38. **Boley, S. J., Sprayregen, S., Sammartano, R. J., Adams, A., and Kleinhaus, S.,** The pathophysiologic basis for the angiographic signs of vascular ectasias of the colon, *Radiology,* 125, 615, 1977.
39. **Galdabini, J. J.,** Case records of the Massachusetts General Hospital; case 36-1974, *N. Engl. J. Med.,* 291, 569, 1974.
40. **Athanasoulis, C. A., Galdabini, J. J., Waltman, A. D., Novelline, R. A., Greenfield, A. J., and Ezpeleta, M. L.,** Angiodysplasia of the colon: a cause of rectal bleeding, *Cardiovasc. Radiol.,* 1, 3, 1978.
41. **Dorland's Illustrated Medical Dictionary,** 23rd ed., W. B. Saunders, Philadelphia, 1974.
42. **Tarin, D., Allison, D. J., Modlin, I. M., and Neale, G.,** Diagnosis and management of obscure gastrointestinal bleeding, *Br. Med. J.,* 2, 751, 1978.
43. Halpern, M., Turner, A. F., and Citron, B. P., Angiodysplasias of the abdominal viscera associated with hereditary hemorrhagic telangiectasia, *Am. J. Roentgenol., Radium Ther. Nucl. Med.,* 102, 783, 1968.
44. **Bentley, P. G.,** The bleeding cecal angioma: a diagnostic problem, *Br. J. Surg.,* 63, 455, 1976.
45. **Waye, J. D.,** Colonoscopy: guidelines and techniques for diagnosis and therapy, in *Progress in Gastroenterology,* Vol. 3, Glass, G. B. L., Ed., Grune & Stratton, New York, 1977, chap. 39.
46. **Gelfand, M. L., Cohen, T., Ackert, J. J., Ambox, M., and Mayadag, M.,** Gastrointestinal bleeding in aortic stenosis, *Am. J. Gastroenterol.,* 71, 30, 1979.
47. **Whitehouse, G. H.,** Solitary angiodysplastic lesions in the ileocaecal region diagnosed by angiography, *Gut,* 14, 977, 1973.
48. **Blackstone, M. O., Rogers, B. H. G., and Baker, A. L.,** A cutaneous and pelvic lymphangioma with varices, lymphangiomas and capillary hemangiomas of the rectosigmoid colon, *Gastrointest. Endosc.,* 23, 39, 1976.
49. **Williams, C. B.,** Diathermy-biopsy: a technique for endoscopic management of small polyps, *Endoscopy,* 5, 215, 1973.
50. **Bigard, M. A., Gaucher, P., and Lassalle, C.,** Fatal colonic explosion during colonoscopic polypectomy, *Gastroenterology,* 77, 1307, 1979.
51. **Nüesch, H. J., Kobler, E., Bühler, H., Jenny, S., Sulser. H., Bonetti, A., Schläpfer, H., and Deyhle, P.,** Angiodysplasien des kolons-diagnose und therapie, *Schweiz. Med. Wochenschr.,* 109, 607, 1979.

52. **Stewart. W. B., Gathright, J. B., Jr., and Ray, J. E.,** Vascular ectasias of the colon, *Surg. Gynecol. Obstet.,* 148, 670, 1979.
53. **Wolff, W. I., Grossman, M. B., and Shinya, H.,** Angiodysplasia of the colon, *Gastroenterology,* 72, 329, 1977.
54. **Salt, W. B., II and Marshall, J. P.,** Angiodysplasia of the cecum (correspondence), *Gastroenterology,* 73, 195, 1977.
55. **Love, J. W., Jahnke, E. J., Zacharias, D., Davidson, W. A., Kidder, W. R., and Luan, L. L.,** Calcific aortic stenosis and gastrointestinal bleeding, (correspondence), *N. Engl. J. Med.,* 302, 968, 1980.
56. **Weaver, G. A., Arquin, P. L., Davis, J. S., and Ramsey, W. H.,** More on aortic stenosis and gastrointestinal bleeding (correspondence), *N. Engl. J. Med.,* 303, 584, 1980.
57. **Bourdette, D. and Greenberg, B.,** Twelve-year history of gastrointestinal bleeding in a patient with calcific aortic stenosis and hemorrhagic telangiectasia, *Dig. Dis. Sci.,* 24, 77, 1979.
58. **Heald, R. J. and Ray, J. E.,** Vascular malformations of the intestine: an important cause of obscure gastrointestinal hemorrhage, *South. Med. J.,* 67, 33, 1974.
59. **Baum, S., Athanasoulis, C. A., and Waltman, A. C.,** Angiographic diagnosis and control of large bowel bleeding, *Dis. Colon Rectum,* 17, 447, 1974.
60. **Gocke, D. J., and Healey, L. A.,** Polyarteritis and other primary vasculitides, in *Immunological Diseases,* Samter, M., Ed., Little, Brown, Boston, 1978, 1087.
61. **Check, W.,** Angiogenesis factor found in eye tumors, (Medical News), *JAMA,* 241, 1559, 1979.

INDEX

A

B

C

D

E

F

G

H

I

J

L

M

N

O

P

Q

R

S

T

U

V

W

X

Y